Public Health and Evidence-Based Healthcare

Public Health and Evidence-Based Healthcare

Edited by **Felix Rohmer**

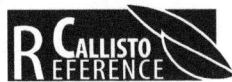

R CALLISTO REFERENCE

New York

Published by Callisto Reference,
106 Park Avenue, Suite 200,
New York, NY 10016, USA
www.callistoreference.com

Public Health and Evidence-Based Healthcare
Edited by Felix Rohmer

Contents

Preface

I am honored to present to you this unique book which encompasses the most up-to-date data in the field. I was extremely pleased to get this opportunity of editing the work of experts from across the globe. I have also written papers in this field and researched the various aspects revolving around the progress of the discipline. I have tried to unify my knowledge along with that of stalwarts from every corner of the world, to produce a text which not only benefits the readers but also facilitates the growth of the field.

Public health refers to building an organized effort towards prevention of diseases, promotion of health and improved life expectancy. It is an interdisciplinary field that encompasses biostatistics, health services and epidemiology. This discipline tries to improve health and quality of life through promotion of healthy habits, scrutinizing cases and health indicators. Evidence-based healthcare is the practice of medicine that tries to optimize the results using evidences from well designed and precisely conducted researches. Both of these work in tandem to create a synergic effect resulting in maximum positive impact. This book includes some of the vital pieces of work being conducted across the world, on various topics related to public health and evidence-based healthcare. The topics included herein are of utmost significance and bound to provide incredible insights to readers. This book presents researches performed by experts across the globe and explains the significance of public health in modern times. It is a resource guide for healthcare experts as well as students.

Finally, I would like to thank all the contributing authors for their valuable time and contributions. This book would not have been possible without their efforts. I would also like to thank my friends and family for their constant support.

Editor

Immigrants' Satisfaction from the National Health System in Greece: In the Quest of the Contributing Factors

Athanassios Vozikis*, Maria Siganou

Economics Department, University of Piraeus, Piraeus, Greece
Email: *avozik@unipi.gr

Abstract

Immigrants deserve special attention as they constitute a very sensitive social group, facing an increasing risk of social exclusion. The access of immigrants to health services is one of the most important factors, which contributes to their integration into the society of induction. The purpose of this study is to track and assess the immigrants' satisfaction from the health services provided by the Greek National Health System (NHS). The satisfaction level assessment is examined in conjunction with demographic and socio-economic characteristics of the study participants, as well as with the characteristics that are related to their personal experience with the National Health System in Greece. The research was conducted from March 2012 to May 2013. The sample of the research comprises of 126 "first-generation" immigrants on legal permit of residence in Greece, who lived in the prefecture of Attica. It is panel study based on "snowball sampling" and the statistical analysis was conducted with the use of the Stata (ver. 11), while the statistical analysis used probit estimation techniques. The demographic and social variables—particularly the variables of gender, "understanding the Greek language", "education", "participation in the community of origin" and "insurance"—the variables of "health" and specifically "long-term diseases" and the variable of "trust" are found to be highly related with immigrants' satisfaction degree from the Greek health system. Our research concludes that health is a fundamental, human right and immigrants' access to health services is essential not only for their instant and effective treatment of their health problems and the improvement of their lives but also for ensuring the public health in Greece. In order to properly incorporate immigrants in Greece in particular, the health policy decision-makers have to pay attention to the contributing factors.

Keywords

National Health System in Greece, Immigrants, Access to Health Services, Satisfaction Level

---

*Corresponding author.

1. Introduction

Immigrants constitute a vulnerable population group, a fact suggesting that they are facing an increased risk of social isolation. Their access to health services is one of the key parameters that contribute to their social inclusion, in the receptive society.

Nowadays, Greece, like all Western countries after all, has a new reality to manage, such as the one formed by the immigrant (and recently the refugees) phenomenon. Immigration to Greece began during the '80s, was limited in terms of the number of immigrants the country could hold and in a legal form, while the majority of immigrants originated from Africa and Asia. During the '90s, after the "Eastern block's" collapse, Greece started receiving a large number of people coming from Central and Eastern Europe, thus, making Greece the country with the highest percentage of immigrants in the EU, in relation to its working force [1].

Since the mid-90s, the increase of immigrant flows toward Greece made the country number one in the percentage increase of incoming immigrants in the whole of Europe, with a large percentage of illegal immigrants. In 2012, of the total number of 10,815,197 residents, 537,273 were legal residents, while the number of illegal immigrants was estimated at 577,900 people [2].

Access of immigrants to health services in the country of reception constitutes a parameter that, on one hand, ensures the basic human rights and, on the other hand, contributes to the immigrants' social inclusion. Formal access of immigrants to the services of Greece's National Health System constitutes their formal employment and legal status. Immigrants, who possess legal rights to residency in Greece (Law. 2910/2001), enjoy the same rights as Greek citizens concerning national insurance and social protection. On the contrary, foreigners who reside in Greece without any legal documents of residency, have no right to access health services. The law excludes underage children and immigrants who are hospitalized as emergency cases (Article. 84, of Law 3386/2005) [3] [4].

However, legal immigrants who reside in Greece, also face significant obstacles when trying to access the health system, such as long waiting time in hospitals, deficient communication with health professionals, high cost (out-of-pocket payments) and complexity of the health system [1]. Additionally, foreigners are faced with financial insecurity at a greater degree than the native population, for the reason that their income is generally lower, while significant barriers are documented in the provision of information, concerning the Medicare and the immigrants' and refugees' ignorance in relation to their rights [5]-[7].

Similar research in Europe, has not detected significant inequalities versus the general population. In their research, Dixon and Woods *et al.* (2005) showed satisfactory immigrant access to Primary Health Care, documenting differentiations between the different ethnic groups [8]. The capacity to understand the language and the lack of sufficient information concerning health services were included within the basic parameters blocking the access.

Respective results of satisfactory access to health services are documented in research done in the Netherlands, where there is a very high percentage of immigrants on a European level [9]-[11].

Hjern *et al.* report equal access of immigrants to primary healthcare in Scandinavian countries, in relation to the native population, although immigrants are more likely to report dissatisfaction, in terms of healthcare needs being met and termination of therapy [12].

Finally, concerning Spain, the study of Carrasco-Gariddo *et al.* provided evidence that immigrants had higher hospitalization percentages than the Spanish population (11.4% versus 8.2%) [13]. Furthermore, the study of Cots *et al.* showed higher ratings for the use of the emergency room by immigrants [14]

Besides the serious issue of the access to health services, another crucial matter, that constitutes a widespread requirement of contemporary developed societies, is the quality for the provided health services.

Measurement of the patients' degree of satisfaction constitutes one of the most important parameters for documenting the quality of the health services and induces many benefits to the health units and, as an extension, to a wider social context.

Donabedian defined patient satisfaction as the outcome index of provided health services [15]. He claims that patient satisfaction reflects her opinion on the quality of healthcare services and represents specific qualitative features that are mainly related to the patient's expectations and values. Patient satisfaction, according to Yucelt, constitutes the confirmation, or not, of pursuit concerning the quality and effectiveness of the services provided [16]. While what a patient requires from a hospital is therapy, the inability to evaluate clinical care leads to a variety of other factors which affect one's judgment, such as the way health services deal with complaints, the health professionals' behavior, the immediacy of healthcare provision, the convenience of the services and, in general, the overall image of the hospital [17].

The main factors that contribute to the patients' satisfaction and that are documented through the questionnaire of the present study are concerned with the demographic features of patients (gender, age, family situation, education, profession, income), the relationship between healthcare professionals and patients, and the amount of the services provided rather than the quality [18] [19].

In contrast to North America and Australia, in Europe one rarely comes across studies that are concerned with recording data for the immigrant populations. (Sweden, the Netherlands and the United Kingdom are exceptions) [20]. However, despite of the fact that there are several reports of health status, access to care, treatment and survival for different minority groups, relatively few reports on patient satisfaction in these minority and immigrant groups are available [21]-[31]. In the USA, the National Quality Forum addressed measurement issues and challenges in reporting health care quality for minority populations and recommended improved race and ethnicity data collection practices for quality measurement [32]. Even if the target of this report was US racial and ethnic minorities, the immigrant population in other countries can also easily be considered as minority groups and thereby as having similar problems.

Our research paper aims at documenting the degree of immigrants' satisfaction with the health services provided to them by the Greek National Health System, through access and utilization of these services in relation to the effect of demographic and socioeconomic features of the participants, as well as the features that are associated with their experience thus far, through personal contact with their national health system.

2. Methods

2.1. Study Population

The present research study is a cross-sectional (**panel**), since the data collected regarded the years 2009-2011, and was conducted from Mars 2012 to May 2013 in Athens, Greece. The study population consisted of 126 immigrants (third country nationals) who were living in area of Athens. Regarding the sampling method, there is no accurate census of immigrants in Greece. Thus, probability or random sampling could not be realized and therefore snowball sampling (a nonprobability sampling method) was applied. Immigrants originated from various countries (of Asian, Africa and East Europe). Initially, we contacted key persons in immigrant communities, such as their leaders or representatives. Those key persons acted as mediators and between investigator and immigrants in order to increase feelings of trust and comfort. The mediators acted as interpreters also. Face-to-face interviews were conducted with immigrants with a mean duration of 15 min. Through the abovementioned research design a high response rate (100%) was achieved.

All participants were over 17 years, residing legally in Greece and were first-generation immigrants. Participants were informed about the study and gave their written consent. Personal data of immigrants were not registered at any stage of the study.

2.2. Measures

A questionnaire was developed including information on sociodemographic characteristics, health status, public health services knowledge and utilization and perception of difficulties in health services access. Sociodemographic characteristics included age, country of origin, years of stay in Greece, gender, marital status, number of children, educational level, health insurance coverage, employment at the time of study, personal and family monthly income, participation in community in the country of origin. Also, we measured immigrants' ability to understand, speak, read and write in Greek in a five-point Likert-type scale. Information about health status included self-reported health status and medication use for chronic diseases. Public health services knowledge was measured on a five-point Likert-type scale. Public health services utilization was measured for the years of study (2009-2011) and the degree of trustfulness the participants had in health professionals on a five-point Likert-type scale.

The final configuration of the questionnaire used, was based on the questionnaire of the previous study "Knowledge and Use of Health Services by Immigrants in Greece", where the study protocol was approved by the ethics committee of the Faculty of Nursing of the University of Athens [3].

2.3. Statistical Analysis

Stata (version 11) data analysis and statistical software was used for statistical analysis.

Our Model encompasses the dependent variable (y) and thirteen independent variables (x_s). The mathematical Model that will be estimated is the following: $y_{it} = f(X, Z, H, T)$, where:

X is a sum that encompasses demographic/social variables.

More specifically:

1) x_1 (gender), 2) x_2 (age), 3) x_3 (country), 4) x_4 (residence), 5) x_5 understanding), 6) x_6 (education), 7) x_7 (job), 8) x_8 (insurance) και 9) x_{10} (community)

Z is a sum that encompasses financial variables and more specifically:

10) x_9 (income), 11) x_{12} (payment)

H is the variable that is concerned with the health condition of the participants. More specifically:

12) x_{11} (disease)

T is the variable that states the degree of trust the sampled immigrants feel toward the Greek Health system. More specifically:

13) x_{13} (trust)

The aforementioned model to be evaluated will be studied as linear. The dependent variable is distinctive and is given values 0 and 1. Consequently, the model we used for the processing and statistical analysis of empirical data is a "**probit**" model and will be evaluated accordingly.

3. Results

Table 1 presents the participants' countries of origin:

Table 2 presents information regarding the immigrants' sociodemographic characteristics, their satisfaction with the NHS, their health status and their speaking level of the Greek language.

Based on the data presented above, the sample of immigrants in our research study tend, on average, to be

Table 1. Countries of origin of participants.

Country of origin of participants	N	%
Afghanistan	2	1.59%
Albania	14	11.11%
Bangladesh	1	0.79%
China	1	0.79%
Cuba	1	0.79%
Georgia	14	11.11%
Ghana	4	3.17%
Egypt	3	2.38%
Eretria	2	1.59%
Ethiopia	25	19.84%
India	4	3.17%
Iran	2	1.59%
Iraq	1	0.79%
Kenya	4	3.17%
Moldova	1	0.79%
Morocco	1	0.79%
Nigeria	16	12.70%
Pakistan	20	15.87%
Sierra Leone	1	0.79%
Syria	3	2.38%
Turkey	1	0.79%
Ukraine	5	3.97%
Total	**126**	**100%**

Table 2. Statistical data description.

Variable	Obs	Mean	Std. Dev.	Min	Max
satisfaction	141	0.6737589	0.4705081	0	1
gender	378	0.452381	0.4983869	0	1
age	378	1.722222	0.4659019	1	3
country	378	11.51058	5.982835	1	22
residence	378	13.43254	8.028056	0	38
understanding	378	2.891534	1.051149	0	4
education	378	2.873016	1.032502	1	5
job	378	1.261905	0.6576855	0	4
insurance	378	0.9206349	0.2657208	0	1
income	378	707.4153	483.1436	0	4000
community	375	0.384	0.4870077	0	1
disease	378	0.2460317	0.4312681	0	1
payment	143	0.1398601	0.348061	0	1
trust	375	2.448	1.047962	0	4

satisfied by the access to the Greek Health system, reside in Greece for about 13 years and, in their majority, are younger than 65 years of age—specifically between the ages of 30 to 64. On average, their understanding of the Greek language is good (=3) and their academic level is of secondary (9 - 12 years of school attendance) and post-secondary (13 - 15 years of school attendance) education. The majority of the immigrants were employed in the private sector, while the overriding majority of the sampled individuals are insured, which is expected given the fact that our sample included immigrants residing legally in Greece and, as aforementioned, security of legal residency requires legal employment and vice versa. On average, immigrants had a monthly income of about 707 €, while the mean number of participants did not belong/participate to a community/cultural organization at their country of origin, nor did any of them suffer from a chronic condition during the 3 years the study was carried out (2009-2011), a fact that would require one's regular visits (at least once every three months) to a healthcare facility.

Finally, on average, sampled immigrants had not been required to pay extra money for health services received by a public hospital during the 3 years of the study. Additionally, the participants expressed that their trust level toward the health professionals (doctors and nurses) of public hospitals and of their insurance carrier was moderate (=2).

From the above data it occurs that the three independent variables:

- x_{10} (community)
- x_{11} (disease)
- x_{13} (trust)

are statistically significant in our model, while chi2 = 0 determines that there is a zero possibility for an incorrect estimation (see **Table 3**).

Table 4 determines that the research's dependent variable and the estimated dependent ŷ (or y_hat) present similarities at about 61.5%. Based on the specific correlation degree, we conclude that the estimated model satisfactorily explains the true data.

To continue with, we express the coefficients of **Table 5** at an odds ratio.

The data of the above table suggest that the variables that determine the degree of the immigrants' satisfaction with the largest odds ratio (OR), are:

- The independent variable of *gender* which, when the condition changes (man to woman and vice versa), the probabilities of y being y = 1, that is the probability that the immigrants are satisfied with the hospital personnel's response to the health problem they faced during the course of the study (2009-2011), are reduced by **51%**. Meaning that, the degree of immigrants' satisfaction concerning the access they gain to the Greek health system, varies according to their sex at a percentage of 51%.
- The independent variable of *understanding*, which puts forward the degree of understanding of the Greek

Table 3. Probit results.

Iteration 0: log likelihood = −87.129444
Iteration 1: log likelihood = −60.919341
Iteration 2: log likelihood = −60.036189
Iteration 3: log likelihood = −60.027714
Iteration 4: log likelihood = −60.027711

Logistic regression

Number of obs = 138
LR chi2(12) = 54.20
Prob > chi2 = 0.0000

Log likelihood = −60.027711

Pseudo R2 = 0.3111

Satisfaction	Coef.	Std. Err.	Z	P > |z|	[95% Conf.	Interval]
gender	−0.7041091	0.5049579	−1.39	0.163	−1.693808	0.2855903
age	−0.0779157	0.5479484	−0.14	0.887	−1.151875	0.9960435
residence	0.0390207	0.0368509	1.06	0.290	−0.0332056	0.1112471
understanding	0.173153	0.2903223	0.60	0.551	−0.3958682	0.7421742
education	0.3657477	0.2705502	1.35	0.176	−0.1645209	0.8960163
job	−0.0639429	0.3931309	−0.16	0.871	−0.8344652	0.7065794
insurance	0.5942555	1.207695	0.49	0.623	−1.772784	2.961295
income	0.0004521	0.0004838	0.93	0.350	−0.0004962	0.0014004
community	−1.261027	0.5418181	−2.33	0.020	−2.322971	−0.1990828
disease	1.357208	0.5409311	2.51	0.012	0.2970021	2.417413
payment	0.1579794	0.834384	0.19	0.850	−1.477383	1.793342
trust	1.420884	0.3287442	4.32	0.000	0.7765572	2.065211
_cons	−5.197037	2.0217	−2.57	0.010	−9.159496	−1.234578

Table 4. Correlation ŷ & y.

. pwcorr satisfaction y_hat		
	satisf~n	y_hat
satisfaction	1000	
y_hat	0.6143	1000

language by the sampled immigrants, which is altered when its status changes, then the probability of y being y = 1 is raised by **19%**. Meaning that, while the level of language understanding is raised, the probability of the immigrants being satisfied by their access to Greece's health system is also raised by 19%

- The independent variable **education**, which represents the educational level of the sampled immigrants, which changes when its status is altered, *i.e.* when the immigrant's educational level is raised by passing from one academic level to the next, then the probability of the immigrant being satisfied with his/her access to the health system is raised by **44%**.

- The independent variable **insurance**, which represents the number of years of insurance of our sample, which when its status is altered, then the probability of y being y = 1 is raised by **80%**. In other words, when uninsured immigrants become insured, then the probability of them being satisfied by the Greek health system is raised by 80%.

- The independent variable **community**, which puts forth the sampled immigrants' participation in communities of their country of origin, which, when its status is altered, the probabilities of y = 1 decrease by **72%**. To wit, when the immigrant transfers from *not belonging to a community of his/her country of origin* (0 = no), into *belonging* (1 = yes), then the probabilities of him/her being satisfied with the Greek health system decrease by 72%.

- When the independent variable **disease**, which represents whether our sampled immigrants are suffering from a chronic disease (0 = no), changes status, then the probabilities of y being y = 1, are raised by **288%**. That is, when the immigrant passes into a condition in which he/she does suffer from a chronic condition (1

Table 5. Probit results (odds ratio).

Iteration 0: log likelihood = −87.129444
Iteration 1: log likelihood = −60.919341
Iteration 2: log likelihood = −60.036189
Iteration 3: log likelihood = −60.027714
Iteration 4: log likelihood = −60.027711

Logistic regression

Number of obs = 138
LR chi2(12) = 54.20
prob > chi2 = 0.0000
pseudo R2 = 0.3111

Log likelihood = −60.027711

Satisfaction	Odds Ratio	Std. Err.	Z	P > |z|	[95% conf.	Interval]
gender	0.494549	0.2497264	−1.39	0.163	0.1838181	1.330547
age	0.9250424	0.5068755	−0.14	0.887	0.3160437	2.707548
residence	1.039792	0.0383172	1.06	0.290	0.9673396	1.117671
understanding	1.189048	−3452071	0.60	0.551	0.6730954	2.100497
education	1.441591	0.3900228	1.35	0.176	0.8483	2.449824
job	0.9380585	0.3687798	−0.16	0.871	0.4341066	2.027046
insurance	1.811682	2.187959	0.49	0.623	0.1698595	19.32297
income	1.000452	0.000484	0.93	0.350	0.999504	1.001401
community	0.2833629	0.1535312	−2.33	0.020	0.0979821	0.819482
disease	3.885329	2.101695	2.51	0.012	1.345818	11.2168
payment	1.171142	0.9771822	0.19	0.850	0.2282342	6.009502
trust	4.140779	1.361257	4.32	0.000	2.173975	7.886959

= yes) and needs to visit a hospital regularly, then the probabilities of him/her being satisfied by his access to the NHS and the related services provided are raised by 288%.

- The independent variable ***trust***, which represents the degree of immigrants' trust toward health professionals (doctors-nurses) who belong to public Health or Insurance carriers, which when its status is altered, that is from no trust at all to some trust, or from a little trust to moderate or a lot and so on, then the probabilities of y being y = 1, *i.e.* the probabilities of the immigrants being satisfied by the personnel's response to the health problem they have encountered during the timeline of the study (2009-2011), are raised by **314%**. Therefore, this suggests that the more trust immigrants feel toward the health professionals, the higher the degree of satisfaction by the Greek health system.

4. Discussion

The findings of our study provide important information on immigrant satisfaction concerning the public health services provided in Greece. It was found that the demographic features of immigrants, and especially the *gender* variable (OR-51%), the *understanding* of the Greek language (OR = 19%), and the *education* variable greatly contribute to the configuration of the degree of immigrant satisfaction concerning the health system.

Other researchers give prominence to the gender variable as a lead factor influencing the level of satisfaction, given that older patients tend to be more easily satisfied in comparison to younger individuals; however, these findings are negated by other studies [33] [34].

It is interesting how the family income of immigrants poses no contribution at all to the degree of their satisfaction with the Greek public health system. The findings of the present study suggest that the income variable does not affect at all (OR = 0%) the modulation of the degree of immigrant satisfaction. This finding demonstrates that the health services are provided by Greek public hospitals without the requirement to submit additional payment (we are referring to insured immigrant patients). Moreover, this finding is entirely differentiated by data derived from other relevant studies, which support that more prosperous individuals receive better healthcare that non-prosperous ones, even within the same service and, thus, are more satisfied in comparison to patients with a lower social status [29]-[31].

Immigrants' participation to a community of their country of origin seems to negatively affect the degree of their satisfaction, to a great extent. Our study findings, suggest that for an immigrant who is a member of a community of his/her country of origin (social, cultural, religious), the probabilities of him/her being satisfied by the Greek NHS), are decreased by 72%. It is possible that this finding is owed to the fact that immigrants' participation to these communities formulates a protected environment, which covers their needs within this community, resulting in the deficient development/reinforcement of skills, such as, for example, learning the Greek language, which may enhance their social incorporation to the receiving country. Therefore, when immigrants need to come in touch with carriers of the Greek society, such as Greek hospitals, they encounter problems such as miscommunication, lack of knowledge concerning where they have to address their health needs, and end up dependent, to a great extent, on other members of their community who assume the role of mediator, interpreter, or escort to the health services, given that, as stated in other relevant studies, the complete lack of interpreters and mediators in public hospitals restricts the safekeeping quality health services [3] [4]. Studies conducted by Carrasquillo [35], Baker [36] and Morales [37], demonstrate the major influence of language knowledge or the provision of interpreters by the health system of the country of reception, on the degree of immigrant satisfaction.

From the findings of the present study, arises that immigrants who are health insured have 80% more probabilities of being satisfied with the health system. The specific finding, in harmony with the Greek legal framework, suggests that immigrant health insurance entails their access to health structures and, thus, constitutes an important factor for their satisfaction with health services. The most important influence on immigrant satisfaction with the health system is placed by the degree of trust that the immigrants themselves feel toward the health professionals of public hospitals and their insurance carrier. As is derived from our study, the more immigrants trust the health professionals, the higher are the probabilities that they will be satisfied by the health system, by an impressive 314%.

Finally, the findings of the present study provide evidence that a 67% of immigrants are satisfied with Greek healthcare services. In a study carried out in the U.K., Dixon-Woods *et al.* (2005) report satisfactory immigrant access to health services [8]. Similar findings resulted from studies carried out in the Netherlands in Scandinavian countries and in Spain [10]-[13]. However, not all studies provide results of a high degree of immigrant satisfaction with the healthcare services provided in the country of reception. More specifically, in a previous study conducted in Greece in 2012 using Russian-speaking sample, a 31.5% of respondents reported moderate satisfaction concerning the health services received in a public hospital, while the 44% was little or not satisfied at all [38]. Studies conducted in Europe [39]-[42], the U.S.A. [43]-[45] and Australia [46] [47], have provided evidence that non-western immigrants were less satisfied than natives. As a matter of fact, in a 2014 Special Eurobarometer, only 26% of Greeks evaluate the quality of healthcare in Greece as being "good" [48].

Similarly, there other studies carried out in Europe [41], the U.S.A. [49] and Australia [47], which report a higher or the same degree of immigrant satisfaction by public health services in relation to natives.

Finally, Kambale places the demographic features of patients, and especially the immigrants' gender, profession, age, income and education level in a high position in relation to the degree of their influence on the patient's satisfaction by the provided health services [50].

There are some limitations in our study. The study population was not a random sample of immigrants in Greece, although an effort was made to include the major groups in proportions similar to those reported by recent statistical data. Additionally, larger scale studies, including rural areas in Greece, should be conducted in order to better understand the degree of satisfaction of immigrants with the Greek NHS.

The present study constitutes one of the very few relevant studies conducted in Greece on the specific issue and, although it was not possible to define a random sample from the whole immigrant population who reside legally in our country, we feel that the final results may satisfactorily represent the general immigrant population who reside legally in Greece and use daily the Greek health system.

5. Conclusions

The results of our study provided evidence that legal immigrants in Greece have access to Greek NHS, while the degree of satisfaction with those services is relatively high (67%). Nevertheless, it must be emphasized that immigrants' reality is a hard one, because it is not enough to have legal residency, as mentioned, but also to be legally employed during periods when governmental and non-carrier research shows very high percentages of illegal employment within the Greek employment field.

Finally, immigrants who do not possess any legal documents constitute another, even more vulnerable and marginal group, which is deprived of the ability to access a series of rights, such as the right to healthcare and requires greater attention and support.

References

[1]　Papadaki, G. and Papapdaki, E. (2011) The Policy of Managing Migration Flows towards the European Union and Greece. *9th National Conference of Hellenic Regional Science Association*, Panteion University, Athens. (In Greek)

[2]　Hellenic Statistical Authority (EL.STAT.) (2012) Resident Population—Census 2011, EL.STAT., Athens.

[3]　Galanis, P., *et al.* (2013) Public Health Services Knowledge and Utilization among Immigrants in Greece: A Cross-Sectional Study. *BMC Health Services Research*, 13, 350 http://dx.doi.org/10.1186/1472-6963-13-350

[4]　Marantou-Alipranti, L. and Gazon, E. (2005) Immigration and Health Care. Assessment of the Current Situation. Challenges and Perspectives. National Center of Social Research—EKKE, Athens.

[5]　Médecins du Monde (2011) Access to Healthcare for Undocumented Migrants in 11 European Countries. Report of the European Observatory, Médecins du Monde, European Observatory on Access to Healthcare, Paris.

[6]　European Commission (2006) Equality in Health: Greek National Report. Edition of Directorate-General for Employment, Social Affairs and Equal Opportunities.

[7]　European Commission (2006) The Demographic Future of Europe—From Challenge to Opportunity, Communication from the Commission, Commission of the European Communities com (2006) 571, Brussels.

[8]　Dixon-Woods, M., Kirk, D., Agarwal, S., Annandale, E., Arthur, T. and Harvey, J. (2005) Vulnerable Groups and Access to Health Care: A Critical Interpretive Review. NCCSDO, London.

[9]　Reijneveld, S.A. (1998) Reported Health, Lifestyles and Use of Health Care of First Generation Immigrants in The Netherlands: Do Socioeconomic Factors Explain Their Adverse Position? *Journal of Epidemiology & Community Health*, 52, 298-304.

[10]　Stronks, K., Ravelli, A.C.J. and Reijneveld, S.A. (2001) Immigrants in the Netherlands: Equal Access for Equal Needs? *Journal of Epidemiology & Community Health*, 55, 701-707.

[11]　Uiters, E., Devillé, W., Foets, M. and Groenewegen, P.P. (2006) Use of Health Care Services by Ethnic Minorities in The Netherlands: Do Patterns Differ? *European Journal of Public Health*, 16, 388-393.

[12]　Hjern, A., Haglund, B., Persson, G. and Rosén, M. (2001) Is There Equity in Access to Health Services for Ethnic Minorities in Sweden? *European Journal of Public Health*, 11, 147-152.

[13]　Carrasco-Garrido, P., Gil De Miguel, A. and Jiménez-García, R. (2007) Health Profiles, Lifestyles and Use of Health Resources by the Immigrant Population Resident in Spain. *European Journal of Public Health*, 17, 503-507.

[14]　Cots, F., Castells, X., García, O., Riu, M., Felipe, A. and Vall, O. (2007) Impact of Immigration on the Cost of Emergency Visits in Barcelona (Spain). *BMC Health Services Research*, 7, 9-21. http://dx.doi.org/10.1186/1472-6963-7-9

[15]　Donabedian, A. (1988) The Quality of Care: How Can It Be Assessed? *The Journal of the American Medical Association*, 260, 1743-1748.

[16]　Yucelt, U. (1994) An Invetsigation of Causes of Patient Satisfaction/Dissatisfaction with Physician Services. *Health Marketing Quarterly*, 12, 11-28. http://dx.doi.org/10.1300/J026v12n02_03

[17]　Kolter, P. and Clarke, R. (1987) Marketing for Health Care Organisation. Prentice-Hall, Inc., Englewood Cliffs.

[18]　Tselepis, C. (2000) Satisfaction of the Health Service Users, Sociological and Psychological Approach of Hospitals. Health Services, Vol. A, Hellenic Open University, Patras, 158-164.

[19]　Mirvis, D.M. (1998) Patient Satisfaction: Can Patients Evaluate the Quality of Health Care? *Tennessee Medicine*, 91, 277-279.

[20]　Mladovsky, P. (2007) Research Note: Migration and Health in the EU. European Commission, Brussels.

[21]　Venema, H.P.U., Garrestsen, H.F.L. and Van der Maas, P.J. (1995) Health of Migrants and Migrants Health Policy. The Netherlands as an Example. *Social Science & Medicine*, 41, 809-818. http://dx.doi.org/10.1016/0277-9536(95)00065-F

[22]　Perez, C.E. (2002) Health Status and Health Behaviours among Immigrants. Supplement to Health Reports. Statistics Canada, Ottawa, 1-12.

[23]　Singh, G.K. and Siahpush, M. (2002) Ethnic-Immigrant Differentials in Health Behaviours, Morbidity and Cause-Specific Mortality in the United States. *Human Biology*, 74, 83-109. http://dx.doi.org/10.1353/hub.2002.0011

[24]　Muennig, P. and Fahs, M.C. (2002) Health Status and Hospital Utilization of Recent Immigrants to New-York City. *Preventive Medicine*, 35, 225-231. http://dx.doi.org/10.1006/pmed.2002.1072

[25] Leduc, N. and Proux, M. (2004) Patterns of Health Services Utilization by Recent Immigrants. *Journal of Immigrant Health*, **6**, 15-27. http://dx.doi.org/10.1023/B:JOIH.0000014639.49245.cc

[26] Khan, S.A. and Ghosh, P. (2005) Medical Needs of Immigrant Populations. *BMJ*, **331**, 418. http://dx.doi.org/10.1136/bmj.331.7514.418

[27] Wang, L. (2007) Immigration, Ethnicity and Accessibility to Culturally Diverse Family Physicians. *Health & Place*, **13**, 656-671. http://dx.doi.org/10.1016/j.healthplace.2006.10.001

[28] Hargreaves, S., Friedland, J.S., Gothard, P., *et al.* (2006) Impact on and Use of Health Services by International Migrants: Questionnaire Survey of Inner City London A&E Attenders. *BMC health Services Research*, **6**, 153. http://dx.doi.org/10.1186/1472-6963-6-153

[29] Mohanty, S.A., Woolhander, S., Himmelstein, D.U., Pati, S., Carrasquillo, O. and Bor, D.H. (2005) Health Care Expenditures of Immigrants in the United States: A Nationally Representative Analysis. *American Journal of Public Health*, **95**, 1431-1438. http://dx.doi.org/10.2105/AJPH.2004.044602

[30] Uiters, E., Devillé, W.L., Foets, M. and Groenewegen, P.P. (2006) Use of Health Care Services by Ethnic Minorities in the Netherlands: Do Patterns Differ? *European Journal of Public Health*, **16**, 388-393.

[31] Jansa, J.M. and Garcia de Olalla, P. (2004) Health and Immigrations: New Situations and Challenger. *Gaceta Sanitaria*, **18**, 207-213.

[32] National Quality Forum (2002) Improving Health Care Quality for Minority Patients: Workshop Proceedings. National Forum for Health Care Quality Measurement and Reporting, Washington DC.

[33] Hall, J.A. and Dornan, M.C. (1988) What Patients Like about Their Medical Care and How Often They Asked: A Meta-Analysis of the Satisfaction Literature. *Social Science & Medicine*, **27**, 935-939. http://dx.doi.org/10.1016/0277-9536(88)90284-5

[34] Khayat, K. and Salter, B. (1994) Patient Satisfaction Surveys as s Market Research' Tool for General Practices. *British Journal of General Practice*, **44**, 215-219.

[35] Carrasquillo, O., Orav, E.J., Brennan, T.A. and Burstin, H.R. (1999) Impact of Language Barriers on Patient Satisfaction in an Emergency Department. *Journal of General Internal Medicine*, **14**, 82-87. http://dx.doi.org/10.1046/j.1525-1497.1999.00293.x

[36] Baker, D.W., Hayes, R. and Fortier, J.P. (1998) Interpreter Use and Satisfaction Interpersonal Aspects of Care for Spanish-Speaking Patients. *Medical Care*, **36**, 1461-1470. http://dx.doi.org/10.1097/00005650-199810000-00004

[37] Morales, L.S., Cunningham, W.E., Brown, J.A., Liu, H. and Hays, R.D. (1999) Are Latinos Less Satisfied with Communication by Health Care Providers? *Journal of General Internal Medicine*, **14**, 409-417.

[38] Kotsioni, I. (2011) Access and Use of Healthcare Services by Migrants. Doctoral Thesis, National and Kapodistrian University of Athens, Medical School, Athens.

[39] Else, L. (2008) Non-Western Immigrants' Satisfaction with General Practitioners' Services in Oslo, Norway. *International Journal for Equity in Health*, **7**, 7. http://dx.doi.org/10.1186/1475-9276-7-7

[40] Borde, T., David, M. and Kentenich, H. (2002) What Turkish-Speaking Women Expect in a German Hospital and How Satisfied They Are with Health Care during Their Stay in a Gynaecological Hospital in Berlin. A Comparative Approach. *Gesundheitswesen*, **64**, 476-485. http://dx.doi.org/10.1055/s-2002-33775

[41] Ogden, J. and Jain, A. (2005) Patients' Experiences and Expectations of General Practice: A Questionnaire Study of Differences by Ethnic Group. *British Journal of General Practice*, **55**, 351-356.

[42] Mygind, A., Norredam, M., Nielsen, A.S., Bagger, J. and Krasnik, A. (2008) The Effect of Patient Origin and Relevance of Contact on Patient and Caregiver Satisfaction in the Emergency Room. *Scandinavian Journal of Public Health*, **36**, 76-83. http://dx.doi.org/10.1177/1403494807085302

[43] Taira, D.A., Safran, D.G., Seto, T.B., *et al.* (1997) Asian-American Patient Ratings of Physician Primary Care Performance. *Journal of General Internal Medicine*, **12**, 237-242. http://dx.doi.org/10.1007/s11606-006-5046-0

[44] Dallo, F.J., Borrell, L.N. and Williams, S.L. (2008) Nativity Status and Patient Perceptions of the Patient-Physician Encounter: Results from the Commonwealth Fund 2001 Survey on Disparities in Quality of Health Care. *Medical Care*, **46**, 185-191. http://dx.doi.org/10.1097/MLR.0b013e318158af29

[45] Ngo-Metzger, Q., Legedza, A.T. and Phillips, R.S. (2004) Asian Americans' Reports of Their Health Care Experiences. Results of a National Survey. *Journal of General Internal Medicine*, **19**, 111-119. http://dx.doi.org/10.1111/j.1525-1497.2004.30143.x

[46] Small, R., Yelland, J., Lumley, J., Brown, S. and Liamputtong, P. (2002) Immigrant Women's Views about Care during Labour and Birth: An Australian Study of Vietnamese, Turkish, and Filipino Women. *Birth*, **29**, 266-277. http://dx.doi.org/10.1046/j.1523-536X.2002.00201.x

[47] McLachlan, H. and Waldenström, U. (2005) Childbirth Experiences in Australia of Women Born in Turkey, Vietnam, and Australia. *Birth*, **32**, 272-282. http://dx.doi.org/10.1111/j.0730-7659.2005.00370.x

[48] European Commission (2014) Patient Safety and Quality of Care. Special Eurobarometer 411 Report. European Commission, Directorate-General for Health and Consumers (DG SANCO), Brussels.

[49] Markova, T., Dean, F. and Neale, A.V. (2007) Health Care Attitudes and Behaviours of Immigrant and US-Born Women in Hamtramck, Michigan: A MetroNet Study. *Ethnicity & Disease*, **17**, 650-656.

[50] Kambale, J.M. (2010) Migrant Patients' Satisfaction with Health Care Services: A Comprehensive Review. *Italian Journal of Public Health*, **7**, 69-81.

2

Exercise and Smoking: A Literature Overview

Maria Hassandra[1], Marios Goudas[2*], Yiannis Theodorakis[2]

[1]University of Jyväskylä, Jyväskylä, Finland
[2]Department of Physical Education and Sport Science, University of Thessaly, Karyes, Greece
Email: maria.m.chasandra@jyu.fi, *mgoudas@pe.uth.gr, theodorakis@pe.uth.gr

Abstract

The purpose of this review is to summarize the more recent research findings regarding the relationship between exercise and smoking behavior. Reviewed studies have been presented according to themes and research design types. Initially cross-sectional and longitudinal epidemiological studies have been reviewed in order to map findings regarding the correlations between those two behaviors. Moreover, studies exploring variables that function as mediators or moderators between smoking and exercise relationship have been included. Then studies examining the possible preventive effects of exercise on smoking behavior for adolescents are reviewed and implications for developing effective preventive intervention programs are provided. Finally, experimental studies examining the acute and long term effects of exercise on smokers are reviewed in order to conclude if exercise can act as a treatment for smokers to manage withdrawal symptoms and help them quit smoking. Overall, exercise seems to have a protective effect against smoking as well as a supportive effect on smoking cessation treatments. The investigation of the underlying mechanisms behind this relationship and the systematic synthesis of new knowledge on this topic can improve our understanding and inform the development of more effective health promotion programs.

Keywords

Physical Activity, Smoking, Prevention, Treatment

1. Introduction

Physical activity and smoking are among those modifiable behaviors with a great impact on health. Regular

---

*Corresponding author.

physical activity enhances prevention of heart-related diseases, hypertension, osteoporosis, diabetes, back pain, respiratory and musculoskeletal problems and metabolic and neurological disorders [1]. Also, depression and anxiety can be reduced through exercise [2] [3]. Regarding smoking, research has shown that it exacerbates the prevalence of various functional problems and leads to serious diseases. According to the World Health Organization, half of regular smokers will die from diseases that are directly attributable to smoking [4].

Research examining physical activity and smoking behaviors concurrently has begun during the 80's [5], with more studies emerging in the last decade. The purpose of this review is to summarize research examining the relationship between exercise and smoking. The reviewed studies are organized along three themes: a) How these behaviors are related? b) Can exercise serve as a preventive factor for future smoking behavior? c) Can exercise be employed as a treatment in smoking cessation programs? It should be noted here that the terms exercise, physical activity and sport have been used interchangeably throughout this review.

The studies are organized in three sections. The first one presents cross-sectional and longitudinal studies examining the relationship between exercise and smoking behaviors in various populations as well as possible mediators or moderators of this relationship. The second section reviews programs for smoking prevention and outlines implications for improving the efficiency of respective programs. Finally, the third section is on exercise as a means to quit smoking and outlines acute and long-term effects of exercise on smokers as well as findings from theory-based respective interventions.

2. The Relation of Exercise with Smoking Behaviors

The relationship between exercise and smoking has been explored employing cross-sectional or longitudinal research designs and by examining the effects of possible moderators or mediators on this relationship.

2.1. Cross Sectional Studies

Cross sectional epidemiological studies show an inverse relationship both for adolescent and adult populations. Regarding adults, an early study of Thorlindsson, Vilhalmsson, & Valgeirsson [6], found that those who took part in various sporting activities smoked less. Similar results were reported by Theodorakis and Hassandra [7] exploring smoking habits in relation to exercise and sport participation of Greek participants, with a mean age of 20.7 years.

Several studies on adolescent populations also showed that physical activity and smoking behavior are inversely related. For example, Marti and Vartiainen [8] reported that frequency of leisure time exercise was inversely related to daily smoking in 1142 Finnish boys and girls 15 years old. Coulson, Eiser and Eiser [9] assessed physical activity and smoking of 932 high school students (12 - 15 years old) with smoking being related to lower levels of physical activity. Similar findings were reported by Holmen, Barrett-Connor, Clausen, Holmen, & Bjermer [10], in a study with 6.811 Norwegian students aged 13 - 19 years old. Another study of Audrain-McGovern, Rodriguez and Moss [11] examined the relationship between changes in physical activity and changes in smoking habits of adolescents. Their results showed that higher physical activity levels of high school students reduced the odds of progressing to smoking. Finally, a more recent study of Leatherdale, Wong, Manske, and Colditz [12], examined how physical activity in youth populations is associated with susceptibility to smoking among never smokers. For the 14.795 students who had never smoked, smoking susceptibility was negatively associated with being highly active. All the above cross sectional studies imply that there is an inversed relationship between smoking and exercise.

A cross sectional approach has several limitations on establishing a clear relationship between measured variables. Studies with a longitudinal design have many advantages in comparison with cross-sectional studies in advancing knowledge, providing information about continuity and prediction, and about within-individual change [13].

2.2. Longitudinal Studies

Longitudinal epidemiological studies indicate that higher levels of physical activity reduced the odds of initiating smoking or increasing smoking [12] and persistent physical inactivity in adolescence relates to adult smoking, even after family-related factors are taken into account [14]. These results imply that higher levels of physical activity may reduce the risk of smoking not only during adolescence but also for later adulthood. A study tracking adolescents' physical activity and smoking behavior [14] concluded that participants who at baseline exhibited high levels both of smoking and physical activity levels, remained high, and those who had low levels retained these. On a more recent study, [15], investigated continuity and change in smoking behavior of Australian young women and associated attributes over a 10-year period. Moderate and high physical activity levels were associated positively with remaining an ex-smoker, implicating that cessation strategies should examine the role of physical activity in relapse prevention.

The inverse relationship between exercise and smoking behaviors derived mainly from epidemiological studies has generated related research questions, for example, since there is a trend which implies that the more you exercise the less you smoke, what other factors possibly mediate or moderate this relationship?

2.3. Mediation-Moderation

Several factors have been identified as either mediators or moderators of the smoking and exercise relationship. Tart, Leyro, Richter, Zvolensky, Rosen field and Smits [16], evaluated whether people who engage in vigorous-intensity exercise are better suited to regulate negative affective states. Negative affect mediated the relationship between vigorous-intensity physical activity and smoking, accounting for about 12% of this relation. Moreover, these relationships were stronger for individuals with high anxiety sensitivity than for those with low anxiety sensitivity.

Motivational variables have also been shown to regulate the relationship between smoking and exercise behavior. A study of Verkooijen, Nielsen and Kremers [17], showed that for males, participation in leisure time physical activity for friendship or competition reasons strengthened the inverse association between physical activity and smoking, whereas, in females, participation for losing weight or gaining self-esteem weakened the inverse association. In addition, enjoyment, health and, for females, friendships and stress relief were associated with less smoking irrespective of participation level, while self-esteem, losing weight and, for males, friendships were unrelated or even positively related to smoking. Thus the association between adolescents' leisure time physical activity and smoking behavior may differ according to the underlying motivation for the activity. Also, Papaioannou, Sagovits, Ampatzoglou, Kalogiannis, and Skordala [18] reported that a personal improvement goal in life was positive predictor of sport and exercise involvement and negative predictor of smoking and truancy two years later.

Global physical self-concept (GPSC), which is defined as a general perception of one's physical self, including appearance and physical activity competence, has been found to have an indirect effect on the relationship between physical activity and smoking to adolescents [19]. This finding suggests that the potential beneficial effects of physical activity on adolescent smoking may depend, in part, on GPSC and an adolescent's perception of his or her physical self may be one important factor to consider in youth smoking interventions.

King, Marcus, Pinto, Emmons, and Abrams, [20], examined the relationship between cognitive–behavioral (self-efficacy, decisional-balance) and motivational mechanisms (stage of change) which have been shown to mediate changes in both exercise and smoking behavior in 332 smokers. They reported that the cognitive mechanisms associated with changes in smoking behavior are related to the cognitive variables (decision balance and self-efficacy) which have been shown to predict changes in exercise behavior. Significant relationships in mediating mechanisms including decisional balance and self-efficacy between smoking and exercise provide preliminary information on how change in one risk behavior may relate to change in another. These associations have implications for future intervention research and for methods research on multiple risk factor interactions.

Overall, negative affect, anxiety sensitivity, emotional vulnerability, reasons for being physically active, personal improvement as a life goal, global physical self-concept, decisional balance and self-efficacy have been detected as mediation or moderation variables on the relationship between physical activity and smoking.

Given the inverse relationship between exercise and smoking and information regarding possible mediators or moderators of this relationship, questions that arise are: a) is it possible to prevent future smoking behavior if we promote exercise, especially in youngsters? and b) can exercise be employed in smoking cessation programs? Most of the above reviewed studies suggest that future youth smoking prevention programs should integrate strategies to promote physical activity in order to prevent smoking (e.g. [11]).

2.4. Exercise for Smoking Prevention

Youth who participate in organized sports at school or in their communities are, in general, less likely to engage in risky behaviors, such as cigarette smoking and drug use, than non-sports participants [21] although the cultural norms related to some forms of organized or competitive sports may be more or less conducive in encouraging and reinforcing tobacco use by adolescents [22]. This implies that the development of a healthy lifestyle in general (including physical activity) might be the main mechanism of smoking prevention (and other unhealthy behaviors e.g.: drugs) and not the activity per se. There is evidence that supports the incompatibility between those two behaviors, indicating that adolescents who participate in greater levels of physical activity are less likely to smoke, or they smoke fewer cigarettes [6] [9] [21] [23] [24].

Despite calls for interventions that address multiple health behaviors concurrently [12] [25] [26] most of the preventive programs for adolescents target solely smoking behavior or smoking related variables. Addressing two health-related behaviors concurrently, Hassandra, Theodorakis, Kosmidou, Grammatikopoulos, and Hatzigeorgiadis [27], applied a smoking prevention program, named "I do not smoke, I exercise", to 210 students of junior high school. The main focus of this program was the promotion of exercise as an alternative behavior to smoking. Results showed that the program succeeded in changing the students' attitudes, but follow-up assessment 12 months later showed that attitudes towards smoking and interest in information relapsed to the pre-intervention levels although knowledge was sustained. A review of 8 successive applications of this program, showed that it had stronger effects for elementary school students, but when additional activities for smoking cessation were added then positive results for high school students were also reported [28].

The Oslo Youth Study [29] targeted three behaviors: eating habits, physical activity, and tobacco smoking. At the end of the program the intervention group experienced a smoking onset rate of 16.5% and the reference group a rate of 26.9%. Additionally, intervention group students had a significantly larger increase in scores on a smoking knowledge index; they also reported a significantly larger increase in frequent exercise and a significantly smaller increase in consumption of alcoholic beverages. Both the above programs had as a long term effect the increased knowledge of experimental group students about smoking. Additionally, in the study of Tell et al. [29] the frequency of exercise was higher in the intervention group. This implies that if students manage to keep their exercise levels high then the probability of adoption of unhealthy behaviors (e.g.: smoking and alcohol) is lower.

Large scale surveys showed that there is a link between tobacco use and other unhealthy behaviors, and that people generally adopt an overall healthy or unhealthy lifestyle [26] [30] [31]. Theodorakis et al. [32] examined the healthy and unhealthy behavioral profiles of Greek high school students. Most of the students were clustered on the healthy profile with high scores on healthy attitudes towards lifestyle behaviors (exercise, healthy eating) whereas, the remaining students adopted an unhealthy profile with positive attitudes towards smoking, drugs and violence. It was concluded that students tend to adopt a group of healthy or unhealthy behaviors and therefore interventions aiming to promote healthy lifestyle should target more than one behavior. Similar conclusions have been offered by Coulson, et al. [9] who suggested adopting an integrated approach for school-based health education programs rather than treat health behaviors in isolation from each other. According to Lippke, Nigg, & Maddock [33], success in one behavior change can be used to facilitate change in another health-related behavior as well.

A related question regards the form of physical activity that may have the best results in preventing smoking. According to a study of Rodriguez and Audrain-McGovern [19], adolescents with decreasing and erratic levels of team sports participation were more likely to smoke than those with high levels of participation. Further, in the Holmen et al. [10] study, participants in individual sports requiring less endurance, especially body-building and fighting sports, were more likely to be daily smokers than nonparticipants. These data suggest that smoking habits associated with different sports should be considered when promoting physical activity for smoking prevention.

There are several intervention programs for adults aiming to raise awareness for the benefits of a physically active style for both physical and mental health and the benefits of quitting smoking on their health. A recent meta-analysis [34] which examined the outcomes of interventions aiming to increase physical activity as part of comprehensive multiple risk factors programs, reviewed 358 reports comprising 99,011 participants. The overall mean effect size for comparisons of treatment groups versus control groups was 0.19 (higher mean for treatment participants than for control participants). Participant characteristics were unrelated to physical activity effect sizes. Exploratory moderator analyses suggested that the characteristics of the most effective interventions were behavioral interventions instead of cognitive interventions, face-to-face delivery versus mediated interventions (e.g., via telephone or mail), and targeting individuals instead of communities.

2.5. Implications for Future Preventive Program Development

The general guidelines of successful interventions aiming to promote healthy behaviors and prevent unhealthy ones apply also to the effectiveness of intervention programs aiming to prevent smoking by promoting physical activity. The combination of program contents, the social setting, and individual dispositional characteristics can have an effect on the effectiveness of the prevention programs and therefore their design and implementation should be sensitive to population characteristics at both the individual and socio cultural levels [35] [36]. A review of reviews of behavioral change interventions aiming to reduce unhealthy behaviors and/or promote healthy behaviors (including physical activity and smoking behavior) concluded that interventions that were most effective across a range of health behaviors included physician advice or individual counselling, and workplace- and school-based activities. Mass media campaigns and legislative interventions also showed small to moderate effects in changing health behaviors [37]. The family status of adolescents also has been found to relate with both smoking and physical activity [30]. Finally, another suggested effective strategy that relates to both physical activity promotion and smoking prevention is the teaching of life skills to intervention groups. According to the World Health Organization [38] an important component of health education programs is a skills-based education including life skills. Therefore the incorporation of skills training especially for school children is necessary in order to effectively promote health related behaviors. Intervention programs who included skills training have reported positive results. For example, in the Sorensen, Gupta, Nagler, and Viswanath [39] study, the intervention group students were significantly more knowledgeable about tobacco and related legislation, reported more efforts to prevent tobacco use among others, and reported stronger life skills and self-efficacy than students in control schools. The life skills component has been used to the smoking prevention program "I do not smoke, I exercise" [27], with positive results, as mentioned earlier.

The need to develop, implement and evaluate public health interventions based on sound health behavioral theories has been well documented [40] [41]. The most popular psychological theories employed to explain the relationship between psychological variables and smoking behavior include: the Social Cognitive Theory [42], the Theory of Planned Behavior [43], the Goal-setting Theory [44], the Health Belief Model [45] the Thranstheoretical model [46], and the Self-Determination Theory [47] [48]. According to all the previous information it is clear that there is a need for awareness programs in order to promote physical activity and prevent smoking initiation especially to young people. School based awareness programs for all educational levels must be developed in order to promote healthy habits in early ages where the lifelong habits are formed. There is also a need to promote awareness in adults, where the awareness programs should be more focused to different targeted groups and develop interventions according to their needs, e.g. workplaces, or special populations.

3. Exercise as Treatment

The last two decades several studies have been published examining the effects of exercise on smoking cessation. Long term effects of smoking cessation programs that used exercise promotion as an additional aid strategy are less reported in the literature. A clearer understanding of the relationship between exercise and smoking cessation outcomes may improve the design and the effectiveness, of future exercise-based smoking cessation interventions. There are two main groups of experimental studies examining the effect of exercise on smoking related variables; those examining the acute effects and the ones examining the long term effects of an exercise program.

3.1. Acute Effects of Exercise on Smokers

Three reviews have been published since 2007 with a focus on the acute effects of exercise on smoking related measures [49]-[51]. Twelve of the 14 studies that were reviewed by Taylor, *et al.* [51] compared a bout of exercise with a passive condition and reported a positive effect on cigarette cravings, withdrawal symptoms and smoking behavior. The two remaining studies compared two intensities of exercise and showed no differences in outcomes between them. In all these studies cigarette cravings, withdrawal symptoms and negative affect decreased rapidly during exercise and remained reduced for up to 50 minutes after exercise. Cravings and withdrawal symptoms were reduced with an exercise intensity from as high as 60% - 85% heart rate reserve (HRR) (lasting 30 - 40 minutes) to as low as 24% HRR (lasting 15 minutes), and also with isometric exercise (for 5 minutes). It was concluded that even relatively small doses of exercise should be recommended as an aid to managing cigarette cravings and withdrawal symptoms.

Haasova, *et al.* [49] examined data from 17 studies which compared participants engaging in physical activity against control group participants using post-intervention measures of strength of desire and desire to smoke with baseline adjustments. Despite a high degree of between-study heterogeneity, their results showed that the effects sizes of all primary studies were in the same direction, with physical activity groups showing a greater reduction in cravings compared with controls, implying strong evidence that physical activity acutely reduces cigarette craving. The latest review of Roberts, *et al.* [50], came up with similar results as the two previous ones: cigarette cravings were reduced following exercise with a wide range of intensities from isometric exercise and yoga to activity as high as 80% - 85% heart rate reserve. However, measures of tobacco withdrawal symptoms (TWS) and negative affect increased during vigorous exercise. The authors pointed out that it remains unclear which is the most effective exercise intensity to reduce cravings and what are the underlying mechanisms associated with these effects.

All the above reviews provide strong evidence that exercise sessions have an acute effect on cigarette cravings, but the mechanisms remain quite unclear. All of the reviewed studies come from the behavioral discipline. There are other studies that come from the physiology discipline which might contribute to the understanding of the physiological mechanisms underlying these effects. The Roberts et al. [50] review grouped the most recent research findings in three hypothetical explanation scenarios: the affect, biological and cognitive hypotheses.

According to the affect hypothesis, several studies support the claim that an increase in positive affect could result in a decreased desire to smoke. However results from different studies are not consistent about which intensity is most likely to create a positive affect [52]. According to Bock, Marcus, King, Borrelli, and Roberts [53] and Harper [54] a bout of vigorous exercise reduced smokers' negative affect and psychological withdrawal symptoms. Whereas, in the Everson, Daley & Ussher [55] study both moderate and vigorous intensities had similar effects on cravings, but there was an adverse effect on mood. However, in non-acute effects interventions where the exercise intensity was gradually increased [53] [55], which allowed the smokers to adapt to exercise gradually the results may be different. Another way to examine the acute effect of different exercise intensities on mood in this context is to allow the participants to choose the intensity themselves during the exercise session according to the positive or negative mood they experience during exercise in relation to TWS. An experiment with this design might therefore give additional information on the Roberts, *et al.*, [50] suggestion to examine the mediating effect of mood on the exercise-craving relationship.

The proposed biological hypothesis as an underlying mechanism on the relation of exercise and TWS is quite equivocal. Some of the biomarkers influenced by both nicotine and exercise include cortisol, autonomic regulation (indexed by heart rate variability), noradrenaline, and adrenaline [56]. The general hypothesis is that exercise acts via the same neurobiological pathway(s) as nicotine to relieve cravings and TWS that cause relapse to smoking [51]. For example, stimulating increases in cortisol with exercise during nicotine depletion could provide an equivalent endogenous endocrine drive as nicotine. If exercise can have an effect in these physiological processes, then perhaps it can reduce the likelihood of smoking relapse, and offer an additional treatment option.

Changes in catecholamines is another area of exploration which is based on previous findings that levels of adrenaline and noradrenaline increase with smoking [57], and smoking cessation results in a decrease of both [58]. Thus, the increase in adrenaline and noradrenaline post-exercise may explain the effect of exercise on cigarette cravings. But, according to Richter and Sutton [59], during single bouts of exercise, the concentration of adrenaline and noradrenaline increases in line with the intensity and duration of exercise, which means that, if the exercise session is short and the intensity is moderate to light then it might be quite difficult for any changes to occur. Lately, this has been partially confirmed by a study which compared the effects of three exercise intensities on the desire to smoke. Findings support the use of vigorous exercise to reduce cigarette cravings, showing potential alterations in a noradrenergic marker [60]. Finally, changes in Heart Rate Variability (HRV) caused by short or long smoking abstinence and how acute bouts of exercise can have an immediate effect on HRV needs to be further examined in future research [61]-[64]. In this direction some later studies are much more supportive, for example, a single session of exercise (e.g.: a self-paced 15-min walk) can attenuate or reduce post-exercise both systolic blood pressure and diastolic blood pressure responses to stress [65] [66]. Korhonen, Goodwin, Miesmaa, Dupuis, and Kinnunen [67], also suggest that even if complete abstinence is not achieved, reduction in tobacco exposure and increase in exercise can improve the cardiovascular risk profile.

The cognitive hypothesis which claims that exercise may influence cognitive demand in such a manner that it acts as a distraction from smoking-related thoughts has not gained support lately since studies showed no effect of distraction on cigarette cravings [54] [68]-[70]. Roberts *et al.*, [50] postulate that expectancy and credibility are two factors that need to be further examined as possible regulating factors to this cognitive hypothesis in future research. Nevertheless, a more recent study showed differing activation towards smoking images following exercise compared to a control treatment and may point to a neuro-cognitive process following exercise that mediates effects on cigarette cravings [71].

It is apparent that in future research examining the acute effects of exercise on TWS, there is a need of integration of different methods and concepts from different disciplines. That way might be possible to avoid the pitfalls of these acute studies in a laboratory setting, where the effects do not necessarily translate to the real world settings.

To that direction it would be interesting to examine how different exercise intensities affect the interaction of physiological, biochemical and psychological mechanisms and what is the optimal level of exercise intensity and physical conditioning which has beneficial effects on physiological (catecholamines, opioids, inflammatory markers) and psychological (perceived self-control, positive mood and levels of feelings of euphoria and pleasure and decreased levels of pressure, stress and depression) indexes? Also, what other variables act as moderators or mediators when participants experience the effects of exercise on TWS from the participants' perspective?

In conclusion, we can postulate that there is strong evidence that an acute bout of exercise reduces cigarette cravings and TWS, although there might be some differences in the magnitude of this effect for light, moderate, or vigorous exercise. The underlying mechanisms associated with the effect of exercise remain unclear. These acute effects should be utilized in smoking cessation programs. Therefore, a review of longer term effects of exercise on smoking cessation follows.

3.2. Long Term Effects of Exercise on Smokers

A narrative review by Ussher, Taylor, and Faulkner [72] on exercise interventions for smoking cessation revealed mixed results. They focused more on studies that provided data for long term effects (more than 6 months). They identified 15 trials, seven of which had fewer than 25 participants in each treatment condition. These studies varied in the timing and intensity of the smoking cessation and exercise programmes. Three studies showed significantly higher abstinence rates in a physically active group versus a control group at the end of the treatment [73]-[75]. One of these studies also showed a significant benefit for exercise versus control on abstinence in a three-month follow up and a benefit for exercise in a 12-month follow up [74]. One study showed significantly higher abstinence rates for the exercise group versus the control group in the three-month follow up but not in the end of treatment or 12-month follow up [76]. An updated review by the same authors [77] concluded that two of the 20 trials offered evidence for exercise aiding smoking cessation in the long term.

In relation to the interventions' components, there is some evidence that additional (to the exercise program) supportive actions are necessary. This support can be either pharmaceutical e.g.: nicotine patches or gums [78]-[80] or counselling sessions, e.g.: cognitive behavioral support [74] [81]. Counselling can help people in organizing their everyday life activities, and direct them to participate in physical activity. Counselling techniques can also be employed to help deal with the desire for smoking and all the associated symptoms, such as sleeping problems, lack of concentration, depression and irritability. Within this approach, the aim of exercise is not necessarily fitness improvement but rather substituting attachment to smoking with attachment to physical activity, which offers a valuable and healthier alternative for smokers who try to quit [82].

It is not clear yet if an exercise program alone is enough to attain long term abstinence. Moreover, there is an on-going debate if the exercise program should start before, at the same time or after a set "quitting day". There are reasonable arguments for all these choices, but it is still unclear what other contributing factors may affect the effectiveness of these different options like, the previous fitness levels, age, motivation or the readiness level. The optimal length and frequency of the intervention sessions is still unclear but according to Marcus, *et al.* [76], at least 110 minutes of activity per week is suggested in order to maintain abstinence.

Regarding the exercise characteristics there are several combinations of type, intensity, frequency and duration that have been tested. Low intensity and frequency e.g.: once per week [76] [83] has provided inconsistent results on abstinence. Moderate and vigorous intensity with a frequency of three times per week for at least 2 months, provided more promising results [73] [84]. However, findings from the longitudinal studies showed that if intensity of exercise is progressively increased through smoking cessation programs smokers tend to adapt better to higher intensities [53] [54].

There is also an argument whether the supervised or unsupervised kind of exercise is more appropriate to achieve both abstinence and exercise adherence [74]. In order to increase the probability of abstinence at the end of an intervention, supervised exercise sessions look more adequate [74] [78]. But if at the same time the goal is to keep the participants active in order to prevent future relapses then, the addition of self-directed exercise looks more promising [79] [83] [85]. Therefore, a combination of both types may be the preferable choice. There is also a need to examine the effect of booster sessions after the end of the intervention (e.g.: via web-based programs, follow-up telephone counselling, mail out printed material, mobile phone SMS) on the long term exercise adherence and cigarette abstinence.

Several types of exercise have been tested, for example, resistance training [78], isometric exercise [86], t'ai chi classes [87] and yoga [88] for their effectiveness. According to Daniel, Cropley, Ussher & West [68], even very brief bouts of exercise (5 minutes) may be useful as an aid to smoking cessation. The positive effects of the different exercise types on quit smoking might suggest that any kind of exercise is effective or that exercise acts as a placebo effect to the quitting effort, because of the expectations. Nevertheless, if the focus of an intervention is exercise adherence then the individual preferences on the type of exercise might be an additional issue to be explored in future research.

Physical fitness is also considered as a contributing factor to the exercise-smoking relationship [89]. Usually low fitness levels act as a barrier when individuals try to exercise and not smoke. However, previous studies aiming to increase the physical conditioning as well, have reported positive results, although they did not provide long-term follow ups [73] [81] [90]. Nevertheless, physical activity as a smoking cessation aid is beneficial for participants in terms of psychological and general health even without any increases in fitness levels [51] [91]. In addition, regular physical activity increases caloric expenditure, and therefore may increase the metabolic rate and reduce the weight gain associated with smoking cessation [15] [82]. It has also been suggested that during therapy, the combination of appropriate exercise intensity and the use of techniques dealing with negative psychological situations are necessary in order to avoid interrupting the quitting efforts [92]. Findings from another study indicate that imagery-based self-talk exercises aimed at increasing self-compassion might facilitate the self-regulation of compulsive behaviors such as smoking [93]. Several studies have used supervised sessions of exercise in combination with cognitive behavioral strategies with satisfactory results. For example, goal setting, self-monitoring, reinforcement, self-monitoring and pedometers have been employed as motivational tools [80] [90] [94] [95]. A relative factor that has not been examined is the fitness level of the participants on the baseline and if this has an effect on the results of the intervention. The majority of the interventions either do not assess the starting fitness level or they target only sedentary participants.

Apart from assessing the behavioral measures related to the intervention programs aiming to achieve smoking abstinence through an exercise program, a series of psychological constructs have also been assessed, showing interesting results. Self-efficacy has been increased on programs, who involved cognitive behavioral strategies [81]. Depression and perceived stress were not affected by exercise, according to Bize, *et al.* [83], but according to Vickers *et al.* [96] depression was lower on women smokers on the exercise group and increased fitness was associated with fewer depressive symptoms on successful smoking abstinence among women [97]. The latest findings seem to be in accordance with the literature, which supports the claim that exercise reduces mood disturbance, stress and anxiety [98]. But, according to earlier research findings [95], there was a significant increase in Profile of Mood States (POMs) tension and anxiety scores for the active group compared with the controls at four months follow up. Schneider, Spring and Pagoto [99] commenting on these contradictory findings about the effects of exercise on negative affect during smoking cessation stated that exercise may help temper negative affect states for women with heightened smoking-specific weight concern.

Finally, physical activity could be promoted as a cessation aid and as part of a holistic lifestyle change consistent with a non-smoker's identity [100]. In a relevant study [101], participants stated that they perceived exercise as a means that helped them manage their feelings of stress and tension during their effort to quit smoking, and as a way to improve their life by adopting a healthier lifestyle.

Overall, the majority of the above studies focus on either physiological or psychological underlying mechanisms. There is a need for studies to explore both psychological and physiological variables in order to give a more holistic explanation of these mechanisms. Based on the above, it seems that understanding the psychological, biochemical, and physiological factors during smokers' exercise could lead to the development and implementation of an intervention program that combines exercise with applied counselling techniques aiming at smoking cessation. Therefore, it would be interesting to investigate how a smoking cessation program which incorporate an optimal intensity exercise program in combination with the more updated applied psychological and counselling techniques will affect the participants' physiological (e.g.: the increase of the levels of VO2), biochemical variables (such as β-endorphin) and psychological measures (increased perceived self-control, positive mood and levels of feelings of euphoria and pleasure and decreased levels of pressure, stress and depression)? In addition, it would be useful to examine at the same time what other moderators and mediators affect the exercise and smoking relationship, as they are reported by the subjects (motivation, significant others influence, attitudes, self-confidence)?

3.3. Theory Based Interventions

Behavior change is a multifaceted task and the attempt to change two behaviors at the same time is much more complicated. The need to build interventions on well theoretical grounded models is essential in order to better understand the most effective mechanisms to achieve long term effects on exercise adherence and smoking abstinence. On the other hand, the efficacy of health behavior change programs addressing a single behavior is questionable, as most people usually adopt multiple unhealthy behaviors [31] [102]. Therefore, targeting two behaviors, like exercise and smoking, in interventions may be more effective than focusing only in one.

There is prior research knowledge, well grounded in theory, on both behavior changes separately, which we can build on and test further on the combination of those two behaviors [103]. A theoretical model that has been extensively used on the prediction and explanation of health behaviors is the Theory of Planned Behavior [TPB, 43]. Central of the TPB is that any behavior is codetermined by behavioral intention and perceived behavioral control and that intention to smoke/to exercise can be predicted by attitudes toward smoking/exercise, subjective norms and perceived behavioral control. Intention reflects an individual's decision to exert effort to perform the behavior. On the other hand, Perceived Behavioral Control (PBC) is the extent to which an individual perceives that the behavior is under his/her control.

According to a meta-analysis of the prospective prediction of health-related behaviors with the TPB, its efficacy varies depending on behavior type, with physical activity best predicted, and abstinence behaviors predicted relatively poorly. The age of participants moderated the relations with student samples providing better predictions for physical activity, and adolescent samples giving better predictions for abstinence behaviors. The length of follow-up measures moderated models' relationships with behavior better predicted in the shorter term. Finally, self-report behavior measures were better predicted than objective behavior measures [104]. Armitage & Conner [105] in a review of 185 studies concluded that the TPB accounted for 27% and 39% of the variance in behavior and intention, respectively. When behavior measures were self-reports, the TPB accounted for 11% more of the variance in behavior than when behavior measures were objective. Attitude, subjective norm and PBC account for significantly more of the variance in individuals' desires than intentions or self-predictions, but intentions and self-predictions were better predictors of behavior. Additionally, according to Shiehotta, Scholz & Schwarzer [106] planning, maintenance self-efficacy and action control may be important volitional variables as they served as mediators between earlier exercise intentions and later physical activity. According to another systematic review of Hardeman et al. [107] the TPB mainly is used to measure process and outcome variables and to predict intention and behavior on interventions aiming to change health behaviors. Persuasion, information and skill development are the most common behavior change methods. All the above support the effectiveness of the TPB as an adequate theoretical background for behavior change interventions. Nevertheless, in smoking behavior the role of exercise has not been examined satisfactory.

4. Conclusion

Based on the studies reviewed in this paper, it seems plausible to state that exercise can be used both for smoking prevention and for smoking cessation. However, preventive programs should focus on an overall healthy lifestyle including exercise, rather than on smoking solely. Moreover, long-term interventions employing exercise to stop smoking should be coupled with respective counselling strategies.

Acknowledgements

This research has been co-financed by the European Union (European Social Fund—ESF) and Greek national funds through the Operational Program "Education and Lifelong Learning" of the National Strategic Reference

Framework (NSRF)—Research Funding Program: THALES. Investing in knowledge society through the European Social Fund.

References

[1]   Dishman, R.K., Heath, G.W. and Washburn, R. (2004) Physical Activity Epidemiology. Human Kinetics, Champaign, IL.

[2]   Petruzzello, S.J., Landers, D.M., Hatfield, B.D., Kubitz, K.A. and Salazar, W. (1991) A Meta-Analysis on the Anxiety-Reducing Effects of Acute and Chronic Exercise. *Sports Medicine*, **11**, 143-182.
http://dx.doi.org/10.2165/00007256-199111030-00002

[3]   Faulkner, G. and Taylor, A.H. (2005) Exercise as Therapy: Emerging Relationships between Physical Activity and Psychological Wellbeing. Routledge Press, Abingdon, Oxon, UK.

[4]   WHO (2015) Tobacco: Fact Sheet N°339. http://www.who.int/mediacentre/factsheets/fs339/en/

[5]   Blair, S.N., Jacobs Jr., D.R. and Powell, K.E. (1985) Relationships between Exercise or Physical Activity and Other Health Behaviors. *Public Health Reports*, 100, 172-180.

[6]   Thorlindsson, T. and Vilhjalmsson, R. (1991) Factors Related to Cigarette Smoking and Alcohol Use among Adolescents. *Adolescence*, **26**, 399-418.

[7]   Theodorakis, Y. and Hassandra, M. (2005) Smoking and Exercise, Part II: Differences between Exercisers and Non-Exercisers. *Inquiries in Sport & Physical Education*, **3**, 239-248.

[8]   Marti, B. and Vartiainen, E. (1989) Relation between Leisure Time Exercise and Cardiovascular Risk Factors among 15-Year-Olds in Eastern Finland. *Journal of Epidemiology Community & Health*, **43**, 228-233.
http://dx.doi.org/10.1136/jech.43.3.228

[9]   Coulson, N.S., Eiser, C. and Eiser, J.R. (1997) Diet, Smoking and Exercise: Interrelationships between Adolescent Health Behaviors. *Child: Care, Health and Development*, **23**, 207-216.
http://dx.doi.org/10.1111/j.1365-2214.1997.tb00964.x

[10]   Holmen, T.L., Barrett-Connor, E., Clausen, J., Holmen, J. and Bjermer L. (2002) Physical Exercise, Sports, and Lung Function in Smoking versus Non-Smoking Adolescents. *European Respiratory Journal*, **19**, 8-15.
http://dx.doi.org/10.1183/09031936.02.00203502

[11]   Audrain-McGovern, J., Rodriguez, D. and Moss, H.B. (2003) Smoking Progression and Physical Activity. *Cancer Epidemiology Biomarkers & Prevention*, **12**, 1121-1129.

[12]   Leatherdale, S.T., Wong, S.L., Manske, S.R. and Colditz, G.A. (2008) Susceptibility to Smoking and Its Association with Physical Activity, BMI, and Weight Concerns among Youth. *Nicotine & Tobacco Research*, **10**, 499-505.
http://dx.doi.org/10.1080/14622200801902201

[13]   Farrington, D.P. (1991) Longitudinal Research Strategies: Advantages, Problems, and Prospects. *Journal of the American Academy of Child and Adolescence Psychiatry*, **30**, 369-74.
http://dx.doi.org/10.1097/00004583-199105000-00003
Kujala, U.M., Kaprio, J. and Rose, R.J. (2007) Physical Activity in Adolescence and Smoking in Young Adulthood: A Prospective Twin Cohort Study. *Addiction*, **102**, 1151-1157. http://dx.doi.org/10.1111/j.1360-0443.2007.01858.x

[14]   Kelder, S.H., Perry, C.L., Klepp, K.I. and Lytle, L.L. (1994) Longitudinal Tracking of Adolescent Smoking, Physical Activity, and Food Choice Behaviors. *American Journal of Public Health*, **84**, 1121-1126.
http://dx.doi.org/10.2105/AJPH.84.7.1121

[15]   McDermott, L., Dobson, A. and Owen, N. (2009) Determinants of Continuity and Change Over 10 Years in Young Women's Smoking. *Addiction*, **104**, 478-487. http://dx.doi.org/10.1111/j.1360-0443.2008.02452.x

[16]   Tart, C.D., Leyro, T.M., Richter, A., Zvolensky, M.J., Rosenfield, D. and Smits, J.A. (2010) Negative Affect as a Mediator of the Relationship between Vigorous-Intensity Exercise and Smoking. *Addictive Behavior*, **35**, 580-585.
http://dx.doi.org/10.1016/j.addbeh.2010.01.009

[17]   Verkooijen, K.T., Nielsen, G.A. and Kremers, S.P.J. (2008) The Association between Leisure Time Physical Activity and Smoking in Adolescence: An Examination of Potential Mediating and Moderating Factors. *International Journal of Behavioral Medicine*, **15**, 157-163. http://dx.doi.org/10.1080/10705500801929833

[18]   Papaioannou, A.G., Sagovits, A., Ampatzoglou, G., Kalogiannis, P. and Skordala, M. (2011) Global Goal Orientations: Prediction of Sport and Exercise Involvement and Smoking. *Psychology of Sport and Exercise*, **12**, 273-283.
http://dx.doi.org/10.1016/j.psychsport.2010.12.001

[19]   Rodriguez, D. and Audrain-McGovern, J. (2004) Team Sport Participation and Smoking: Analysis with General Growth Mixture Modeling. *Journal of Pediatric Psychology*, **29**, 299-308. http://dx.doi.org/10.1093/jpepsy/jsh031

[20] King, K.T., Marcus, B.H., Pinto, B.M., Emmons, K.M. and Abrams, D.B. (1996) Cognitive-Behavioral Mediators of Changing Multiple Behaviors: Smoking and a Sedentary Lifestyle. *Preventive Medicine*, **25**, 684-691. http://dx.doi.org/10.1006/pmed.1996.0107

[21] Pate, R.R., Trost, S.G., Levin, S. and Dowda, M. (2000) Sports Participation and Health-Related Behaviors among US Youth. *Archives of Pediatrics & Adolescent Medicine*, **154**, 904-911. http://dx.doi.org/10.1001/archpedi.154.9.904

[22] deRuiter, W. and Faulkner, G. (2006) Tobacco Harm Reduction Strategies: The Case for Physical Activity. *Nicotine & Tobacco Research*, **8**, 157-168. http://dx.doi.org/10.1080/14622200500494823

[23] Aaron, D.J., Dearwater, S.R., Anderson, R., Olsen, T., Kriska, A.M. and Laporte, R.E. (1995) Physical Activity and the Initiation of High-Risk Health Behaviors in Adolescents. *Medicine and Science in Sports and Exercise*, **27**, 1639-1645. http://dx.doi.org/10.1249/00005768-199512000-00010

[24] Abrams, K., Skolnik, N. and Diamond, J.J. (1999) Patterns and Correlates of Tobacco Use among Suburban Philadelphia 6th- through 12th-Grade Students. *Family Medicine*, **31**, 128-132.

[25] Wilson, D.B., Smith, B.N., Speizer, I.S., Bean, M.K., Mitchell, K.S., Uguy, L.S. and Fries, E.A. (2005) Differences in Food Intake and Exercise by Smoking Status in Adolescents. *Preventive Medicine*, **40**, 872-879. http://dx.doi.org/10.1016/j.ypmed.2004.10.005

[26] Theodorakis, Y., Natsis, P., Papaioannou, A. and Goudas, M. (2003) Greek Students' Attitudes toward Physical Activity and Healthrelated Behavior. *Psychological Reports*, **92**, 275-283. http://dx.doi.org/10.2466/pr0.2003.92.1.275

[27] Hassandra, M., Theodorakis, Y., Kosmidou, E., Grammatikopoulos, V. and Hatzigeorgiadis, A. (2009) I Do Not Smoke—I Exercise: A Pilot Study of a New Educational Resource for Secondary Education Students. *Scandinavian Journal of Public Health*, **37**, 372-379. http://dx.doi.org/10.1177/1403494809103910

[28] Theodorakis, Y., Kosmidou, E., Hassandra, M. and Goudas, M. (2008) Review of the Applications of a Health Education Program "I Do Not Smoke I Exercise" to Elementary, Junior High School and High School Students. *Inquiries in Sports and Physical Education*, **6**, 181-194.

[29] Tell, G.S., Klepp, K.I., Vellar, O.D. and McAlister, A.L. (1984) Preventing the Onset of Cigarette Smoking in Norwegian Adolescents: The Oslo Youth Study. *Preventive Medicine*, **13**, 256-275. http://dx.doi.org/10.1016/0091-7435(84)90083-5

[30] Theodorakis, Y., Papaioannou, A. and Karastogianidou, K. (2004) Relations between Family Structure and Students' Health-Related Attitudes and Behaviors. *Psychological Reports*, **95**, 851-858. http://dx.doi.org/10.2466/pr0.95.7.851-858

[31] Theodorakis, Y., Papaioannou, A., Chatzigeorgiadis, A. and Papadimitriou, E. (2005) Patterns of Health-Related Behaviors among Hellenic Students. *Hellenic Journal of Psychology*, **2**, 225-242.

[32] Theodorakis, Y, Natsis, P., Papaioannou, A. and Goudas, M. (2002) Correlation between Exercise and Other Health Related Behaviors in Greek Students. *International Journal of Physical Education*, **XXXIX**, 30-34.

[33] Lippke, S., Nigg, C.R. and Maddock, J.E. (2012) Health-Promoting and Health-Risk Behaviors: Theory-Driven Analyses of Multiple Health Behavior Change in Three International Samples. *International Journal of Behavioral Medicine*, **19**, 1-13. http://dx.doi.org/10.1007/s12529-010-9135-4

[34] Conn, V.S., Hafdahl, A.R. and Mehr, D.R. (2011) Interventions to Increase Physical Activity among Healthy Adults: Meta-Analysis of Outcomes. *American Journal of Public Health*, **101**, 751-758. http://dx.doi.org/10.2105/AJPH.2010.194381

[35] Hanson, M.D. and Chen, E. (2007) Socioeconomic Status and Health Behaviors in Adolescence: A Review of the Literature. *Journal of Behavioral Medicine*, **30**, 263-285. http://dx.doi.org/10.1007/s10865-007-9098-3

[36] Johnson, C.A., Cen, S., Gallaher, P., Palmer, P.H., Xiao, L., Olson, A.R. and Unger, J.B. (2007) Why Smoking Prevention Programs Sometimes Fail. Does Effectiveness Depend on Sociocultural Context and Individual Characteristics? *Cancer Epidemiology Biomarkers Prevention*, **16**, 1043-1049. http://dx.doi.org/10.1158/1055-9965.EPI-07-0067

[37] Jepson, R.G., Harris, F.M., Platt, S. and Tannahill, C. (2010) The Effectiveness of Interventions to Change Six Health Behaviors: A Review of Reviews. *BMC Public Health*, **10**, 538. http://dx.doi.org/10.1186/1471-2458-10-538

[38] WHO (2015) The World Health Organization's Information Series on School Health (Document 9), Skills for Health. http://www.who.int/school_youth_health/media/en/sch_skills4health_03.pdf

[39] Sorensen, G., Gupta, P.C., Nagler, E. and Viswanath, K. (2012) Promoting Life Skills and Preventing Tobacco Use among Low-Income Mumbai Youth: Effects of Salaam Bombay Foundation Intervention. *PLoS ONE*, **7**, e34982. http://dx.doi.org/10.1371/journal.pone.0034982

[40] Glanz, K., Rimer, B.K. and Viswanath, K. (2008) Health Behavior and Health Education: Theory, Research, and Practice. John Wiley and Sons, Hoboken.

[41] Glanz, K. and Bishop, D. (2010) The Role of Behavioral Science Theory in Development and Implementation of Public Health Interventions. *Annual Review of Public Health*, **31**, 399-418. http://dx.doi.org/10.1146/annurev.publhealth.012809.103604

[42] Bandura (1986) Social Foundations of Thought and Action: A Social Cognitive Theory. Prentice-Hall, Englewood Cliffs.

[43] Ajzen, I. (1991) The Theory of Planned Behavior. *Organizational Behavior and Human Decision Processes*, **50**, 179-211. http://dx.doi.org/10.1016/0749-5978(91)90020-T

[44] Locke, E.A. and Latham, G.P. (1990) A Theory of Goal Setting and Task Performance. Prentice Hall, Englewood Cliffs.

[45] Rosenstock, I. (1974) Historical Origins of the Health Belief Model. *Health Education & Behavior*, **2**, 328-335.

[46] Prochaska, J.O. and DiClemente, C.C. (1983) The Stages and Processes of Self-Change in Smoking: Towards an Investigative Model of Change. *Journal of Consulting and Clinical Psychology*, **51**, 390-395. http://dx.doi.org/10.1037/0022-006X.51.3.390

[47] Deci, E.L. and Ryan, R.M. (1985) Intrinsic Motivation and Self-Determinaton in Human Behavior. Plenum, New York. http://dx.doi.org/10.1007/978-1-4899-2271-7

[48] Deci, E.L. and Ryan, R.M. (2000) The "What" and "Why" of Goal Pursuits: Human Needs and the Self-Determination of Behavior. *Psychological Inquiry*, **11**, 227-268. http://dx.doi.org/10.1207/S15327965PLI1104_01

[49] Haasova, M., Warren, F.C., Ussher, M., Janse Van Rensburg, K., Faulkner, G., Cropley, M., Byron-Daniel, J., Everson-Hock, E.S., Oh, H. and Taylor, A.H. (2012) The Acute Effects of Physical Activity on Cigarette Cravings: Systematic Review and Meta-Analysis with Individual Participant Data (IPD). *Addiction*, **108**, 26-37. http://dx.doi.org/10.1111/j.1360-0443.2012.04034.x

[50] Roberts, V., Maddison, R., Simpson, C., Bullen, C. and Prapavessis, H. (2012) The Acute Effects of Exercise on Cigarette Cravings, Withdrawal Symptoms, Affect, and Smoking Behavior: Systematic Review Update and Meta-Analysis. *Psychopharmacology*, **222**, 1-15. http://dx.doi.org/10.1007/s00213-012-2731-z

[51] Taylor, A.H., Ussher, M.H. and Faulkner, G. (2007) The Acute Effects of Exercise on Cigarette Cravings, Withdrawal Symptoms, Affect and Smoking Behavior: A Systematic Review. *Addiction*, **102**, 534-543. http://dx.doi.org/10.1111/j.1360-0443.2006.01739.x

[52] Elibero, A., Janse Van Rensburg, K. and Drobes, D.J. (2011) Acute Effects of Aerobic Exercise and Hatha Yoga on Craving to Smoke. *Nicotine Tobacco Research*, **13**, 1140-1148. http://dx.doi.org/10.1093/ntr/ntr163

[53] Bock, B.C., Marcus, B.H., King, T.C., Borrelli, B. and Roberts, M.R. (1999) Exercise Effects on Withdrawal and Mood among Women Attempting Smoking Cessation. *Addictive Behaviors*, **24**, 399-410. http://dx.doi.org/10.1016/S0306-4603(98)00088-4

[54] Harper, T.M. (2011) Mechanisms behind the Success of Exercise as an Adjunct Quit Smoking Aid. Electronic Thesis and Dissertation Repository. Paper 198. http://ir.lib.uwo.ca/etd/198

[55] Everson, E.S., Daley, A.J. and Ussher, M. (2008) The Effects of Moderate and Vigorous Exercise on Desire to Smoke, Withdrawal Symptoms and Mood in Abstaining Young Adult Smokers. *Mental Health and Physical Activity*, **1**, 26-31. http://dx.doi.org/10.1016/j.mhpa.2008.06.001

[56] Brunzell, D.H. (2007) Neurochemistry of Nicotine Addiction. In: Karch, S.B., Ed., *Drug Abuse Handbook*, CRC Press, New York, 23-38.

[57] Laustiola, K.E., Kotamaki, M., Lassila, R., Kllioniemi, O.P. and Manninen, V. (1991) Cigarette Smoking Alerts Sympathoadrenal Regulation by Decreasing the Density of *β*2 Adrenoceptors. A Study of Monitored Smoking Cessation. *Journal of Cardiovascular Pharmacology*, **17**, 923-928. http://dx.doi.org/10.1097/00005344-199106000-00010

[58] Ward, K.D., Garvey, A.J., Bliss, R.E., Sparrow, D., Young, J.B. and Landsberg, L. (1991) Changes in Urinary Catecholamine Excretion after Smoking Cessation. *Pharmacological Biochemical Behavior*, **40**, 937-940. http://dx.doi.org/10.1016/0091-3057(91)90109-F

[59] Richter, E.A. and Sutton, J.R. (1994) Hormonal Adaptation to Physical Activity. In: Bouchard, C., Shephard, R.J. and Stephens, T., Eds., *Physical Activity and Health: International Proceedings and Consensus Statement*, Human Kinetics, Champaign, 331-342.

[60] Roberts, V., Gant, N., Sollers III, J.J., Bullen, C., Jiang, Y. and Maddison, R. (2015) Effects of Exercise on the Desire to Smoke and Physiological Responses to Temporary Smoking Abstinence: A Crossover Trial. *Psychopharmacology*, **232**, 1071-1081. http://dx.doi.org/10.1007/s00213-014-3742-8

[61] Lucini, D., Bertocchi, F., Malliani, A. and Pagani, M. (1996) A Controlled Study of the Autonomic Changes Produced by Habitual Cigarette Smoking in Healthy Subjects. *Cardiovascular Research*, **31**, 633-639. http://dx.doi.org/10.1016/0008-6363(96)00013-2

[62] Niedermaier, O.N., Smith, M.L., Beightol, L.A., Zukowskagrojec, Z., Goldstein, D.S. and Eckberg, D.L. (1993) Influence of Cigarette-Smoking on Human Autonomic Function. *Circulation*, **88**, 562-571. http://dx.doi.org/10.1161/01.CIR.88.2.562

[63] Daniel, J.Z., Cropley, M., Ussher, M. and West, R. (2004) Acute Effects of a Short Bout of Moderate versus Light Intensity Exercise versus Inactivity on Tobacco Withdrawal Symptoms in Sedentary Smokers. *Psychopharmacology*, **174**, 320-326. http://dx.doi.org/10.1007/s00213-003-1762-x

[64] Stein, P.K., Rottman, J.N. and Kleiger, R.S. (1996) Effect of 21 mg Transdermal Nicotine Patches and Smoking Cessation on Heart Rate Variability. *American Journal of Cardiology*, **77**, 701-705. http://dx.doi.org/10.1016/S0002-9149(97)89203-X

[65] Hamer, M., Taylor, A.H. and Steptoe, A. (2006) The Effect of Acute Aerobic Exercise on Blood Pressure Reactivity to Psychological Stress: A Systematic Review and Meta-Analysis. *Biological Psychology*, **71**, 183-190. http://dx.doi.org/10.1016/j.biopsycho.2005.04.004

[66] Taylor, A. and Katomeri, A. (2006) Effects of a Brisk Walk on Blood Pressure Responses to the Stroop, a Speech Task and a Smoking Cue among Temporarily Abstinent Smokers. *Psychopharmacology*, **184**, 247-253. http://dx.doi.org/10.1007/s00213-005-0275-1

[67] Korhonen, T., Goodwin, A., Miesmaa, P., Dupuis, E.A. and Kinnunen, T. (2011) Smoking Cessation Program with Exercise Improves Cardiovascular Disease Biomarkers in Sedentary Women. *Journal of Women's Health*, **20**, 1051-1064. http://dx.doi.org/10.1089/jwh.2010.2075

[68] Daniel, J.Z., Cropley, M. and Fife-Schaw, C. (2006) The Effect of Exercise in Reducing Desire to Smoke and Cigarette Withdrawal Symptoms Is Not Caused by Distraction. *Addiction*, **101**, 1187-1192. http://dx.doi.org/10.1111/j.1360-0443.2006.01457.x

[69] Ussher, M., Nunziata, P., Cropley, M. and West, R. (2001) Effect of a Short Bout of Exercise on Tobacco Withdrawal Symptoms and Desire to Smoke. *Psychopharmacology*, **158**, 66-72. http://dx.doi.org/10.1007/s002130100846

[70] Daniel, J.Z., Cropley, M. and Fife-Schaw, C. (2007) Acute Exercise Effects on Smoking Withdrawal Symptoms and Desire to Smoke Are Not Related to Expectation. *Psychopharmacology*, **195**, 125-129. http://dx.doi.org/10.1007/s00213-007-0889-6

[71] Janse Van Rensburg, K., Taylor, A.H., Hodgson, T. and Benattayallah, A. (2012) The Effects of Exercise on Cigarette Cravings and Brain Activation in Response to Smoking-Related Images. *Psychopharmacology*, **221**, 659-666. http://dx.doi.org/10.1007/s00213-011-2610-z

[72] Ussher, M.H., Taylor, A. and Faulkner, G. (2012) Exercise Interventions for Smoking Cessation. *Cochrane Database Systematic Review*, No. 4, CD002295.

[73] Marcus, B.H., Albrecht, A.E., King, T.K., Parisi, A.F., Pinto, B.M., Roberts, M., *et al.* (1999) The Efficacy of Exercise as an Aid for Smoking Cessation in Women: A Randomised Controlled Trial. *Archives of Internal Medicine*, **159**, 1229-1234. http://dx.doi.org/10.1001/archinte.159.11.1229

[74] Marcus, B.H., Albrecht, A.E., Niaura, R.S., Abrams, D.B. and Thompson, P.D. (1991) Usefulness of Physical Exercise for Maintaining Smoking Cessation in Women. *American Journal of Cardiology*, **68**, 406-407. http://dx.doi.org/10.1016/0002-9149(91)90843-A

[75] Martin, J.E., Kalfas, K.J. and Patten, C.A. (1997) Prospective Evaluation of Three Smoking Interventions in 205 Recovering Alcoholics: One-Year Results of Project SCRAP-Tobacco. *Journal of Consulting and Clinical Psychology*, **65**, 190-194. http://dx.doi.org/10.1037/0022-006X.65.1.190

[76] Marcus, B.H., Lewis, B.A., Hogan, J., King, T.K., Albrecht, A.E., Bock, B., *et al.* (2005) The Efficacy of Moderate-Intensity Exercise as an Aid for Smoking Cessation in Women: A Randomized Controlled Trial. *Nicotine & Tobacco Research*, **5**, 871-880. http://dx.doi.org/10.1080/14622200500266056

[77] Ussher, M.H., Taylor, A. and Faulkner, G. (2014) Exercise Interventions for Smoking Cessation. *Cochrane Database of Systematic Reviews*, No. 8, Article No.: CD002295. http://dx.doi.org/10.1002/14651858.cd002295.pub5

[78] Ciccolo, J.T., Dunsiger, S.I., Williams, D.M., Bartholomew, J.B., Jennings, E.G., Ussher, M.H., *et al.* (2011) Resistance Training as an Aid to Standard Smoking Cessation Treatment: A Pilot Study. *Nicotine & Tobacco Research*, **13**, 756-760. http://dx.doi.org/10.1093/ntr/ntr068

[79] Ussher, M., West, R., McEwen, A., Taylor, A. and Steptoe, A. (2003) Efficacy of Exercise Counselling as an Aid for Smoking Cessation: A Randomized Controlled Trial. *Addiction*, **98**, 523-532. http://dx.doi.org/10.1046/j.1360-0443.2003.00346.x

[80] Kinnunen, T., Leeman, R.F., Korhonen, T., Quiles, Z.N., Terwal, D.M., Garvey, A.J., *et al.* (2008) Exercise as an Adjunct to Nicotine Gum in Treating Tobacco Dependence among Women. *Nicotine & Tobacco Research*, **10**, 689-703. http://dx.doi.org/10.1080/14622200801979043

[81] Prapavessis, H., Cameron, L., Baldi, J.C., Robinson, S., Borrie, K., Harper, T., *et al.* (2007) The Effects of Exercise and Nicotine Replacement Therapy on Smoking Rates in Women. *Addictive Behaviors*, **32**, 1416-1432. http://dx.doi.org/10.1016/j.addbeh.2006.10.005

[82] Taylor, A. and Ussher, M. (2005) Effects of Exercise on Smoking Cessation and Coping with Withdrawal Symptoms and Nicotine Cravings. In: Faulnkner, G. and Taylor, A., Eds., *Exercise, Health and Mental Health*, Routledge, London, 135-158. http://dx.doi.org/10.4324/9780203415016_chapter_8

[83] Bize, R., Willi, C., Chiolero, A., Stoianov, R., Payot, S., Locatel, I. and Cornuz, J. (2010) Participation in a Population-Based Physical Activity Programme as an Aid for Smoking Cessation: A Randomised Trial. *Tobacco Control*, **19**, 488-494. http://dx.doi.org/10.1136/tc.2009.030288

[84] Williams, D.M., Whiteley, J.A., Dunsiger, S., Jennings, E.G., Albrecht, A.E., Ussher, M.H., *et al.* (2010) Moderate Intensity Exercise as an Adjunct to Standard Smoking Cessation Treatment for Women: A Pilot Study. *Psychology of Addictive Behaviors*, **24**, 349-354. http://dx.doi.org/10.1037/a0018332

[85] McKay, H.G., Danaher, B.G., Seeley, J.R., Lichtenstein, E. and Gau, J.M. (2008) Comparing Two Web-Based Smoking Cessation Programs: Randomized Controlled Trial. *Journal of Medical Internet Research*, **10**, e40. http://dx.doi.org/10.2196/jmir.993

[86] Al-Chalabi, L., Prasad, N., Steed, L., Stenner, S., Aveyard, P., Beach, J. and Ussher, M. (2008) A Pilot Randomised Controlled Trial of the Feasibility of Using Body Scan and Isometric Exercises for Reducing Urge to Smoke in a Smoking Cessation Clinic. *BMC Public Health*, **8**, 349. http://dx.doi.org/10.1186/1471-2458-8-349

[87] Gryffin, P.A. and Chen, W.C. (2012) Implications of T'ai Chi for Smoking Cessation. *Journal of Alternative and Complementary Medicine*, **19**, 141-145.

[88] Bock, B.C., Morrow, K.M., Becker, B.M., Williams, D.M., Tremont, G., Gaskins, R.B., *et al.* (2010) Yoga as a Complementary Treatment for Smoking Cessation: Rationale, Study Design and Participant Characteristics of the Quitting-in-Balance Study. *BMC Complementary & Alternative Medicine*, **10**, 14. http://dx.doi.org/10.1186/1472-6882-10-14

[89] Macera, C.A., Aralis, H.J., Macgregor, A.J., Rauh, M.J., Han, P.P. and Galarneau, M.R. (2011) Cigarette Smoking, Body Mass Index, and Physical Fitness Changes among Male Navy Personnel. *Nicotine Tobacco Research*, **13**, 965-971. http://dx.doi.org/10.1093/ntr/ntr104

[90] Taylor, C.B., Houston-Miller, N., Haskell, W.L. and Debusk, R.F. (1988) Smoking Cessation after Acute Myocardial Infarction: The Effects of Exercise Training. *Addictive Behaviors*, **13**, 331-334. http://dx.doi.org/10.1016/0306-4603(88)90039-1

[91] Pate, R.R., Heath, G.W., Dowda, M. and Trost, S.G. (1996) Association between Physical Activity and Other Health Behaviors in a Representative Sample of U.S. Adolescents. *American Journal of Public Health*, **86**, 1577-1581. http://dx.doi.org/10.2105/AJPH.86.11.1577

[92] Irvin, J.E., Bowers, C.A., Dunn, M.E. and Wang, M.C. (1999) Efficacy of Relapse Prevention: A Meta-Analytic Review. *Journal of Consulting and Clinical Psychology*, **67**, 563-570. http://dx.doi.org/10.1037/0022-006X.67.4.563

[93] Kelly, A.C., Zuroff, D.C., Foa, C.L. and Gilbert, P. (2010) Who Benefits from Training in Self-Compassionate Self-Regulation? A Study of Smoking Reduction. *Journal of Social and Clinical Psychology*, **29**, 727-755. http://dx.doi.org/10.1521/jscp.2010.29.7.727

[94] Hill, J.S. (1985) Effect of a Program of Aerobic Exercise on the Smoking Behavior of a Group of Adult Volunteers. *Canadian Journal of Public Health*, **76**, 183-186.

[95] Russell, P.O., Epstein, L.H., Johnson, J.J., Block, D.R. and, Blair, E. (1988) The Effects of Exercise as Maintenance for Smoking Cessation. *Addictive Behaviors*, **13**, 215-218. http://dx.doi.org/10.1016/0306-4603(88)90016-0

[96] Vickers, K.S., Patten, C.A., Lewis, B.A., Clark, M.M., Ussher, M., Ebbert, J.O., *et al.* (2009) Feasibility of an Exercise Counseling Intervention for Depressed Women Smokers. *Nicotine & Tobacco Research*, **11**, 985-995. http://dx.doi.org/10.1093/ntr/ntp101

[97] Williams, D.M., Lewis, B.A., Dunsiger, S., King, T.K., Jennings, E. and Marcus, B.H. (2008) Increasing fitness Is Associated with Fewer Depressive Symptoms during Successful Smoking Abstinence among Women. *International Journal of Fitness*, **4**, 39-44.

[98] Taylor, A.H. (2000) Physical Activity, Stress and Anxiety: A Review. In: Biddle, S.J.H., Fox, K. and Boutcher, S., Eds., *Physical Activity and Psychological Well-Being*, Routledge, London, 10-45.

[99] Schneider, K.L., Spring, B. and Pagoto, S.L. (2007) Affective Benefits of Exercise While Quitting Smoking: Influence of Smoking-Specific Weight Concern. *Psychology of Addictive Behaviors*, **21**, 255-260. http://dx.doi.org/10.1037/0893-164X.21.2.255

[100] Everson-Hock, E.S., Taylor, A.H. and Ussher, M. (2010) Readiness to Use Physical Activity as a Smoking Cessation aid: A Multiple Behavior Change Application of the Transtheoretical Model among Quitters Attending Stop Smoking Clinics. *Patient Education and Counseling*, **79**, 156-159. http://dx.doi.org/10.1016/j.pec.2009.09.016

[101] Hassandra, M., Kofou, G., Zourbanos, N., Gratsani, S., Zisi, V. and Theodorakis, Y. (2012) Initial Evaluation of a Smoking Cessation Program Incorporating Physical Activity Promotion to Greek Adults on Anti-Smoking Clinics. *Evaluation & the Health Professions*, **35**, 323-330. http://dx.doi.org/10.1177/0163278712445202

[102] Laaksonen, M., Luoto, R., Helakorpi, S. and Uutela, A. (2002) Associations between Health-Related Behaviors: A 7-Year Follow-Up of Adults. *Preventive Medicine*, **34**, 162-170. http://dx.doi.org/10.1006/pmed.2001.0965

[103] Faulkner, G., Taylor, A.H., Urban, S., Ferrence, R., Munreo, S. and Selby, P. (2006) Exercise Science and the Development of Evidence-Based Practice: A Better Practices' Frameworks. *European Journal of Sport Sciences*, **6**, 117-126. http://dx.doi.org/10.1080/17461390500528568

[104] McEachan, R.R.C., Conner, M.T., Taylor, N.J. and Lawton, R.J. (2011) Prospective Prediction of Health-Related Behaviors with the Theory of Planned Behavior: A Meta-Analysis. *Health Psychology Review*, **5**, 97-144. http://dx.doi.org/10.1080/17437199.2010.521684

[105] Armitage, C.J. and Conner, M. (2001) Efficacy of the Theory of Planned Behavior: A Meta-Analytic Review. *British Journal of Social Psychology*, **40**, 471-499. http://dx.doi.org/10.1348/014466601164939

[106] Sniehotta, F.F., Scholz, U. and Schwarzer, R. (2005) Bridging the Intention-Behavior Gap: Planning, Self-Efficacy, and Action Control in the Adoption and Maintenance of Physical Exercise. *Psychology & Health*, **20**, 143-160. http://dx.doi.org/10.1080/08870440512331317670

[107] Hardeman, W., Johnston, M., Johnston, D., Bonetti, D., Wareham, N. and Kinmonth, A.L. (2002) Application of the Theory of Planned Behavior in Behavior Change Interventions: A Systematic Review. *Psychology & Health*, **17**, 123-158. http://dx.doi.org/10.1080/08870440290013644a

3

Health Related Lifestyle Behaviors among Students at a Vocational Education Center in Turkey

Melis Naçar[1]*, Fevziye Çetinkaya[1], Zeynep Baykan[1], Gökmen Zararsiz[2], Gülay Yilmazel[3], Mehmet Sağiroğlu[1]

[1]Department of Medical Education, School of Medicine, Erciyes University, Kayseri, Turkey
[2]Department of Biostatistics, School of Medicine, Erciyes University, Kayseri, Turkey
[3]Department of Nursery, School of Health, Hitit University, Çorum, Turkey
Email: *mnacar@erciyes.edu.tr

Abstract

Background: This study assessed health promoting lifestyle behaviors (HPLP) among apprentices trained in the Kayseri Turkey Vocational Education Center. Methods: This descriptive study was performed in 2012 in a province of Turkey. The study group included a cohort of 332 students attending the Vocational Education Center. All data were collected by using a 54-item (6-item related with socio-demographic and 48 item related with HPLP Scale) questionnaire. Data were evaluated by independent t test, One-Way Anova and Multiple logistic regression analyses. Results: In the study group, 88.0% were male and 12.0% were female. The mean age of participants was 17.1 ± 1.5 years. The mean HPLP scale score was 111.2 ± 22.0. The mean sub-scale scores were as follows: self-actualization 34.6 ± 7.5, interpersonal relations 18.6 ± 4.3, exercise 9.4 ± 3.0, nutrition 13.9 ± 3.5, stress management 16.2 ± 4.0, and health responsibility 18.6 ± 5.7. Age groups, regular payment and job satisfaction were significant variables for sub-scales of HPLP. In the regression analysis, job satisfaction had a significant impact on HPLP sub-scale scores. Conclusions: Healthy lifestyle behaviors were moderate level among students. Physical activity and health responsibility scores were the lowest scores. "Health Protection and Development" should be included as a standard component of vocational education.

Keywords

Health Promotion, Apprentice, Healthy Life, Education, Scale

---

*Corresponding author.

1. Introduction

The development of health consciousness, or the perception that personal health is an important part of daily life, inevitably enhances protection from disease and injury through the avoidance of risky behaviors [1] [2].

Health enhancement includes not only the prevention of illness, but also the promotion of general health and wellbeing [3] [4]. A healthy lifestyle consists of accepting personal responsibility for one's own health, self-fulfillment, health screenings, stress management, healthy diet and regular exercise [5]. Previous studies have suggested that lifestyle choices may account for as much as 50% of preventable deaths; lifestyle factors during childhood, adolescence, and adulthood are major factors in human disease [6] [7]. Behavior patterns are typically established during adolescence [8]; instruction of children and adolescents in health consciousness is more effective than alteration of adult behavior patterns. The extent to which childhood labor, living conditions, and harmful occupational environments affect the establishment of a healthy lifestyle remains unknown.

Dust, toxic chemical agents, lighting, heating, crowded workplaces, humidity, smell, ionizing radiation and other elements of harmful occupational environments threaten youth health [9]. It is vital that all individuals are knowledgeable regarding disease prevention and management in these environments. Childhood labor may lead to the slowing of normal development and growth, therefore, it is critically important that all underage laborers possess the health related knowledge that may provide protection from disease throughout life.

In Turkey, an apprentice is defined as one who receives knowledge, skills and on-the-job training in accordance with an apprenticeship agreement. An apprentice must be at least 14 years old, a primary school graduate, and healthy enough to meet the responsibilities and requirements of the workplace. An apprentice attends school one day per week and works five days a week.

A limited number of studies have been conducted on the lifestyle choices of working youth in Turkey; therefore, there is an urgent need for studies that can help assist in establishing health consciousness in this population.

This study aims to evaluate lifestyle instruction in working youth and to study the factors that influence these behaviors.

2. Material and Method

The research protocol was drafted in accordance with the Helsinki principles and Erciyes University reviewed and approved the study protocol. All participating students provided informed consent documentation. A written administrative permit was obtained from the Kayseri Provincial Directorate for National Education to conduct a survey in the Occupational Education Center.

2.1. Study Design

This study was conducted between January and February of 2012 at an Occupational Education Center attended by 3735 students.

2.2. Sample

The study recruitment goal was 400 students, or approximately 10% of the student body. The students were selected at random for participation in the study. Of the 400 students contacted by the researchers, 68 were withdrawn from the study due to refusal to participate or an inability to contact the student. The final study group included 332 students (83%).

2.3. Survey

The data was collected by survey. Participating students completed the survey under the supervision of a researcher. The first section of the survey examined the socio-demographic attributes of the participants (age, gender, education status of their parents, students' jobs, places they have spent the most of their lives) and self-reported economic status, perceptions regarding personal health, pre-existing disease, weight, height, apprenticeship, and workplace environment. The total period of study varies according to training program (two or three years for elementary school graduates; reduced by half for high school graduates). The classrooms are divided by grade.

The second part of the survey was adapted from Walker, Sechrist and Pender in 1987 [5], with a Turkish validation study conducted by Esin [10] in 1997. This study is referred to as the "Health Promoting Lifestyle Profile (HPLP) Scale". The coefficient of internal consistency (Cronbach Alpha) was reported as 0.91.

The questionnaire included the following subgroups: self-development, health responsibility, exercise, nutrition, interpersonal support and stress management.

2.4. Measures

Responses were scored using a four point Likert-type scale, with "Anytime" = 1 point, "Sometimes" = 2 point, "Often" = 3 points, and "Regularly" = 4 points.

The self-development component (range: 13 - 52), consisting of 13 questions, determines an individual's life goals and self-fulfillment. The health responsibility component (range: 10 - 40), consisting of ten questions, determines the extent to which an individual participates in their own health. The exercise component (range: 5 - 20), consisting of five questions, evaluates the degree to which an individual practices regular exercise. The nutrition component (range: 6 - 24), consisting of six questions, evaluates an individual's food consumption. The interpersonal support component (range: 7 - 28), consisting of seven questions, determines an individuals' level of engagement with family and friends. The stress management component (range: 7 - 28), consisting of seven questions, evaluates an individual's ability to recognize and manage sources of stress. Overall, the HPLP Scale (range: 48 - 192) consists of 48 unique questions.

According to the World Health Organization, a Body Mass Index (BMI) of less than 18.5 is defined as underweight, BMI of 18.5 - 24.9 is defined as normal, BMI of 25.0 - 29.9 is overweight, and BMI of 30.0 and greater is defined as obese [11].

2.5. Statistical Analysis

IBM SPSS Statistics 20.0 (IBM Inc., Chicago, IL, USA) was used for all data analysis. The Shapiro-Wilk's Test was used to determine conformation with the normal distribution. Multiple Regression Analysis was conducted to evaluate the influence of variables such as gender, rank, age, pre-existing chronic disease, and employment status on the healthy lifestyle scale score or on sub-scale scores. Age and daily work hours were treated as continuous variables. The threshold of statistical significance was set at $p < 0.05$.

3. Results

The average age of the apprentices participating in the study was 17.1 ± 1.5 years, with 88.0% of the study group composed of males and females accounting for 12% of the study group. A total 39.8% of the apprentices were in the first year of study. The participants reported that 63.0% of their fathers and 68.1% of their mothers were primary school graduates. 71.6% of the participating apprentices indicated that their fathers are working and 15.4% retired; 16.6% indicated that their mothers are working and 4.5% retired. 59.9% of study participants had spent the majority of their life living in urban areas.

The socio-demographic characteristics of the students are given in **Table 1**.

The average age at which the participants started apprenticeships was 15.4 ± 1.7 years (range: 10 - 28 years). 41.9% of the students indicated that their term of employment had been two years or less; 75.3% of participants indicated that they were paid regularly; 15.4% of participants were provided with insurance by their employer. 15.6% of the students were underweight and 71.0% of students had normal body weight. The mean Body Mass Index (BMI) was 21.7 ± 3.5. A total of 7.5% of participants had been diagnosed with a chronic disease.

Distribution and healthy lifestyle behavior scale scores of students are given in **Table 2**. The average overall HPLP scale score was 111.2 ± 22.0 and the average subgroup scale scores were 34.6 ± 7.5 for self-fulfillment, 18.6 ± 4.3 for support among individuals, 9.4 ± 3.0 for exercise, 13.9 ± 3.5 for nutrition, 16.2 ± 4.0 for stress management, and 18.6 ± 5.7 for health responsibility (**Table 2**).

Health Promoting Lifestyle Profile Scale and Subscale scores of students according to some characteristics are given in **Table 3**. There was no difference among male students and female students in terms of the HPLP scores. Class and chronic disease diagnosis were not associated with significant differences in HPLP scores. Gender, rank, age group, pre-existing chronic disease, employment status and job satisfaction were not associated with differences in exercise sub-scale scores. Gender, rank, age group, and pre-existing chronic disease were not associated with significant differences in nutrition sub-scale scores, although job satisfaction was associated with higher nutrition sub-scale scores compared to individuals who reported being unsatisfied with their current employment (**Table 3**).

Table 1. The socio-demographic characteristics of the students.

Characteristics	n	%
Gender		
Male	292	88.0
Female	40	12.0
Grade		
First year	132	39.8
Last year	200	60.2
Age Groups		
15 - 17	213	64,2
18 and ↑	119	35.8
Mothers education		
illiterate/literate	31	9.3
Primary or secondary school	226	61.8
At least high school	75	22.6
Fathers Education		
Illiterate/literate	15	4.5
Primary or secondary school	209	63.0
At least high school	108	32.5
Mothers occupation		
Working	55	16.6
Retired	15	4.5
Housewife	262	78.9
Fathers occupation		
Working	238	71.6
Retired	51	15.4
Not working	43	13.0
The place mostly lived in		
Rural area	133	40.1
Urban area	199	59.9
Economic status (according to their evaluation)		
Good	137	41.3
Moderate	169	50.9
Bad	26	7,8
Presence of chronic disease		
Yes	25	7.5
No	307	92,5
Perception of health situation		
Very good	72	21.7
Good	156	47.0
Moderate/Bad	104	31.3

Table 2. Distribution and healthy lifestyle behavior scale scores of students.

HPLP and subscales	Items	Range of obtainable scores (min-max)	Mean score ± SD	Items mean score ± SD*
Self-actualization	13	13 - 52	34.6 ± 7.5	2.7 ± 0.6
Interpersonal relations	7	7 - 28	18.6 ± 4.3	2.7 ± 0.6
Physical activity	5	5 - 20	9.4 ± 3.0	1.9 ± 0.6
Nutrition	6	6 - 24	13.9 ± 3.5	2.3 ± 0.6
Stress management	7	7 - 28	16.2 ± 4.0	2.3 ± 0.6
Health responsibility	10	10 - 40	18.6 ± 5.7	1.9 ± 0.6
Total Score	48	48 - 192	111.2 ± 22.0	2.3 ± 0.5

*The highest possible score in each item four.

Table 3. Health promoting lifestyle profile scale scores of students according to some characteristics.

Variables	n	Health Promoting Lifestyle Profile Scale Scores						
		Self-actualization	Health responsibility	Physical activity	Nutrition	Interpersonal relations	Stress management	Total
		X ± SD	X ± SD	X ± SD	X ± SD	X ± SD	X ± SD	X ± SD
Gender								
Male	292	34.6 ± 7.6	18.6 ± 5.7	9.5 ± 3.1	14.0 ± 3.4	18.7 ± 4.4	16.3 ± 4.1	111.6 ± 22.5
Female	40	34.5 ± 6.7	19.0 ± 5.3	8.7 ± 2.5	13.1 ± 3.5	17.5 ± 3.1	15.6 ± 3.7	108.3 ± 18.0
		p = 0.933	p = 0.712	p = 0.120	p = 0.095	p = 0.087	p = 0.311	p = 0.385
Grade								
First year	132	34.8 ± 7.0	18.8 ± 4.8	9.6 ± 3.0	14.0 ± 3.2	18.5 ± 4.2	16.5 ± 3.9	112.0 ± 20.3
Last year	200	34.4 ± 7.9	18.5 ± 6.2	9.3 ± 3.0	13.9 ± 3.6	18.7 ± 4.4	16.0 ± 4.1	110.6 ± 21.2
		p = 0.677	p = 0.640	p = 0.419	p = 0.692	p = 0.767	p = 0.254	p = 0.581
Age Groups								
15 - 17	213	34.9 ± 7.2	18.0 ± 5.7	9.5 ± 3.0	14.1 ± 3.4	18.6 ± 4.2	16.6 ± 4.0	112.2 ± 21.2
18 and ↑	119	34.1 ± 8.0	18.2 ± 5.7	9.2 ± 3.0	13.6 ± 3.5	18.6 ± 4.5	15.6 ± 4.0	109.3 ± 23.4
		p = 0.377	p = 0.248	p = 0.388	p = 0.154	p = 0.6998	**p = 0.045**	p = 0.262
Presence of chronic disease								
Yes	25	33.1 ± 8.7	19.1 ± 6.7	10.1 ± 3.4	13.3 ± 4.2	18.2 ± 4.8	15.8 ± 4.9	109.6 ± 28.8
No	307	34.7 ± 7.4	18.6 ± 5.6	9.3 ± 3.0	14.0 ± 3.4	18.6 ± 4.3	16.3 ± 4.0	111.3 ± 21.4
		p = 0.317	p = 0.659	p = 0.239	p = 0.359	p = 0.601	p = 0.544	p = 0.706
Regular pick up fees								
Yes	260	34.9 ± 7.5	18.8 ± 5.7	9.5 ± 3.1	14.2 ± 3.4	18.8 ± 4.2	16.3 ± 4.0	112.3 ± 21.8
No	72	33.4 ± 7.4	17.8 ± 5.4	8.8 ± 2.9	12.9 ± 3.5	17.8 ± 4.4	15.6 ± 4.1	105.9 ± 21.8
		p = 0.143	p = 0.204	p = 0.084	**p = 0.009**	**p = 0.019**	p = 0.211	**p = 0.033**
Job satisfaction								
Satisfied	270	35.6 ± 7.4	19.0 ± 5.8	9.5 ± 3.0	14.2 ± 3.5	18.9 ± 4.2	16.4 ± 4.0	113.4 ± 21.7
Undecided	42	30.0 ± 6.9	17.2 ± 5.0	9.5 ± 2.8	13.0 ± 2.9	17.6 ± 4.1	15.0 ± 3.8	101.9 ± 21.6
Not satisfied	20	30.3 ± 6.0	16.3 ± 4.3	8.1 ± 3.0	11.8 ± 3.0	16.1 ± 5.1	16.0 ± 4.4	99.3 ± 18.1
		p = 0.0001	**p = 0.029**	p = 0.157	**p = 0.002**	**p = 0.005**	p = 0.091	**p = 0.0001**

Job satisfaction was the most significant independent predictor of self-fulfillment, health responsibility, interpersonal support, stress management and total score; both job satisfaction and daily work status were significant predictors of nutrition sub-scale score. Job satisfaction accounted for 8.4% of variation in the self-fulfillment sub-scale score, 2.0% of the variation in health responsibility sub-scale score, 5.4% of the variation in nutrition sub-scale score (along with daily work status), 2.7% of variation in interpersonal support sub-scale score, 1.2% of the variation in stress management, sub-scale score, and 4.7% of the variation in total healthy lifestyle scale score (**Table 4**).

In an effort to model the relationship between job satisfaction and daily work variables with individual sub-scale scores, a linear regression analysis was performed. The analysis revealed the following relationships:

Self-actualization = 30.049 + (5.564 × Job Satisfaction)

Health responsibility = 16,933 + (2.085 × Job Satisfaction)

Nutrition = 14.942 + (1.619 × Job Satisfaction) + (2.085 × Daily work)

Interpersonal relations = 17.083 + (1.846 × Job Satisfaction)

Stress management = 15.306 + (1.138 × Job Satisfaction)

Total HPLP = 101.069 + (12.315 × Job Satisfaction)

All of the regression equations produced were found to be statistically significant ($p < 0.05$). The relationship between the scale score and the job satisfaction was positive (Beta > 0), while the relationship between the scale score and daily work status was negative (Beta < 0). Satisfaction with the current job increased self-fulfillment score by 28.9%, health responsibility score by 14.2%, nutrition scale score by 18.2%, group support score by 16.6%, stress management score by 11.1%, and increased total scale score by 21.6% (**Table 4**).

4. Discussion

The present study evaluated health-related behavior among a population of young workers who are at high risk

Table 4. Evaluation of healthy lifestyles of various variables impact on the scale and subscale scores with multiple linear regression analysis in the study group.

Variable	b_i	$S(b_i)$	BETA	t	p
Self-actualization					
Constant	30.049	0.924	-	32.517	**<0.001**
Job satisfaction	5.564	1.025	0.289	5.427	**<0.001**
$s = 7.217, R^2 = 0.084$ ($F = 29.453, p < 0.001$)					
Health responsibility					
Constant	16.933	0.724	-	23.390	**<0.001**
Job satisfaction	2.085	0.800	0.142	2.605	**0.010**
$s = 5.608, R^2 = 0.020,$ ($F = 6.788, p = 0.010$)					
Nutrition					
Constant	14.942	1.081	-	13.825	**<0.001**
Job satisfaction	1.619	0.491	0.182	3.297	**0.001**
Daily work	−0.217	0.090	−0.134	-2.415	**0.016**
$s = 3.347, R^2 = 0.054,$ ($F = 8.793, p < 0.001$)					
Interpersonal relations					
Constant	17.083	0.549	-	31.094	**<0.001**
Job satisfaction	1.846	0.607	0.166	3.040	**0.003**
$s = 7.217, R^2 = 0.027,$ ($F = 9.240, p = 0.003$)					
Stress management					
Constant	15.306	0.508	-	30.104	**<0.001**
Job satisfaction	1.138	0.564	0.111	2.016	**0.045**
$s = 4.004, R^2 = 0.012,$ ($F = 4.065, p = 0.045$)					
Total					
Constant	101.069	2.825	-	35.779	**<0.001**
Job satisfaction	12.315	3.121	0.216	3.946	**<0.001**
$s = 21.513, R^2 = 0.047,$ ($F = 15.572, p < 0.001$)					

of developing chronic disease. Students at the Apprenticeship Education Center scored 111.2 ± 22.0 out of 192 possible points on the HPLP scale; expressed as a four-point scale, this corresponds to 2.3 ± 0.5 (**Table 2**).

Our results were lower than results reported in a previous study [12] (117.43 ± 19.5) of adolescent workers and lower (118.5 ± 21.4) than the average for Higher Education Occupational Schools in Kayseri. The health responsibility (1.9 ± 0.6) and exercise (1.9 ± 0.6) sub-scores were the lowest scoring categories in the present study (**Table 2**).

In a previous study of Turkish high school students [13], the health responsibility (1.9 ± 0.5) and exercise (2.2 ± 0.7) sub-scores were also the lowest scoring categories. These results are similar to the results of other studies that have applied the HPLP scale [14] [15].

Apprentices in the present study reported the highest scores for group support (2.7 ± 0.6) and self-fulfillment sub-groups (2.7 ± 0.6) (**Table 2**). This result was similar to previous reports, both internationally and domestically, using the same scale in comparable populations [13] [16]-[18]. Gender, grade, age, and existence of a chronic disease were not associated with meaningful differences in HPLP scale scores. However, regular pay and job satisfaction were associated with higher HPLP scores. Regression analysis revealed that job satisfaction was a significant factor in total HPLP Scale and the sub-scale points, however other variables were not found to be meaningful (**Table 3**, **Table 4**). There was no difference in HPLP score or sub-scores between freshman students and those who were enrolled in advanced classes. The inclusion of health and behavioral instruction in apprenticeship training is important for the improvement of health outcomes in this population. There was no age-dependent difference in total HPLP score, self-fulfillment, health responsibility, exercise, nutrition, interpersonal support subs-scores. This is consistent with the published literature [17]. Age was not a significant factor in the multiple regression analysis. Total HPLP score and sub-scale scores increased with age, similar to previous studies [12] [19]. However, the stress management sub-scale score for students' age 15 - 17 was significantly higher relative to students aged 18 and over. Thus, while overall healthy behavior does not increase with age, stress management ability generally decreases. Job satisfaction affects the organizational behavior of employees. The characteristics of a job influence job satisfaction, motivation and self-fulfillment behavior [20] [21]. The self-fulfillment sub-scores were much higher among individuals who reported high levels of job satisfaction. In the present study, the healthy responsibility sub-scores were significantly higher among participants who reported being satisfied with their current jobs. Self-responsibility that develops during childhood and adolescence persists during adulthood.

In this study, male apprentices attending the first grade, who were diagnosed with a chronic disease, who got paid regularly, and who reported being pleased with their jobs scored higher in the exercise sub-scale. Exercise scores decreased with increasing age (p < 0.05). Previous studies conducted in Turkey support these findings [12] [22] [23]. Physical activity decreases over time, particularly among adolescents [24]. Regular exercise during childhood and adolescence has a positive influence on long-term health. Regular exercise is associated with reduced risk of coronary artery disease, improved blood pressure, enhanced immunity, reduced risk of osteoporosis, and longevity [1]. Hence, regular exercise is vital for apprentices and other adolescent populations. Healthy growth and development requires adequate and balanced nutrition. General nutritional requirements increase during adolescence. The additional expenditure of calories in the workplace further increases nutritional requirements. Nutritional inadequacies inevitably slow development and decrease workplace productivity [25]. Gender, rank, age group, and pre-existing chronic disease did not significantly influence the nutrition sub-scale score. In our study, nutrition sub-scale scores were higher among participants who reported regular pay and satisfaction with their job.

Group support plays a key role in comfortable assimilation to new work conditions [26]. Communicating with others is a part of a healthy lifestyle. Group support has a positive effect on physical health and the absence of group support may contribute to depression and other diseases [27]. In the present study, group support sub-scores were higher among individuals who reported good job satisfaction. In a previous study conducted in China, poor social support was shown to be associated with dissatisfaction [28]. Job satisfaction is a significant variable affecting quality of life [29]. In a study evaluating the relationship between job satisfaction and quality of life among factory employees in Japan, employees with higher job satisfaction also reported a higher quality of life [30]. Other studies have supported the conclusion that job satisfaction leads to better quality of life [29] [31]. A number of studies performed around the world and in Turkey support these findings [12] [16] [19] [28].

Negative conditions at a work place have a negative impact on the health of employees [32]. In a study conducted with a similar population attending the Zonguldak Occupational Education Center located in northern

Turkey [33], 17.1% of apprentices stated that an inadequate work environment affected their psychological health in a negative way. A stress-free life is an unrealistic goal; however, the weight of stress due to low socioeconomic conditions and harsh conditions is obvious. Therefore, the need for stress management instruction is clear, especially in apprentices age 18 and older. In a study of high school students [13], education in stress management improved stress management knowledge. The development of methods to cope with stress effectively is essential for the minimization of the negative effects of work on the psychological health in young adults.

5. Conclusion

In conclusion, HPLP scale evaluation revealed moderate health behavioral awareness among adolescent apprentices, with health responsibility and exercise identified as specific areas in need of improvement. Future studies should promote increased exercise and educate individuals regarding health responsibility. Job satisfaction was the most significant variable influencing HPLP scale scores. Therefore, training in healthy lifestyle practices should be included in all occupational education programs.

References

[1] Kivelä, K., Elo, S., Kyngäs, H. and Kääriäinen, M. (2014) The Effects of Health Coaching on Adult Patients with Chronic Diseases: A Systematic Review. *Patient Education & Counseling*, **97**, 147-157. http://dx.doi.org/10.1016/j.pec.2014.07.026

[2] Sauter, S.L. (2013) Integrative Approaches to Safeguarding the Health and Safety of Workers. *Industrial Health*, **51**, 559-561. http://dx.doi.org/10.2486/indhealth.MS5106ED

[3] Paredes-López, O., Cervantes-Ceja, M.L., Vigna-Pérez, M. and Hernández-Pérez, T. (2010) Berries: Improving Human Health and Healthy Aging, and Promoting Quality Life—A Review. *Plant Foods for Human Nutrition*, **65**, 299-308. http://dx.doi.org/10.1007/s11130-010-0177-1

[4] Buranatrevedh, S. and Sweatsriskul, P. (2005) Model Development for Health Promotion and Control of Agricultural Occupational Health Hazards and Accidents in Pathumthani, Thailand. *Industrial Health*, **43**, 669-676. http://dx.doi.org/10.2486/indhealth.43.669

[5] Walker, S.N., Sechrist, K.R. and Pender, N.J. (1987) The Health-Promoting Lifestyle Profile: Development and Psychometric Characteristics. *Nursing Research*, **36**, 76-81. http://dx.doi.org/10.1097/00006199-198703000-00002

[6] Fish, C. and Nies, M.A. (1996) Health Promotion Needs of Students in a College Environment. *Public Health Nursing*, **13**, 104-111. http://dx.doi.org/10.1111/j.1525-1446.1996.tb00227.x

[7] Spear, H.J. and Kulbok, P.A. (2001) Adolescent Health Behaviors and Related Factors: A Review. *Public Health Nursing*, **18**, 82-93. http://dx.doi.org/10.1046/j.1525-1446.2001.00082.x

[8] Velsor, F.B. (2001) Adolescent School Health. *Journal of Pediatric Nursing*, **16**, 194-196. http://dx.doi.org/10.1053/jpdn.2001.24877

[9] Ferguson, K.T., Cassells, R.C., MacAllister, J.W. and Evans, G.W. (2013) The Physical Environment and Child Development: An International Review. *International Journal of Psychology*, **48**, 437-468. http://dx.doi.org/10.1080/00207594.2013.804190

[10] Esin, M.N. (1999) Sağlıklı yaşam biçimi davranışları ölçeğinin Türkçeye uyarlanması. *Hemşirelik Bülten*, **2**, 87-96.

[11] Centers for Disease Control and Prevention (CDC) (2014) About Body Mass Index for Adults. http://www.cdc.gov/healthyweight/assessing/bmi/adult_bmi/index.html

[12] Ünalan, D., Şenol, V., Öztürk, A., *et al.* (2007) A Research on the Relation between the Healthy Life Style Behaviors and Self-Care Levels of the Students in Health and Social Programs of Vocational Collages. *Journal of Turgut Özal Medical Center*, **14**, 101-109.

[13] Geckil, E. and Yıldız, S. (2006) Adolescent Health Behaviors and Problems. *Journal of Hacettepe University School of Nursing*, **25**, 26-34.

[14] Nacar, M., Baykan, Z., Cetinkaya, F., *et al.* (2014) Health Promoting Lifestyle Behaviours in Medical Students: A Multicentre Study from Turkey. *Asian Pacific Journal of Cancer Prevention*, **15**, 8969-8974. http://dx.doi.org/10.7314/APJCP.2014.15.20.8969

[15] Felton, G.M., Parsons, M.A., Misener, T.R. and Oldaker, S. (1997) Health Promoting Behaviors of Black and White Collage Women. *Western Journal of Nursing Research*, **19**, 654-666. http://dx.doi.org/10.1177/019394599701900506

[16] Can, H.O., Ceber, E., Sogukpinar, N., Saydam, B.K., Otles, S. and Ozenturk, G. (2008) Eating Habits, Knowledge about Cancer Prevention and the HPLP Scale in Turkish Adolescents. *Asian Pacific Journal of Cancer Prevention*, **9**,

569-574.

[17] Ulla Díez, S.M. and Pérez-Fortis, A. (2010) Socio-Demographic Predictors of Health Behaviors in Mexican College Students. *Health Promotion International*, **25**, 85-93. http://dx.doi.org/10.1093/heapro/dap047

[18] Hendricks, C.S., Murdaugh, C., Tavakoli, A. and Hendricks, D.L. (2000) Health Promoting Behaviors among Rural Southern Early Adolescents. *ABNF Journal*, **11**, 123-128.

[19] Al-Kandari, F., Vidal, V.L. and Thomas, D. (2008) Health Promoting Lifestyle and Body Mass Index among College of Nursing Students in Kuwait: A Correlational Study. *Nursing & Health Sciences*, **10**, 43-50. http://dx.doi.org/10.1111/j.1442-2018.2007.00370.x

[20] Chen, L.H. (2008) Job Satisfaction among Information System (IS) Personnel. *Computers in Human Behavior*, **24**, 105-118. http://dx.doi.org/10.1016/j.chb.2007.01.012

[21] Tatsuse, T. and Sekine, M. (2013) Job Dissatisfaction as a Contributor to Stress-Related Mental Health Problems among Japanese Civil Servants. *Industrial Health*, **51**, 307-318. http://dx.doi.org/10.2486/indhealth.2012-0058

[22] Yılmazel, G., Çetinkaya, F. and Nacar, M. (2013) Hemşirelik öğrencilerinde sağlığı geliştirme davranışları. *TAF Preventive Medicine Bulletin*, **12**, 261-270.

[23] Yılmaz, U. and Bayat, M. (2005) Oto tamirhanelerinde çalışan çocuk işçilerin sağlıklarını koruyucu davranışları ile iş ortamı ve çalışma koşullarının değerlendirilmesi. *Journal of Health Science*, **14**, 37-44.

[24] Dumith, S.C., Gigante, D.P., Domingues, M.R. and Kohl, H.W. (2011) Physical Activity Change during Adolescence: A Systematic Review and a Pooled Analysis. *International Journal of Epidemiology*, **40**, 685-698. http://dx.doi.org/10.1093/ije/dyq272

[25] Ceylan, S.S. and Metin, Ö. (2009) Working Condition Children Who Work in Industry and Educated at Apprenticeship Education Center. *Fırat Sağlık Hizmetleri Dergisi*, **4**, 87-101.

[26] Gunnarsdottir, S. and Björnsdottir, K. (2003) Health Promotion in the Workplace: The Perspective of Unskilled Workers in a Hospital Setting. *Scandinavian Journal of Caring Sciences*, **17**, 66-73. http://dx.doi.org/10.1046/j.1471-6712.2003.00122.x

[27] Jocelyn, O.T.M. and Shaunqula, A.W. (2006) Religious Orientation and Social Support on Health Promoting Behaviors of African American College Students. *Journal of Community Psychology*, **34**, 105-115. http://dx.doi.org/10.1002/jcop.20086

[28] Gu, G.Z., Yu, S.F. and Zhou, W.H. (2011) Relationship between Job Satisfaction and Occupational Stress in the Workers of a Thermal Power Plant. *Chinese Journal of Industrial Hygiene and Occupational Diseases*, **29**, 893-897.

[29] Erbay Dündar, P., Bilge, B., Baydur, H., *et al.* (2006) Quality of Life and Some Related Factors among Young Students of Apprentice School in Manisa. *TAF Preventive Medicine Bulletin*, **25**, 24-29.

[30] Maruyama, S., Sata, H. and Morimoto, K. (1991) Relationship between Working-Life Satisfaction, Health Practices and Primary Symptom/Problem. *Nippon Eiseigaku Zassi*, **45**, 1082-1094. http://dx.doi.org/10.1265/jjh.45.1082

[31] Lerner, D.J., Levine, S., Malspeis, S. and D'Agostino, R.B. (1994) Job Strain and Health-Related Quality of Life in a National Sample. *American Journal of Public Health*, **84**, 1580-1585. http://dx.doi.org/10.2105/AJPH.84.10.1580

[32] Kawakami, N. and Haratani, T. (1999) Epidemiology of Job Stress and Health in Japan: Review of Current Evidence and Future Direction. *Industrial Health*, **37**, 174-186. http://dx.doi.org/10.2486/indhealth.37.174

[33] Sala Razı, G., Kuzu, A., Yıldız, A.N., Ocakcı, A.F. and Çamkuşu Arifoğlu, B. (2009) Self Esteem Communication Skills and Cooping with Stress of Young Workers. *TAF Preventive Medicine Bulletin*, **8**, 17-26.

4

Poverty and Nutritional Health of the Child: Some Evidence from 2005 Demographic and Health Survey of Congo

Samuel Ambapour[1], Jean Christophe Okandza[2], Hylod Armel Moussana[1]

[1]Institut National de la Statistique, Brazzaville, République du Congo
[2]Faculté des Sciences Economiques, Université Marien Ngouabi, Brazzaville, République du Congo
Email: ambapour_samuel@yahoo.fr, jcokandza@gmail.com, hylodmoussana@yahoo.fr

Abstract

The objective of this study is to identify the ways in which poverty could affect the nutritional health of the child and to analyze the strength of these links. On the whole, it appears that the relationship between poverty (measured by the wealth index) and health of the child (measured by an anthropometric index) is positive and highly significant.

Keywords

Wealth Index, Nutritional Health of the Child, Height for Age, Z-Score

1. Introduction

The relationship between health and poverty is often described in the literature as very complex, still poorly identified and reciprocal. In the particular case that interests us, this relationship has a dual aspect [1]. On one hand, economic growth (which is assumed to be able to eradicate poverty) led to reducing malnutrition. On the other hand, nutrition is a key ingredient of human capital, considered as a fundamental factor of economic growth. In this paper, we are particularly concerned about the nutritional health of children under five years of age. In fact, protecting health during childhood is necessary because compromised health at a young age may have consequences during adulthood: lower productivity and income, reduced social participation, no visible "return" on the family's investment in the child's health [2].

To characterize the health status of children, previous research used anthropometric data (size, children's weight); because these data are simple, accurate, and have been the subject of a consensus for estimating the malnutrition of children. In this anthropometric approach, we have focused on the delayed growth factor as measured by the long term indicator of height for age. With regard to poverty, a non-monetary approach is used: a wealth index is built using durable goods owned by households. The indicator thus obtained is considered as a proxy for long-term household income.

In a study of the determinants of the health of the child, the empirical work shows that there is a positive link between household resources and the nutritional status of the child. However, the intensity of this connection may vary from one country to another: for example, it is strong in the case of Benin [3], moderate in Bangladesh [4] and low in Mali [5]. In the case of Congo, this relationship will be analyzed in two phases. In a first phase, we present the results of the direct relationship between poverty and the nutritional status of the child, and in a second phase, the results of the determinants of this status, following the introduction of control variables.

This text is set forth as follows: The following chapter presents the origin of the data; it also describes in detail the variables of the study. In the third chapter, we specify the model chosen to study the relationship between poverty and nutritional health of the child. The fourth chapter provides the results of the econometric estimates.

2. Data and Variables

2.1. Data

This work is based on the Demographic and Health Survey of Congo carried out in 2005 by the National Centre for Statistics and Economic Studies with technical assistance from ORC Macro, an American cooperating institution in support of this type of investigation [6]. The overall objective of this first demographic and health survey was to determine the demographic and health indicators essential to the establishment of policies and programs, and more particularly to finalize the Poverty Reduction Strategy Paper and to follow-up on the Millennium Development Goals. This investigation, which is a rich source of information, appears limited, however, when it comes to studying monetary poverty. In these conditions, the relationship between poverty and the nutritional health of the child will be based on a non-monetary conceptualisation of poverty.

This being said, during the study, all children under five years present in the household selected, had to be weighed and measured. Thus, the results on the nutritional status are based on a sample of 4472 children.

2.2. Specification of Variables

We begin by first defining the nutritional status of the child, then by identifying the main determinants of this state grouped into three categories.

2.2.1. The Nutritional Status of the Child

There is no single indicator of the nutritional status *per se*. We generally use approximate measures which provide information on the nutritional status through their involvement in various processes or physiological functions [7]. In relation to young children, it is based on the anthropometric measures [8]-[10] considered as objective health status indicators [11]. In this case, we can typically identify three indices: height in relation to age; weight compared to height and weight in relation to age. Each index is expressed in terms of the number of standard deviation units (SD) in relation to the median of the international reference population of NCHS/CDC/WHO.

In our study, we have focused on the height for age index1. This index is considered by specialists [7] as a stable, complex indicator, which allows you to judge on the basis of the evolution of a more concise set of factors of family life, and it is for that reason, it gradually supplanted the other two. This is a key indicator of the quality of life in developing countries [12] [13]. Therefore, it will be considered here as a proxy for the nutritional status of the child and is used as a variable explained in our model.

Table 1 presents the percentage of children with malnutrition measured by the anthropometric index heightage and against some sociodemographic characteristics. Below, the sample that we will consider is composed of 3824 children under five years of age, of which 1851 are girls and 1973 are boys and for who we have the complete data.

2.2.2. The Individual Characteristics of the Child

Among the variables specific to the child we have retained a number (depending on the availability of data) that

---

1In this text, the following terms are considered equivalent: nutritional status, height for age, z-score.

Table 1. Children nutritional status: percentage of children under five years of age, with malnutrition (as defined by anthropometric index height/age) and distribution of socio-demographic characteristics.

Socio-demographic Characteristics	Height by Age		Number of children	Socio-demographic Characteristics	Height by age		Number of children
	Percentage of <−3SD	Percentage of <−2SD			Percentage of <−3SD	Percentage of <−2SD	
Children Age				**Weight at birth**			
<6	1.5	4.7	**470**				
6 - 9	3.0	10.2	**359**	Very small	24.1	40.8	**85**
10 - 11	3.2	17.4	**136**	Small	14.4	35.7	**250**
12 - 23	16.1	34.3	**858**	Normal o big	9.2	23.6	**3477**
24 - 35	11.0	28.1	**959**	Not defined	17.9	34.4	**183**
36 - 47	13.9	30.1	**910**				
48 - 59	11.5	30.9	**780**				
Sexe				**Place of residence**			
Masculine	12.3	27.6	**2279**	Urban	9.2	22.1	**2045**
Feminine	9.3	24.3	**2194**	Rural	12.1	29.2	**2427**
Order of birth				**Region**			
1	11.9	27.1	**950**	Brazzaville	11.7	23.7	**1218**
2 - 3	8.7	23.2	**1627**	Pointe Noire	5.0	19.2	**592**
4 - 5	9.6	25.2	**851**	South	11.5	27.6	**1723**
6+	13.5	28.2	**581**	North	11.9	30.3	**940**
Mother's Age				**Mothers' level of education**			
15 - 19	10.2	26.0	**1051**	None	19.4	33.9	**385**
20 - 24	13.2	28.5	**1176**	Primary	12.2	29.3	**1502**
25 - 29	9.8	24.4	**914**	Secondary 1st cycle	7.7	21.2	**2193**
30 - 34	8.3	22.4	**689**	Secondary 2d cycle or above	5.6	22.0	**66**
35 - 49	11.5	27.4	**643**				
Period between births (in months)				**Quintiles of economic wellbeing**			
First born	12.0	27.2	960	Poorest	13.5	31.9	1041
<24	13.0	30.1	388	Second Q	9.9	27.2	1034
24 - 47	11.5	27.0	1546	Medium	11.3	24.6	927
48+	6.3	19.6	1115	Fourth Q	10.8	23.7	780
				richest	7.3	19.7	690
				Total	**10.8**	**26.0**	**4472**

we propose to define[2].

1) The age and gender of the child

For a child of a given gender, age is an important determinant of the individual growth. As age increases, the nutritional status of children in the developing countries deteriorates because of the cumulative effects of the lack of nutritional intake [14]. Generally, we seek to test the hypothesis that, up to a certain age, malnutrition tends to intensify, and beyond this age the trend reverses with the change in food intake.

Recent research [15] suggests that the gender of a child has important and extended effects on parental behaviours and family results. Abundant literature indicates a preference for male children in many developing countries and particularly in Asia [16] [17]. Malnutrition is therefore more frequent among girls than among boys [18]. In Africa, according to a study conducted by the OECD [19], and contrary to what one might imagine, girls are almost always preferred. We will therefore test this hypothesis of the absence of discrimination against girls [20] in our sample which is composed of 48.4% girls and 51.6% boys.

2) The birth rank

Some studies take into account the order of births as an explanatory factor of child malnutrition [4] [14] [16]. It is suggested that the birth rank seems to have a significant effect on the quality of life, including on infant mortality [17]. However, it may be noted that the expected effect of birth order is ambiguous. Some argue that the first-born often have an advantage. Others, on the contrary argue that children of lower rank are sometimes underweight [21]. In addition, some research demonstrates that children of higher rank are poorly fed. The rela-

---

[2]In developing countries, breastfeeding plays an important role in the child's growth. Unfortunately, lacking comprehensive data, this variable is not taken into account in our study.

tionship between the nutritional status of the child and birth order is therefore complex [14] [18] [22] and may depend on household resources (how they are spread over time), biological and cultural factors.

3) The interval of births

A short interval between births can cause a physiological impairment of the mother, such that the child may have a delay in weight and size at birth. The more closely spaced the births, the lower the breast milk quality, particularly under the effect of physical exhaustion of the mother. It is obvious that mothers who must raise two children at the same time give them less care. Accordingly, it is therefore expected that the interval of birth can have a significant impact on the levels of malnutrition.

4) The presence of a twin

It has been found that the absence of a twin significantly improves size. We explain this biological fact in the following manner: each twin often suffers at birth from a handicap that must be compensated for by food and appropriate care [19].

5) The number of children in the household

We want to know if the integration of the child with its siblings has an impact on its growth. To this effect, two variables are tested: the number of children under five years of age and the number of children in the household[3]. A priori, the expected effect of an increase in these variables would be to deteriorate the child's health. The presence of a high number of children under five years of age increases the mother's load in terms of care and therefore should have a negative impact. However, one could imagine, in the case of the variable "number of children in the household" that the older children can take care of the younger children when they are not yet working, providing resources for parents if they work [23]. In this case, this variable should have a positive influence.

2.2.3. The Characteristics of the Parents and the Household

1) The mother's age at the first birth

The expected effect of the mother's age at the first birth upon the size of the child and on its probability of having a normal growth is ambiguous. From a biological point of view, one would assume that the physical conditions of a young mother are better than those of an older mother. In these conditions, a positive relationship is suspected. If age is considered as a variable approached from the accumulation of experience in terms of care, one might think that a mother who is too young is probably less mature and less experienced. In this case, one can expect a negative relationship[4].

2) The mother's health

Among the variables characterising the state of the mother's health, certain previous work continues [24] [25], among other things, the body mass index as an explanatory factor favourable to the child's growth. It is defined by weight in kilograms divided by the square of height in meters. According to Fogel [26], the extreme values of this index (less than 18.5 a sign of chronic energy deficiency or more than 30 a sign of obesity) are for the mother, respectively indicators of poor health or early morbidity. Grira [4] indicates that this index could reflect the availability of food within the household and that a reduction in the supply of food would result in a lower body mass index for the mother and therefore an elevated risk of malnutrition for the child.

3) The mother's family situation

Three situations are distinguished: the monogamous family, the polygamous family and the single parent family (the mother lives alone). Concerning the polygamous family, one might suspect a negative impact of this variable on the nutritional status of the child. In effect, one might think that polygamous fathers would have more of a burden than others, meaning many more children and adults to feed. One could also imagine a woman living alone has fewer resources. In this case, one might expect a negative impact on the growth of the child. However, in the study already cited, Morrison and Liskens [19] note that in most countries, mothers who live alone are usually fewer in number and are distinguished from others by a higher level of education or the possession of durable goods. In these conditions, a positive impact on the growth of the child cannot be ruled out.

4) The parents' education

There is extensive literature on the positive role of parents' education of on the health of children. With respect to the work of Schult [27], we see five main channels of influence of parental education on the children's

---

[3]The variable "number of children born before the child considered" is sometimes used.

[4]In this respect, there is also the effect of the composition of the household in which the mother resides. It is quite frequent, including in the Congo, that children are primarily supported by their grand-mothers in cases where the mother is of a very young age.

health [8] [24] [28] [29]. Firstly, education has a direct effect on the acquisition of knowledge in the field of health and hygiene. Secondly, education increases general skills in reading and logical thinking, which enables one to fully understand instructions from the nursing staff and to better manage diseases by taking initiatives. Thirdly, education increases the probability of obtaining a job, of increasing the total income, which in the end allows one to improve infant health. Fourthly, a better education increases the opportunity cost of work time and thus reduces the time spent caring for the children and breastfeeding. Finally, education can affect the preferences of parents. They may decide to limit the number of births in order to have only children in good health.

In this study, we chose the mother's education, because many studies have shown that the number of years of education of the husband/spouse had little effect on the health of the child. Moreover in Africa, it is the mother who has the primary responsibility for childcare. In fact, the most decisive aspect for the mother is that she knows how to read and write. If this is the case, there would be no correlation between the child's health and the mother's educational level. This hypothesis will therefore be tested. Its non-acceptance would mean that an educated woman would develop greater capability for childcare in particular if she has training in nutrition. In this context, we have introduced a variable of the mother's access to information (access to at least one media). This variable enables checking the likely knowledge of the mother in the area of nutrition and childcare.

5) Household income

Income is the central variable (or variable of interest) of our study. This is one of the most significant variables of child health [16] [30] [31] and, to a certain extent, it determines the amount of other inputs (food, shelter clothing, health care, etc.). The relationship between the child's nutritional status, represented by the height for age and income, has been the subject of many studies having led to very mixed results [32]. Unfortunately income and household consumption is not available to us. Instead, we use a wealth index as a proxy for the long-term income of households. This index has been constructed using the information relating to durable goods owned by households[5]. The aggregation methodology[6] is based on the approach of multiple correspondence analysis [33] [34]. Subsequently, this index is broken down into five socio-economic classes (poorest, poor, average, rich, richest) as a function of goods owned. These classes correspond respectively to the first, second, third, fourth and fifth quintile. The resulting breakdown could enlighten us as to whether or not structural changes exist with respect to variation in the height for age based on the household resources [4].

2.2.4. The Characteristics of the Environment or the Community

The effects of the environment (or the community) on the child's health are well documented in the theoretical literature. The famous model of Mosley-Chen [35], the economic model of the family by Becker [36] and the production function of health by Grossman [37] have shown the direct or indirect impact of community factors on infant health. In our case, in light of the available data, the essentials are access to drinking water, electricity, housing: the presence or absence of a modern toilet, type of floor (cement). There are many studies that have highlighted the importance of these infrastructures for childhood pathologies, and subsequently for malnutrition, on the health of the child. For example, access to drinking water, and the existence of modern toilets and a cement floor to avoid many diseases, particularly intestinal, which affect the child's growth [19]. In addition, there are also the variables of spatial localisation such as the place or region of residence. The environment is different from one region to another; and, in many developing countries, there is often an unequal distribution of the social and health infrastructures between rural and urban areas. Some studies have also taken into account this aspect and analyses have been done based sometimes on separate samples: urban, rural and national.

3 Method of Analysis

3.1. Functional Forms

Two functional forms are often used. In the first, the probability for a child of having a risk to growth is described by a logistic model: $\Pr(z_i = 1) = \dfrac{\exp(x_i\beta)}{1+\exp(x_i\beta)}$ and $\Pr(z_i = 0) = 1 - \Pr(z_i = 1)$; where $z_i = 1$ if the child i has a delay of growth and $z_i = 0$ otherwise. The second form is the following linear model:

---

[5]The following variables were excluded from the wealth index: access to water and electricity, type of toilet and the type of floor. They are taken into account separately because they are related to both the collective facilities and to the heritage of the household.
[6]Principal component analysis is used by numerous researchers.

$z_i = x_i \beta + e_i$; x_i is the vector of explanatory variables that may be exogenous or endogenous. In this study, only the second functional form is considered.

3.2. Selection Bias and Empirical Specification

The linear model can be estimated by ordinary least squares. However, this regression suffers from a few statistical problems likely to create bias in the estimates. In fact, in our sample, only the children alive at the time of the survey could have been measured: there is therefore a selection bias to the extent that it can be assumed that there is no total independence between the fact of being alive and health status [19]. In a country like Congo where infant and child mortality is high, it is possible that some children from our database could have been dying of hunger. It could be said the children in our sample possess particular features: more resistant, better fed, taller, which might distort the estimates. The mechanism of selection assumes that the empirical fact of surviving (s) is determined by a latent variable (non-observable) s^* as follows:

$$S_i = \begin{cases} 1 & \text{if } s_i^* \geq 0 \\ 0 & \text{if } s_i^* < 0 \end{cases} \quad \text{with} \quad s_i^* = w_i \gamma + u_i$$

where w_i is a vector of explanatory variables of survival and u_i an error term. That being so, the estimation of the linear model is therefore conditioned by the survival of the child, *i.e.* $s_i = 1$, which causes the bias. An empirical strategy exists for correcting this bias [29]. We use the following selection model:

$$s_i^* = w_i \gamma + u_i$$

$$s_i = 1 \left[s_i^* \geq 0 \right]$$

$$z_i = x_i \beta + e_i, \text{ observed if } s = 1$$

As can be seen, one is confronted with a system of simultaneous equations, in which one of them can only be estimated on a sub-sample depending on a system determined by the other. By involving a fully parametric characterisation of the system, assuming the joint normality of error terms of the two equations, the model can be estimated by the maximum-likelihood method [38]. Nevertheless, we often use the Heckman two step estimation procedure instead [39].

4. Results

It should first be noted that we used the Nakamura test, to check the endogeneity of some variables. The lack of necessary instruments has led us to consider some of them as exogenous. This is, for example, the case of the variables related to the household composition. The endogenous nature of other variables has been taken into account by applying the two stage regression procedure. Moreover, the problem of heteroscedasticity has been resolved using White's correction. Finally, the Heckit procedure in Stata software has allowed us to reject the hypothesis of a selection bias in our sample. In the analysis of the results, it can be seen that the explanatory powers of the models measured by R^2 are low but consistent with those found in previous works, taking into account the fact that the health status of a population is difficult to measure [8].

4.1. Direct Relationship between Poverty and the Child's Nutritional Health

Table 2 gives the results of the regression between the wealth index and the height for age, for all the children and by gender. As can be seen, the impact of the wealth index is positive and highly significant, showing that an increase in the household wealth of 10%, would reduce chronic malnutrition by 6.3%. It can also be noted that the household resources seem to favour girls a little more than boys. The breakdown of the wealth index gives quite interesting results (**Table 3**). The fact that the child belongs to a very poor household as opposed to a very rich household increases malnutrition. The same observation can be made for poor and intermediate classes. The regression coefficients (in absolute value) tend to decrease when we go from the poorest class to the richest class.

If one takes into account the breakdown of the index by gender, and for significant values (at the threshold of 1%), particularly for the poorest class, one sees a substantial gap between the coefficient of the girls and that of the boys. In effect, an increase of one unit of the wealth index deteriorates the height for age of 0.56 units for boys and by 0.44 units among girls.

Table 2. Relationship height for age index—wealth index.

	All		Boys		Girls	
	Coeff.	t-stat	Coeff.	t-stat	Coeff.	t-stat
Wealth index	0.6345185	6.06***	0.6270308	4.43***	0.6472413	4.15***
Constant	−0.9181392	33.53***	−9,803,026	−25.68***	−0.8517949	−21.67***
	N = 3824		N = 1 973		N = 1851	
	F(1, 3822) = 36.69		F(1, 1971) = 19.62		F(1, 1849) = 17.23	
	R^2 = 0.0089		R^2 = 0.0089		R^2 = 0.0091	

***, **, * represent significant coefficients at the 1%, 5% and 10% respectively.

Table 3. Relationship between height for age index and the classification based on the wealth index

	All		Boys		Girls	
	Coeff.	t-stat	Coeff.	t-stat	Coeff.	t-stat
Poorest	−0.5036724	−4.91***	−0.5622544	−3.98***	−0.4381149	−2.93***
Poor	−0.2899294	−2.83***	−0.4450123	−3.16***	−0.1259365	−0.84
Average	−0.2983505	−2.53**	−0.4338292	−2.71***	−0.1463372	−0.84
Rich	−0.0588918	−0.52	−0.2567768	−1.66*	0.1481544	0.88
Constant	−0.6220886	−6.90***	−0.5676048	−4.62***	−0.6831544	−5.15***
	N = 3824		N = 1973		N = 1851	
	F(4, 3819) = 10.04		F(4, 1968) = 4.72		F(4, 1846) = 6.65	
	R^2 = 0.0101		R^2 = 0.0088		R^2 = 0.0142	

***, **, * represent significant coefficients at the 1%, 5% and 10% respectively.

4.2. The Determinants of the Child's Nutritional Health

In what will follow, we want to assess the net effect of poverty on the child's nutritional health. To do this, we introduced other known control variables. These are in fact the characteristics of the child, the parents, or of the household, community and the environment that we have previously specified. Three regression models are proposed (**Table 4**).

4.2.1. The Characteristics of the Child

The results obtained for the age are consistent with the literature. We found the coefficients significant at the 1% threshold: negative for the age and positive for age squared. As regards the gender, one obtains significant negative coefficients at the threshold of 1%. This result thus confirms the results of Svedberg on the absence of bias against girls.

We found that the presence of a twin significantly deteriorates the size. This result is consistent with those of previous works.

An interval between the birth of the child studied and that of the previous child, has a significant and positive effect on its size.

Our study shows that the birth rank has no impact on the child's size. Finally, we note that the integration of the child with its siblings has no impact on its growth.

4.2.2. Characteristics of the Parents and the Household

With respect to the characteristics of the mother, the mother's state of health represented by body mass index, has a significant negative impact on the child's growth index. This could reflect the fact that household food security is not guaranteed and deteriorates accordingly the child's nutritional status.

Virtually all the works confirmed the role of the mother's education. This is also the case in our research where this variable has a very significant positive effect on the child's health. An increase of one year in the mother's years of education increases the growth score, all other things being equal, by 0.04. Moreover, it must be emphasized that the fact that the mother knows how to read has no effect on the child's nutritional status: the coefficient of this variable is negative and non-significant (regression model 2). One can interpret this result as

Table 4. Relationship between height for age index, wealth index and the control variables.

	Model 1		Model 2		Model 3	
	Coeff.	t-stat	Coeff.	t-stat	Coeff.	t-stat
Characteristics of children						
Child's age in months	−0.0603463	−10.02***	−0.0602642	−10.01***	−0.0603277	−100.01***
Square of the child's age in months	0.0006875	6.80***	0.0006859	6.79***	0.000689	6.81***
Child's gender	−0.1347898	−2.56**	−0.1355429	−2.57**	−0.1314197	−2.49**
Child's birth rank	−0.0169985	−0.25	−0.0165796	−0.24	−0.013153	−0.19
Interval in months separating the child considered from the next oldest child	0.004184	3.72***	0.0041986	3.73***	0.0041768	3.70***
The presence of a twin	−0.8650292	−5.23***	−0.8665762	−5.23***	−0.8491915	−5.12***
The number of children in the household	0.0004628	0.03	0.0004461	0.03	−0.0003524	−0.02
The number of children under age 5 in the household	−0.0328394	−0.65	−0.0324841	−0.65	−0.0315158	−0.63
Characteristics of the household						
Mother's education (years of studies)	0.0361313	3.98***	0.0344436	3.63***	0.0362409	3.99***
The wife has access to at least one media	0.033885	0.45			0.0174828	0.23
The wife knows how to read			−0.0258781	−0.35		
The mother's age at the first birth	0.0131173	1.09	0.013266	1.11	0.0136326	1.13
The mother's age (at the time of the birth)	0.0030219	0.31	0.0027995	0.29	0.0030985	0.32
The mother's health status (body mass index)	−0.0043082	−2.53**	−0.0043145	−2.54**	−0.0041726	−2.46**
Family situation (single parent family)	−0.0545196	−0.75	−0.0547773	−0.75	−0.0486887	−0.67
Family situation (polygamous family)	−0.0924776	−1.15	−0.0918426	−1.14	−0.0917358	−1.13
Wealth index (household income)	0.4357158	2.86***	0.4432275	2.91***		
Socio-economic classification						
Poorest					−0.2930593	−2.19**
Poor					−0.1416679	−1.12
Average					−0.1607942	−1.26
Rich					0.0144374	0.12
Characteristics of environment/community						
The household has access to drinking water	−0.0776559	−1.05	−0.0768514	−1.04	−0.070348	−0.95
The household has electricity	−0.0828471	−1.06	−0.0813175	−1.05	−0.0594063	−0.76
Type of toilet in the household	0.1608071	2.10**	0.161577	2.10**	0.1723039	2.26**
Type of floor in the household	0.0404869	0.54	0.0394338	0.53	0.0284875	0.38
- Place of residence						
Rural	−0.269182	−2.88***	−0.2713925	−2.91***	−0.2618085	−2.81***
- Region of residence						
Brazzaville	−0.1898967	−2.33**	−0.188974	−2.32**	−0.2012345	−2.47**
South	0.2215025	2.17**	0.2223461	2.17**	0.2082142	0.04**
North	0.1044212	0.97	0.1065899	0.99	0.0796651	0.74
Constant	−0.0858426	−0.29	−0.0380752	−0.13	0.0489823	0.15
	N = 3824		N = 3824		N = 3824	
	F(24, 3799) = 17.48		F(24, 3799) = 17.45		F(27, 3796) = 15.61	
	$R^2 = 0.0948$		$R^2 = 0.0949$		$R^2 = 0.0953$	

***, **, * represent significant coefficients at the 1%, 5% and 10% respectively.

follows: "knowing how to read and write in a language without attending a formal school is not enough to put into practise the lessons received in the area of nutrition and child care".

By including the variable "access to at least one media", we wanted to confirm the argument of Thomas, Strauss and Henriques [12] according to which, the influence of maternal education may be interpreted by a better understanding and reception of the information necessary to improve the child's health; and in this case, given the mother's level of education and the household resources, access to different media should play a positive role. This hypothesis is rejected in the case of our sample. The variable access to the media has a positive effect, however, it is not significant (Model 2 and 3).

We found that the family status of women does not intervene in the child's development. The fact that the woman lives alone, or in a polygamous union, has no impact on the child's nutritional status.

The wealth index always appears as a major determinant of the child's nutritional status. Its coefficient remains high and very significant. As of now, an increase in the household wealth of 10%, would reduce chronic malnutrition by 4.3%. This result is close to that obtained by [3], for Benin (4%), but very much higher than that found by [4] for Bangladesh, namely 0.8%. It will also be noted, that the effect of the wealth index has a great impact on that of education.

4.2.3. The Characteristics of the Environment (or the Community)

Some studies have found a reasonably solid connection between access to water and electricity and the nutritional status of the child. In contrast to these studies, in the sample from the Demographic and Health Survey of Congo, these two variables are not significant factors in the child's growth. Most of the coefficients on these two variables are negative, that is to say they do not have the expected sign. It should be noted that access to safe drinking water and electricity depends in general on the state through their national companies for distribution of water and electricity. One can therefore be connected to these distribution networks and not have water or electricity during a good period of the year.

With regard to the two variables on the housing, characterising the household living conditions, only the provision of a modern toilet has a positive and significant impact on the child's growth. The coefficient of the variable type of floor (cement), although having the expected signs is not significant at the thresholds selected.

We found that the children in rural areas are disadvantaged in size by 0.3 SD compared to those in an urban environment.

Finally, we note the existence of a regional dimension of malnutrition. If you take the city of Pointe-Noire (economic capital of the country) as a reference, we found that the children living in the southern part of the country are favoured. An opposite effect is observed in Brazzaville (political capital of the country) whose children are disadvantaged by 0.2 SD compared to those in Pointe-Noire.

5. Conclusions and Recommendations

The objective of this study was to explore the relationship between poverty and the nutritional health of the child based on the data from the first Demographic and health survey of Congo carried out in 2005. Beyond this relationship, we wanted to analyze the determinants of the child's nutritional status and to base it on the specific characteristics of the child, the household and the parents, and on the characteristics of the environment or the community. To this effect, regression models have been proposed and have shown that several variables had a significant impact on the child's nutritional status. The public authorities could therefore take advantage of these results to, in particular, combat malnutrition of children and, in general, fight against poverty. From this study, and in view of the econometric tests performed, we could draw the main conclusions as follows:

- firstly, the study has shown that an increase of the wealth index of households very significantly improved the nutrition of children; that this strong improvement will benefit girls a little more than boys. In the light of the breakdown of this index, it could be suggested that a public policy of transfer, that is to say, which would alter the distribution of income in favour of the poorest (the poorest quintile) could be most effective;

- secondly, the results of the study suggest reflections focused on the health and education of women. First, the study has highlighted the negative role of the mother's health (through the body mass index) on the child's growth, testifying to the importance of household food insecurity. We know that the repetition of closely spaced births weakens the mother. Increasing the gaps between the births would therefore be a fundamental element for improving the health of the child and the dissemination of contraception means would be a key objective in this case. Then, the study has confirmed the role of maternal education in reducing child malnutrition because an educated mother better understands the teachings on child nutrition. The public authorities could therefore improve the living conditions of children by adopting a well-targeted policy concerning certain expenditures for health and education; finally, the study revealed a regional dimension of malnutrition. A policy of intervention aimed at improving the conditions of community life in rural areas and Brazzaville would be desirable.

References

[1]   Linnemayr, S. and Aldeman, H. (2006) Determinants of Malnutrition in Senegal: Individual, Household, Community Variables, and Their Interaction. World Bank, Washington DC.

[2]   Appaix, T. (2003) Impact économique de l'investissement dans la santé de l'enfant, Communication pour les XXVI-èmes journées des économistes français de la santé.

[3]   Ahovey, E.C. and Vodounou, C. (2004) Pauvreté multidimensionnelle et santé de l'enfant: Quelques évidences de l'enquête démographique et de santé du Bénin de 2001. INSAE, Bénin.

[4]   Grira, H. (2007) Les déterminants du statut nutritionnel au Matlab: Une analyse empirique. Centre d'Economie de la Sorbonne, CES Working Paper No. 39.

[5]   Penders, C.L. Staatz, J.M. and Teft, J.F. (2000) How Does Agricultural Development affect Child Nutrition in Mali? Policy Synthesis. Global Bureau, Office of Agriculture and Food Security, USAID.

[6]   CNSEE and ORC Macro (2005) Enquête Démographique et de Santé du Congo, Calverton, Maryland, USA.

[7]   Maire, B. Delpeuch, F. Martin-Prevel, Y. and Fouéré, T. (2001) Nutrition et Pauvreté. Bilan comparatif des enquêtes anthropométriques en Afrique Subsaharienne au cours des deux dernières décennies. In: *Inégalités et politiques publiques en Afrique*: *Pluralité des normes et jeux d'acteurs*, IRD, Karthala.

[8]   Behrman, J.R. and Deolalikar, A.B. (1988) Health and Nutrition. In: Chenery, H. and Srinivan, T.N., Eds., *Handbook of Development Economics*, Amsterdam, North Holland, 1, 631-711.

[9]   Gibson, J. (2000) Child Height, Household Resources, and Household Survey Method. University of Waikato, Waikato.

[10] Strauss, J. and Thomas D. (1995) Human Resources: Empirical Modeling of Household and Family Decisions. In: Behrman, J. and Srinivasan, T.N., Eds., *Handbook of Development Economics*, Elsevier, Amsterdam, 3A, 1883-2023. http://dx.doi.org/10.1016/s1573-4471(05)80006-3

[11] Waterlow, J.C., Buzina, R., Keller, W., Lane, J.M., Nichman, M.Z. and Tanner, J.M. (1977) The Presentation and Use of Height and Weight Data for Comparing the Nutritional Status of Groups of Children under the Age of Ten Years. *Bulletin of the World Health Organisation*, **55**, 489-498.

[12] Thomas, D., Strauss, J. and Henriques, M.-H. (1990) Child Survival, Height for Age and Household Characteristics in Brazil. *Journal of Development Economics*, **33**, 197-234. http://dx.doi.org/10.1016/0304-3878(90)90022-4

[13] Glewwe, P. (1999) Why Does Mother's Schooling Raise Child Health in Developing Countries? Evidence from Morocco. *The Journal of Human Resources*, **34**, 124-159. http://dx.doi.org/10.2307/146305

[14] Horton, S. (1988) Birth Order and Nutritional Status: Evidence from Philippines. *Economic Development and Cultural Change*, **36**, 341-354. http://dx.doi.org/10.1086/451655

[15] Lefebvre, P. (2006) Discrimination sexuelle dans les dépenses des ménages: Survol de littérature et évidences empiriques pour le Canada. *L'actualité Economique*, **32**, 119-153. http://dx.doi.org/10.7202/013467ar

[16] Pal, S. (1999) An Analysis of Childhood Malnutrition in Rural India: Role of Gender, Income and Other Characteristics. *World Development*, **27**, 1151-1171. http://dx.doi.org/10.1016/S0305-750X(99)00048-0

[17] Gangadharan, L. and Maitra, P. (2000) Does Child Mortality Reflect Gender Biais? Evidence from Pakistan, University of Melbourne, Parkville.

[18] Behrman, J.R. (1988) Nutrition, Health, Birth Order and Seasonality. Intrahousehold Allocation among Children in Rural India. *Journal of Development Economics*, **28**, 43-62. http://dx.doi.org/10.1016/0304-3878(88)90013-2

[19] Morrisson, C. and Linskens, C (2000) Les facteurs explicatifs de la malnutrition en Afrique subsaharienne. OCDE, Document de travail No. 167.

[20] Svedberg, P. (1990) Undernutrition in Sub-Saharan Africa: Is There a Sex Bias? *Journal of Development Studies*, **26**, 469-489. http://dx.doi.org/10.1080/00220389008422165

[21] Arif, G.M. (2004) Child Health and Poverty in Pakistan. *The Pakistan Development Review*, **43**, 211-238.

[22] Birdsall, N. (1991) Birth Order Effects and Time Allocation. *Research in Population Economics*, **7**, 191-213.

[23] Handa, S. (1999) Maternal Education and Child Height. *Economic Development and Cultural Change*, **47**, 421-439. http://dx.doi.org/10.1086/452408

[24] Barrera, A. (1990) The Role of Maternal Schooling and Its Interaction with Public Health Programs in Child Health Production. *Journal of Development Economics*, **32**, 69-91. http://dx.doi.org/10.1016/0304-3878(90)90052-D

[25] Strauss, J. (1990) Households, Communities, and Preschool Children's Nutrition Outcomes: Evidence from Rural Cote d'Ivoire. *Economic Development and Cultural Change*, **38**, 232-261. http://dx.doi.org/10.1086/451791

[26] Fogel, R. (1994) Economic Growth Population Theory and Physiology: The Bearing of Long Term Processes on the Making of Economic Policy. *American Economic Review*, **84**, 369-375.

[27] Schultz, T.P. (1984) Studying the Impact of Household Economic and Community Variables on Child Mortality. In: Mosley, W.H. and Chen, L.C., Eds., *Child Survival: Strategies for Research*, Population and Development Review, Vol. 10, Population Council, New York, 215-235. http://dx.doi.org/10.2307/2807962

[28] Charasse, C. (1999) La mesure et les déterminants de l'état de santé en Afrique du Sud. *Revue d'Economie du Développement*, **4**, 9-37.

[29] Shariff, A. and Ahn, A. (1995) Mother's Education Effect on Child Health: An Econometric Analysis of Child Anthropometry in Uganda. *Indian Economic Review*, **30**, 203-222.

[30] Behrman, J.R. and Wolfe, B.L. (1987) How Does Mother's Schooling Affect Family Health, Nutrition, Medical Care Usage, and Household Sanitation? *Journal of Econometrics*, **36**, 185-204. http://dx.doi.org/10.1016/0304-4076(87)90049-2

[31] Thomas, D., Strauss, J. and Henriques, M.-H. (1991) How Does Mother Education Affect Child Height? *The Journal of Human Resources*, **26**, 183-211. http://dx.doi.org/10.2307/145920

[32] Gibson, J. (2000) How Can Women's Education Aid Economic Development? The Effect on Child Stunting in Papua New Guinea. University of Waikato, Waikato.

[33] Benzécri, J.-P. (1993) Correspondence Analysis Handbook. Marcel Dekker, CRC Press, New York.

[34] Asselin, L.-M. (2009) Analysis of Multidimensional Poverty. Theory and Case Studies. Springer, New York. http://dx.doi.org/10.1007/978-1-4419-0843-8

[35] Mosley, W.H. and Chen, L.C. (1984) An Analytical Framwork for the Study of Child Survival in Developing Countries. In: Mosley, W.H. and Chen, L.C., Eds., *Child Survival: Strategies for Research*, Population and Development Review, Vol. 10, Population Council, New York, 25-48.

[36] Becker, G. (1991) A Treatise on the Family. Harvard University Press, Cambridge.

[37] Grossman, G. (1972) On the Concept of Health Capital and Demand of Health. *Journal of Political Economy*, **80**, 224-225. http://dx.doi.org/10.1086/259880

[38] Greene, W. (1997) LIMDEP Version 7.0 User's Manuel. Revised Edition, Econometric Software, Inc., Plainview.

[39] Heckman, J.J. (1979) Sample Selection Bias as a Specification Error. *Econometrica*, **47**, 153-161. http://dx.doi.org/10.2307/1912352

5

Global Standards and Local Policies for School Diabetes Care

María J. Miranda Velasco[1], Maria Gloria Solís Galán[2], Enma Domínguez Martín[3]

[1]Department of Educational Sciences, University of Extremadura, Coordinator of Research Group Education and Health Innovation, Cáceres, Spain
[2]Department of Educational Sciences, University of Extremadura, Research Group Education and Health Innovation, Cáceres, Spain
[3]Research Group Education and Health Innovation, Cáceres, Spain
Email: mirandav@unex.es, glsolisg@unex.es, edominguezmartin86@gmail.com

Abstract

Objectives: The purpose of this study is to analyse the practical implementation of regional and national policies through the *Protocol of Care of Children and Adolescents in School* (2010) in Extremadura Region (Spain), and to compare its contents with the international standards of diabetes care at school defined by American Diabetes Association and International Diabetes Federation. The measures not only affect the security and diabetes care, but also inclusion and the right to health. Methods: A documental comparative analysis between the local and international standards about diabetes care in school setting is carried out. This analysis is framed in a larger project focused on the study of health promoting school and diabetes education, in which perceptions of children and adolescents with diabetes, their parents and school staff were studied. Results: The *Protocol of Care of Children and Adolescents in School* (2010) contains some international recommendations about the care of T1DM at school, but in other cases the measures are non-specific. The distribution of responsibilities for care at school is unclear and no monitoring and evaluation indicators are defined. Some elements are identified to be implemented in the tool to favour the security, management of T1DM care and wellbeing. In general, these elements refer to school plan for diabetes care, school organization and teachers, and school community training. Conclusion: It is required to develop specific policies and decisive action to ensure the right to health of children with diabetes and the full application of international standards for diabetes care at school.

Keywords

Health Policy, Childhood and Adolescents, Diabetes Care, School Setting, Inclusion

1. Introduction

The daily self-management of children and adolescents with T1DM is complex and variable [1] [2]. Besides the inherent requirement of the illness treatment in this period of life, the changes during the development of maturity require continuous adjustments in the treatment plan [3], and the aspects which affect the quality of childhood life need to be considered [4] [5].

Since children spend a significant part of the day in school [3], it is required to bring in their daily care measures into their school routine to accomplish an adequate metabolic control and the optimal development of treatment [6] [7]. At the same time, they should have the possibility of being fully and safely involved in all school activities [8]-[11].

The needs of children and adolescents with diabetes in school have been specifically identified in the main care standards [12]-[14]. These needs are based on the features of the treatment management (insulin therapy, blood glucose control, acute complications treatment and urgency situations and nutritional therapy) [6]-[10] [12].

Scientific literature, in line with current standards, underlines the importance of the training of the teachers and the educational school staff to acquire the basic knowledge about diabetes and the treatment of possible health emergencies [12] [14], to be able to guarantee the school work standardisation and the reduction of absenteeism related to diabetes [15]. Care of children with diabetes in school is an internationally shared concern, as it is shown in the continuous revisions of the care standards, guidelines and position statements from organisations like American Diabetes Association (ADA), American Association of Diabetes Educators (AADE), International Diabetes Federation (IDF) and International Society for Pediatric and Adolescent Diabetes (ISPAD), inter alia. However, there are very different legal and administration structures about diabetes care in school all around the world [16], despite having the American model as reference. Besides, the implementation in practice of recommendations is not being carried out in the desirable way as evidences the scientific literature reviewed [3] [5] [16]-[18]. Nowadays, the discrimination of children with diabetes in school continues to be a problem [8]-[10].

Despite the lack of comparative studies about the T1DM care policy and legal regulation in Europe, the international study "DAWN Youth" (2007-2009) reveals the existence of a great dispersion in terms of diabetes care policy and regulation measures in school in European countries studied [16].

In Spain, there are education policies that highlight the inclusion goals and the attention to student diversity [19] [20]. However, they only provide general prescriptive recommendations without specifying diabetic students' protection in school. Similarly, neither do they include evaluation indicators that guarantee the accomplishment of the objectives of care and educational inclusion.

In the health area, the *National Diabetes Strategy* (2012) recommends to promote the integration of children with diabetes through the design and development of a protocol of T1DM in school in all the Spanish Autonomous Communities.

The Community Autonomous of Extremadura has a *Comprehensive Plan of Diabetes*, which includes the national recommendations and proposes for the elaboration of the *Protocol of Care of Children and Adolescents in School* (2010) [21]. This *Protocol* is one of the few existing in Spain. It is the result of coordinated work held between the Regional Ministry of Education and the Regional Ministry of Health. The *Protocol* is proposed as a strategic solution to meet the care needs of the pediatric population with diabetes in the school setting. Its main objective is:

"*To establish and promote specific measures of attention to children and adolescents with diabetes mellitus in the educational environment, and support for the entire educational community to promote their physical, social and emotional adjustment to illness as well as ensuring the control, security and equality opportunities of children and adolescents with DM in education*" [21].

Currently, it has been implemented in 101 schools and involving a total of 171 children and adolescents with diabetes [22].

In our broader study about the needs and the quality of life of childhood and adolescence with diabetes [4], we wonder what the problem between educational policies and practices of care at school setting is.

The analysis and comparison of this regional document with the international care standards and recommendations are shown in the following paragraphs.

The objective of this study is to analyze the impact of international standards and recommendations of the diabetes care at school in the regional health policy of Extremadura (Spain) through the measures defined in the instrument created for diabetes care at school called Protocol of Care of Children and Adolescents at School [21].

2. Methods

This is a descriptive study. Data collection was conducted through a documental analysis of the actual Spanish educational policy in relation to diabetes care at school. Specifically, the content of the *Protocol of Care of Children and Adolescents at School* (2010) [21], which has been developed by the Regional Ministry of Health of the Autonomous Community of Extremadura, was compared with the international standards and recommendations for diabetes care in childhood at school setting taken as reference in the document analyzed [9] [10] [23]. This study is part of a broader evaluation research related the diabetes education in children and adolescents carried out in Extremadura region, Spain (PRI09A156).

Specifically, it is discussed all necessary measures for diabetes care and safety, inclusion, family involvement, teachers training, school responsibilities, included in the tool in relation the international standards and recommendations of DM care in childhood and adolescence. The purpose is to support the decision-making process for the improvement of the effectiveness of the instruments created within the framework of the policies of Public Health administrations, at the service of the health and welfare of citizens from the international consensus and scientific evidences.The content analysis of the current legislation was made in 2013, after the implementation of the Protocol and the analysis of empirical study on which this paper is framed.

Analyzed dimensions and variables, according to the studied documents, are listed in **Table 1** [9] [10] [23].

3. Results

Table 2 and **Table 3** show the comparative analysis of the political document analysed between the *Protocol of the Care of Children and Adolescents with diabetes in Schools of Extremadura Region* [21] and the international standards by ADA and the IDF recommendations for diabetes care at school setting for Children and Adolescents. Implementation proposals are based in the family and the school responsibilities in the diabetes care [8]-[10] [23] [24].

Table 1. Analyzed dimensions and variables.

Dimension: Family responsibilities	Dimension: School responsibilities
Variables: Key aspects of diabetes care at school	**Variables:** Key aspects of diabetes care at school
1. Participation in the development and implementation of personalized School Care Plan	1. Medical and educational records policy
2. Provision and use of diabetes care supplies	2. Staff training in diabetes care
3. Maintenance of supplies	3. Specification of minimum training content
4. Disposal of materials	4. Medical treatment delivery and self-management policy
5. Health information registration	5. Accommodation and privacy for self-management
6. Transmission of blood glucose values from school to parent/guardian	6. Food school policy
7. Specification of necessary supplies	7. Access to health services
8. Information delivery and training responsibilities	8. Food classroom policy
9. Resources for action in medical emergencies	9. Absence management policy
10. Food policy and family-school collaboration	10. Free access to water and toilet
11. Information policy and justification of absences for medical reasons	11. Medical supplies storage
	12. Food and nutritional information policy
	13. Free access to medical supplies and participation in school activities

Table 2. Family responsibilities in diabetes care at school.

ADA 2004	ADA 2008	IDF 2005	Protocol for the Care of Adolescent Children with Diabetes in School (2010) Extremadura, (Spain)
1. **Collaboration with the student's diabetes health care team to develop a personal** *Diabetes Medical Management Plan*		1. **Collaboration with** the healthcare providers, school personnel, and the student for devised a *Diabetes Healthcare Plan* 1.1. **Transmitting** the *Diabetes Healthcare Plan* and an *emergency plan* to the school	1. **To inform the educational center about the diagnosis of the T1DM. Collaborate in the elaboration of a children and adolescents with diabetes personal plan** (It is not specified who with, what or how)
2. **All materials and equipment necessary for diabetes care tasks**, including blood glucose testing, insulin administration (if needed), and urine or blood ketone testing		2. **Bringing diabetes supplies**	2. **Only after the needed care for the diabetes in school has been authorised by the School Board will all materials and essential equipment for the diabetes care be provided** 2.1. Someone to go to administer insulin or other necessities when required by the school staff, and when the child/adolescent cannot do it by himself.
3. The parent/guardian is **responsible for the maintenance of the blood glucose testing equipment.**		3.--------------------------	3. The parent is responsible for the maintenance of the blood glucose testing equipment.
4. Must provide materials necessary to ensure **proper disposal of materials.**		4.--------------------------	4. The **proper disposal of materials in a small container** should be ensured **working together with the reference nurse in DM.**
5. A separate **logbook** should be kept at school with the diabetes supplies for the staff or student to record test results.		5.--------------------------	5. **To collaborate in the update of the student with DM's health card**
6. **Blood glucose values should be transmitted** to the parent/guardian for review as often as requested.		6.------------------------------------	6.------------------------------------
7. Supplies to treat hypoglycaemia, including a source of glucose and a glucagon emergency kit, if indicated in the Diabetes Health Care Plan		7.------------------------------------	7.------------------------------------
8. Information about diabetes and the performance of diabetes-related tasks		8. Transmitting diabetes information to the school	8. **Transmitting information about diabetes to school. Collaborating on everything required to control your son/daughter DM, with the teachers and the health professionals.**
9. Emergency phone numbers for the parent/guardian and the diabetes care team so that the school can contact these individuals with diabetes-related questions and/or during emergencies		9.------------------------------------	9.------------------------------------
10. Information about the student's meal/snack schedule. The parent should work with the school to coordinate this schedule with that of the other students as closely as possible. For young children, instructions should be given for when food is provided during school parties and other activities.		10.------------------------------------	10. **Collaborating on everything required to control your children's DM, with the teachers and the health professionals.**
11. In most locations and increasingly, a signed release of confidentiality from the legal guardian will be required so that the health care team can communicate with the school. Copies should be retained both at school and in the diabetes offices and health care professionals' offices.		11.------------------------------------	11. To inform teachers and school staff, at the discretion of the centre and under the family's authorization, about any student with DM. 11.1. To supply the student's medical and nurse reports relating to a student's illness, when they are required by the professionals who attend the child/adolescent. 11.2. To supply the teacher proof of student's absenteeism when it is due to the attendance of doctor or nurse's appointment or other reasons related to DM.

Table 3. School responsibilities in the management of diabetes care.

ADA 2004	ADA 2008	IDF 2005	Protocol for the Care of Adolescent Children with Diabetes in School (2010) Extremadura, (Spain)
1.--------------------------------		1.-------------------------------	1. An individual Plan of diabetes care for the child or adolescent should be attached to the student academic record.
			2.--------------------------------
2. **Training** to all adults who provide education/care for the student on the symptoms and treatment of hypoglycaemia and hyperglycemia and other emergency procedures.	2. **Training** of an adequate number of personnel		2.1. It is only recommended an increase in the Regional Teaching training Plan, the number of educational activities in Health Education related to DM (obesity, physical exercise promotion, healthy eating, diabetes education.
3. An adult and back-up adult(s) trained to 1) perform fingerstick blood glucose monitoring and record the results; 2) take appropriate actions for blood glucose levels outside of the target ranges as indicated in the student's Diabetes Medical Management Plan; and 3) test the urine or blood for ketones, when necessary, and respond to the results of this test.		3--------------------------	3.-----------------------------
4. Immediate accessibility to the treatment of hypoglycaemia **by a knowledgeable adult**			4. To request emergency health care
4.1. The student should remain supervised until appropriate treatment has been administered, and 4.2. **The treatment should be available as close to where the student is as possible**.		4. Supervision or execution of diabetes tasks	4.1. To encourage the child/adolescent to be accompanied by a teacher or a social educator when he has to carry out a glycemic control, insulin administration or when a hypoglucemic situation is suspected.
4.3. An adult and back-up adult(s) trained to administer glucagon, in accordance with the student's Diabetes Medical Management Plan.			4.2.----------------------------
4.4. If indicated by the child's developmental capabilities and the Diabetes Medical Management Plan, an adult and back-up adult(s) trained in insulin administration.			4.3.----------------------------- 4.4.-----------------------------------
5. **A location in the school to provide privacy** during testing and insulin administration, if desired by the student and family, or permission for the student to check his or her blood glucose level and to take appropriate action to treat hypoglycaemia in the classroom or anywhere the student is in conjunction with a school activity, if indicated in the student's Diabetes Medical Management Plan.		5--------------------------------	5 -------------------------------------
6. **An adult and back-up adult(s) responsible for the student** who will know the schedule of the student's meals and snacks and work with the parent/guardian to coordinate this schedule with that of the other students as closely as possible. This individual also will notify the parent/ guardian in advance of any expected changes in the school schedule that affect the student's meal times or exercise routine. Young children should be reminded of snack times.		6--------------------------------	6----------------------------------
7. Permission for the student to see school medical personnel, school nurse and other trained school personnel upon request.		7----------------------------------	7. Permission for the attendance to external medical appointments or other reasons related to DM
8. Permission for the student to eat a snack anywhere, including the classroom or the school bus, if necessary to prevent or treat hypoglycaemia.		8--------------------------------	8. Permission, only when this is integrated in the Organisation and Operation Regulations in schools, to eat or to have a drink in class only to avoid a possible hypoglycaemia It is considered bad monitoring when the frequency of this behaviour is high and the family must be reported.

Continued

9. Permission to miss school without consequences for required medical appointments to monitor the student's diabetes management. This should be an excused absence with a doctor's note, if required by usual school policy.	9-------------------------------	9. Permission to allow the academic tests performance (exams, work handling, etc.) to be carried out later if the child/adolescent with DM condition requires and always when it is justified by document: hyperglycemia or hypoglycaemia, review medical appointments, etc.)
10. Permission for the student to use the restroom and have access to fluids (*i.e.*, water) as necessary.	10-----------------------------	10. Only when these circumstances have been added to the Organisation and Operation Regulations in schools will permission be granted.
11. An appropriate location for insulin and/or glucagon storage, if necessary.	11-----------------------------	11. Only after getting from the School Board the permission for the admission of materials related to DM, will they count on a small refrigerator.
12. Information on serving size and caloric, carbohydrate, and fat content of foods served in the school (27).	12-----------------------------	12. There is no specific information about the nutrients. It is only indicated that alternative elaboration menus should be ensured in the case that the student with DM uses the school cafeteria.
13. The student with diabetes should have immediate access to diabetes supplies at all times, with supervision as needed. 13.1. Provisions similar to those described Above must be available for field trips, extracurricular activities, other school-sponsored events, and on transportation provided by the school or day care facility to enable full participation in school activities.	13. Accessibility to supplies (particularly for hypoglycemic emergencies)	13. Only with the School Board permission can the admission of materials related to DM be authorised. 13.1. To encourage the child/adolescent to take part in all school activities, including days out and excursions, not specifying measures

The categories analysed in **Table 2** refers to family/guardian responsibilities in the care of diabetes in school setting, Personal *Diabetes Medical Management Plan*, materials and equipment necessary for diabetes care tasks, information to the family, emergency phone numbers for the parent/guardian and the diabetes care team, and the emergency kit.

The categories analysed in **Table 3** refers to the organizational school setting for provide the management of diabetes treatment, security, wellbeing; provider professional at school, educational responsibilities in the management of diabetes care, permissions for children at school, inclusion, and educational staff training.

4. Discussion

4.1. The Regulation of Diabetes in the School Context

The concern about the regulation of diabetes in school is a worldwide problem, where there is no unanimity in the management and each country has adopted different measures [16].

In the first DAWN Youth meeting in 2006, the educational centres were already identified as a priority objective for improvement; however, the current situation reveals that we are still at the same stage as we were years ago, as the evidence about the existence of structural, organisational, educational and attitudinal barriers are shown [16]

In general, in Spain, as it occurs in other countries, there are no state or community measures (administration or legal regulations) that guarantee the implementation and evaluation of the implementation of diabetes care in school.

4.2. Protocol of Attention to Adolescent Children with Diabetes at School

In Extremadura Region, the named *Protocol of attention to adolescent children with diabetes in School* [21] is considered the main reference for diabetes care in the school context. The results of the research carried out reveal that in most cases it is an unknown measure by the school personnel, and as it is designed, the safety and well-being of children with diabetes in school cannot be guaranteed despite being theoretically grounded in the standards of the ADA and the IDF.

The *Protocol* exposes that the approval of the fundamental measures related to diabetes treatment is due to the decision of the school itself. Therefore, the care and safety of children with diabetes are conditioned by the authorisation of the School Board in each centre, above their arising needs from the care and control of the illness. The decisions taken by this governing team consisting of representants of the educational and non-educational local community, affect the stocks and storage of the materials for the diabetes care in school, the administration of drugs, the meal intake in class and the reception of the specific refrigerator for the appropriate conservation of insulin and glucagon.

Another important gap in this *Protocol* is the lack in operability. The implementation is not monitored because there are no measures, nor indicators that guarantee it. On the other hand, the monitoring and the evaluation of it are totally unspecific.

In many cases establishing the roles of all involved does not identify the particular figure in charge of implementing actions or define the specific procedures to materialise them. The supporting functions of the diabetes care are defined ambiguously, not showing the differences between the responsibilities of the professionals and the education and health administration.

Training for diabetes care in school is neither guaranteed for teachers or non-teaching staff, it is only suggested as an increase to the general offers of training actions unspecified from the Teachers and Resources Centres. In practice, this fact is confirmed previous results from the largest study. Besides, recommending the cooperation of the associations of patients with DM and the associations of parents of students. Informative material is referred to as being be available to recipients; in any case this material is specific about T1DM in children and adolescents.

Versus the absence of a school nurse, the *Protocol* proposes the appointment of two people in charge of the care coordination in school: a nurse reference in diabetes in every health area and a reference person in diabetes in each school. The assumption of responsibility by this second figure, however, is voluntary. Previous training of both reference figures in the T1DM care is not established as a pre-requirement. Total or partial lack of a nurse in educational centres is a situation that affects most of the countries studied [6] [16] [17]. Therefore student attendance is devolved to teaching and administration staff [6], particularly to the family [25]. The role of a Credentialed Diabetes Educator in other countries like Australia and United States of America is considered as the ideal figure to provide the support required in the school environment [6].

Planning and implementation of specific measures like the *Protocol* is a step forward in the defense of the rights of children with diabetes, bur still shows important gaps. Regarding the fulfilment of the international care standards, to include control, evaluation and monitoring measures of treatment management in school to guarantee the safety and well-being of children with T1DM, besides ensuring a suitable academic performance [6] [8]-[10] [26]. Along the same line, other authors propose the implementation of auditing and/or feedback systems within an evaluation process orientated to improve quality [17].

Some contents of the *Protocol* seems more oriented as a means of protection against hypothetical legal responsibility of the school, instead of being a useful instrument to guarantee the safety, inclusion and sharing responsibilities. A contradiction is detected between child safety and inclusion objectives, care conditions at school, and the measures established.

The last International DAWN Youth study highlights the need to develop legislation measures to guarantee the distribution of responsibilities, the enforcement of care planning and the treatment management in the educational environment [16]. In another recent study carried out in the UK it is suggested that the policy and the legislative framework related to the diabetes management is not sufficient to ensure schools offer optimal care to children with diabetes [27]. The ambiguity of policies regarding the responsibilities in schools, leads to different care practice of diabetes in school [27].

4.3. Practice and the Reality in Schools

The models in the United States, Sweden, UK, the policies should make clear the role in school, identify the responsibilities for the care and the provision of medical care to support the optimal management of diabetes in schools [27]. Although, more investigation is required to provide more evidence about the reasons for the different diabetes treatment in different schools of the same country and in the world, the international policies of diabetes management in school should be developed to improve the consistency of care and ensure the equity for all children with diabetes [6].

It is recommended an interdisciplinary perspective and measures to guarantee the participation and collaboration between children, parents, educational staff and medical team to ensure the welfare [14], the integration of diabetes care in the school routine and establish a safe learning environment [6]-[11] [16].

5. Relevance and Limitations of the Study

The implications of the findings highlight the need to design systems for evaluating the practical implementation of policies related to health and educational care of children and adolescents with diabetes mellitus at school setting. The implementation measures must ensure the full inclusion of children with diabetes at school, welfare, security and optimal self-care and management of their treatment. In addition, the participation and coordination of all care settings are required.

These international care goals require continuous school staff training in health promoting school and specifically in diabetes care, a certain school organization based on a comprehensive model of education and new political commitments.

Limitations of the study are due to the analysis of the *Protocol* that has been focusing on specific documents relating to the care standards and guidelines of ADA and IDF used by the *Protocol* in their background and justification. Future editions of the *Protocol* must be analysed on the basis of their latest reviews. Also, the comparative analysis of the various documents existing in other regions or countries can provide a broader vision of care policy and legal regulation of diabetes care at school.

Acknowledgements

The Government of Extremadura and Funds FEDER (European Union) for funding the PRI09A156 Project: *Virtual Platform to Support Diabetes Education in Childhood and Adolescence (PAED)*.

References

[1]   Schwartz, F.L., Denham, S., Heh, V., Wapner, A. and Shubrook, J. (2010) Experiences of Children and Adolescents With Type 1 Diabetes in School: Survey of Children, Parents, and Schools. *Diabetes Spectrum*, **23**, 47-55. http://dx.doi.org/10.2337/diaspect.23.1.47

[2]   Faro, B., Ingersoll, G., Fiore, H. and Ippolito, K.S. (2005) Improving Students' Diabetes Management through School-Based Diabetes Care. *Journal of Pediatric Health Care* **19**, 301-308. http://dx.doi.org/10.1016/j.pedhc.2005.03.004

[3]   Tolbert, R. (2009) Managing Type 1 Diabetes at School: An Integrative Review. *The Journal of School Nursing*, **25**, 55-61. http://dx.doi.org/10.1177/1059840508329295

[4]   Miranda Velasco, M.J., Domínguez Martín, E., Arroyo Díez, F.J., Méndez Pérez, P. and González de Buitrago Amigo, J. (2012) [Health Related Quality of Life in Type 1 Diabetes Mellitus]. *Anales de Pediatría*, **77**, 329-233.

[5]   MacLeish, S.A., Cuttler, L. and Koontz, M.B. (2013) Adherence to Guidelines for Diabetes Care in School: Family and School Nurse Perspectives. *Diabetes Care*, **36**, e52. http://dx.doi.org/10.2337/dc12-2083

[6]   Marks, A., Wilson, V. and Crisp, J. (2013) The Management of Type 1 Diabetes in Primary School: Review of the Literature. *Issues in Comprehensive Pediatric Nursing*, **36**, 98-119. http://dx.doi.org/10.3109/01460862.2013.782079

[7]   American Association of Diabetes Educators (2008) Management of Children with Diabetes in the School Setting. AADE Position Statement. *The Diabetes Educator*, **34**, 439-443. http://dx.doi.org/10.1177/0145721708317873

[8]   American Diabetes Association (2014) Diabetes Care in the School and Day Care Setting. *Diabetes Care*, **37**, S91-S96.

[9]   American Diabetes Association (2008) Diabetes Care in the School and day Care Setting. *Diabetes Care*, **31**, S79-S86.

[10] American Diabetes Association (2004) Diabetes Care in the School and Day Care Setting. *Diabetes Care*, **27**, S122-S128.

[11] American Diabetes Association (2005) Care of Children and Adolescents with Type 1 Diabetes: A Statement of the American Diabetes Association. *Diabetes Care*, **28**, 186-212. http://dx.doi.org/10.2337/diacare.28.1.186

[12] American Diabetes Association (2009) Standards of Medical Care in Diabetes—2009. *Diabetes Care*, **32**, S13-S61. http://dx.doi.org/10.2337/dc09-S013

[13] International Diabetes Federation (2011) Global IDF/ISPAD Guideline for Diabetes in Childhood and Adolescence. http://web.ispad.org/sites/default/files/idf-ispad_diabetes_in_childhood_and_adolescence_guidelines_2011.pdf

[14] Pihoker, C., Forsander, G., Fantahun, B., Virmani, A., Luo, X., Hallman, M., Wolfsdorf, J. and Maahs, D.M. (2014) ISPAD Clinical Practice Consensus Guidelines 2014. The Delivery of Ambulatory Diabetes Care to Children and Adolescents with Diabetes. *Pediatric Diabetes*, **15**, 86-101. http://dx.doi.org/10.1111/pedi.12181

[15] Gregg, E.W. and Albright, A.L. (2009) The Public Health Response to Diabetes—Two Steps Forward, One Step Back. *JAMA*, **301**, 1596-1598. http://dx.doi.org/10.1001/jama.2009.519

[16] Lange, K., Jackson, C. and Deeb, L. (2009) Diabetes Care in Schools—The Disturbing Facts. *Pediatric Diabetes*, **10**, 28-36. http://dx.doi.org/10.1111/j.1399-5448.2009.00613.x

[17] Edwards, D., Noyes, J., Lowes, L., Haf Spencer, L. and Gregory, J.W. (2014) An Ongoing Struggle: A Mixed-Method Systematic Review of Interventions, Barriers and Facilitators to Achieving Optimal Self-Care by Children and Young People with Type 1 Diabetes in Educational Settings. *BMC Pediatrics*, **14**, 228. http://dx.doi.org/10.1186/1471-2431-14-228

[18] Lewis, D.W., Powers, P.A., Goodenough, M.F. and Poth, M.A. (2003) Inadequacy of In-School Support for Diabetic Children. *Diabetes Technology & Therapeutics*, **5**, 45-56. http://dx.doi.org/10.1089/152091503763816463

[19] Ley orgánica 2/2006, de 3 de mayo, de Educación. In: BOD, ed. num. 106, 04-May-2006.

[20] Ley 4/2011, de 7 de marzo, de educación de Extremadura. Comunidad Autónoma de Extremadura. In: DOE, ed. num. 47, 9-March-2011. https://www.boe.es/buscar/pdf/2011/BOE-A-2011-5297-consolidado.pdf

[21] Government of Extremadura (2010) Protocol of Care of Children and Adolescents in School (Protocolo de atención al niño/a y adolescente con diabetes en la escuela). Regional Ministry of Health and Dependency-Regional Ministry of Education, Government of Extremadura, Mérida, Extremadura.

[22] Government of Extremadura (2013) Extremadura Health Plan 2013-2020. Mérida, Extremadura.

[23] International Diabetes Federation (2005) The Rights of the Child with Diabetes in the School—Unsafe at School. Position Statement—Rights of Child with Diabetes in the School. http://www.unsafeatschool.ca/the-rights-of-the-child-with-diabetes-in-the-school

[24] American Diabetes Association (2013) Diabetes Care in the School and Day Care Setting. *Diabetes Care*, **36**, S75-S79.

[25] Bodas, P., Marín, M. and Amillategui, B. (2008) Diabetes in the School. Perceptions of Children and Adolescents with Type 1 Diabetes. *Avances en Diabetología*, **24**, 51-55.

[26] Dabelea, D., Mayer-Davis, E.J., Saydah, S., Imperatore, G., Linder, B., Divers, J., Bell, R., Badaru, A., Talton, J.W., Crume, T., Liese, A.D., Merchant, A.T., Lawrence, J.M., Reynolds, K., Dolan, L., Liu, L.L. and Hamman, R.F. (2014) Prevalence of Type 1 and Type 2 Diabetes among Children and Adolescents from 2001 to 2009. *JAMA*, **311**, 1778-1786. http://dx.doi.org/10.1001/jama.2014.3201

[27] Marshall, M., Gidman, W. and Callery, P. (2013) Supporting the Care of Children with Diabetes in School: A Qualitative Study of Nurses in the UK. *Diabetic Medicine*, **30**, 871-877. http://dx.doi.org/10.1111/dme.12154

6

Effects of a Revised Moderate Drinking Program for Enhancing Behavior Modification in the Workplace for Heavy Drinkers: A Randomized Controlled Trial in Japan

Koji Harada[1]*, Michiko Moriyama[2], Mariko Uno[2], Toshio Kobayashi[2], Takefumi Yuzuriha[3]

[1]Graduate School of Health Sciences, Hiroshima University, Hiroshima, Japan
[2]Institute of Biomedical & Health Sciences, Hiroshima University, Hiroshima, Japan
[3]Hizen Psychiatric Center, Saga, Japan
Email: *dddd116639@hiroshima-u.ac.jp

Abstract

This study examined the effects of the Hizen Alcoholism Prevention Program (HAPPY) and the revised version of HAPPY (HAPPY Plus), and also compared the two programs to determine whether the HAPPY Plus achieved better outcomes for heavy drinkers in the workplace. The HAPPY Plus designed to strengthen participants' recruitment, perception of threat, stress management, behavior modification by self-monitoring using a calendar-based diary, and to prevent dropout by telephone and e-mail follow-up by a trained nurse. Participants were men and women who consumed at least 20 g and 10 g of alcohol daily, respectively, and had not been diagnosed with alcohol dependence. A group intervention, 3-month randomized controlled trial was conducted. The control and intervention groups received the HAPPY and HAPPY Plus, respectively. The primary endpoint was average daily alcohol consumption. The Alcohol Use Disorders Identification Test (AUDIT), weight, body mass index, blood pressure, liver function, goal achievement rate, self-efficacy, and self-esteem were also measured. Out of 88 recruited employees, 83 (intervention group: 40; control group: 43) completed the study (completion rates were 100% and 93.4% respectively). As a result, average daily alcohol consumption decreased significantly in both groups ($p < 0.001$), but did not differ between groups. Even though behavior change rate was higher, and self-efficacy and confidence increased in the intervention group, AUDIT decreased in both groups but was significant only in the control group. Physiological indicators in the intervention group improved, but were not significant between the groups. Against the program revision, this study did not prove

---

*Corresponding author.

superiority of HAPPY Plus to the HAPPY regarding the indicators. However, better behavior modification and lower dropout were observed in the HAPPY Plus. Therefore, after further improvement is made, this group intervention program is applied to the workplace.

Keywords

Heavy Drinkers, Harmful Use of Alcohol, Moderate Drinking Program, Behavior Modification, Workplace

1. Introduction

Harmful alcohol use is a risk factor affecting not only drinkers' health but also the risk of traffic accidents, violence, suicide, and injury, which leads to premature death or disability. Despite the fact that these events could be avoided via interventional strategies designed to prevent or reduce harmful alcohol use, global provision of such strategies is inadequate, and there is a need for the involvement of several fields such as primary care, workplace, and school settings [1].

According to the International Classification of Diseases-10 [2], alcohol-related disorders are divided into two categories, for which treatment responses differ. Alcohol dependence is treated as a psychiatric condition, with treatment based on abstinence and rehabilitation, while treatments for harmful use are based on improving health behaviors (e.g., drinking moderation). The World Health Organization (WHO) reported that harmful alcohol use is an important risk factor for noncommunicable diseases such as mental and neurological disorders, cardiovascular disease, cirrhosis of the liver, and various types of cancer. Despite the possibility of risk prevention, there were approximately 2.5 million alcohol-related deaths globally in 2004 [1].

In Japan, drinking has been strongly implicated in the incidence of lifestyle-related diseases [3]-[5], depression and other mental and neurological disorders [6], many types of accidents and injuries, and death due to hypothermia [7]. In addition, companies incur rising medical costs due to increases in lifestyle-related diseases involving drinking, absenteeism, and presenteeism [8].

These alcohol related problems are considered to be caused by consumption of 6 or more alcoholic drinks (60 g of alcohol) per day. The amount of alcohol consumed in Japan represents the consumption by an estimated 8% of the adult population: 2.4 million extremely heavy drinkers and 8.6 million heavy drinkers with average daily pure alcohol intake of at least 120 g and 60 g, respectively [9] [10]. Despite implementation of the 10-year "Health Japan 21" project, which was initiated in 2000 to extend the nation's healthy life expectancy, to reduce the supply of alcohol, increase knowledge, and limit the hours during which alcohol could be sold, the numbers of male and female heavy drinkers increased from 4.1% to 4.8% and 0.3% to 0.4%, respectively [11].

A brief intervention (BI) was developed in the 1980s, and a cross-national collaborative research project driven by WHO had been underway, mainly in Europe, to reduce the number of alcohol-related deaths [12]. The probability that alcohol consumption would decline over a 6 - 12 months period had been found to double in drinkers who received the BI [13]. Some studies have demonstrated the effectiveness of the BI in reducing alcohol consumption, and its use has been recommended in diagnosis and treatment guidelines for harmful drinking in various countries [12] [14]-[16]. On the other hand, other studies have shown that one of the limitations of BI is that the intervention period is short, preventing the provision of evidence of long-term effectiveness [16] [17].

The BI is used mainly in primary care [12] and designed to encourage intrinsic motivation centered on 2 - 3 counseling sessions, each lasting 10 - 15 minutes and including feedback, advice, and goal setting, provided by trained medical and counseling staff. From medical viewpoint, Yuzuriha developed the Hizen Alcoholism Prevention Program (HAPPY) in Japan in 2001, which included feedback, responsibility, advice, a menu, empathy, and self-esteem [18]. In addition, 1) the inclusion of an educational video to present medical information (the effects of drinking on the body) was considered a BI weakness; 2) to amplify the perception of threat, the Japanese version of the Alcohol Use Disorders Identification Test (AUDIT) [19] was administered, with information regarding risk, based on score results, provided for participants as a first assessment; 3) to reinforce self-determined behavior modification [20], a "drinking diary" was included to provide feedback to ensure that participants could view a record of their day-to-day behavior changes and review them with their medical staff; and 4) these diaries were integrated into the program to ensure that it could be implemented consistently. Moreover, in contrast to the BI, which mainly consisted of individual counseling in a primary care setting, the HAPPY was developed to allow implementation for groups in the workplace.

One study showed that the HAPPY significantly reduced the number of days on which heavy drinking occurred and significantly increased the number of alcohol-free days [21]; in addition, it significantly reduced γ-glutamyltranspeptidase (γ-GT) in another study [22]. The first study, however, did not include a control group, and small sample size was an issue for both studies.

Japan does not have a general practitioner system, and the implementation of BIs is not common practice. Because of the low take-up rate (46.2%) in those eligible for specific lifestyle-related disease checkups in their communities [23], it is extremely difficult to use the regional healthcare system framework to identify people whose drinking could be considered harmful. In addition, amid the opportunistic drinking that is customary in the workplace, many employees could be considered to engage in harmful alcohol use. Further, because workplace health checkup take-up rates are high, and the workplace has been linked to the primary prevention of alcohol abuse [24], inclusion of these programs in company-provided health services is considered as both necessary and effective.

Therefore, an improved version of the HAPPY, the HAPPY Plus, was developed, and the purpose of this study was to measure its effectiveness and compare it with that of the HAPPY in employees in the workplace whose drinking qualified as harmful use.

In companies that aim to reduce their healthcare costs, resolving the issue of heavy drinking contributes to this management via primary prevention of alcohol related lifestyle diseases; ultimately controls healthcare costs related to chronic diseases [25]. It is a preventative measure for psychological problems such as depression, insomnia, and social problems, which include absenteeism, presenteeism, and drunken driving; and is connected to controlling the progression of drinking toward alcohol dependence.

2. Methods

2.1. Study Design and Sample

A randomized controlled trial was conducted, with the HAPPY and HAPPY Plus provided for the control and intervention groups, respectively.

Participants were selected from employees of 10 companies that had agreed to collaborate in the study, who provided informed consent and fulfilled the following eligibility criteria: (1) aged over 20 years, (2) average daily alcohol intake of 2 drinks (20 g) for men and 1 drink (10 g) for women, and (3) no diagnosis of alcohol dependence.

Regarding the sample size, given an effect size of 0.33 for the BI [26], a significance level of 5%, and calculation of significant differences with statistical power of 80%, the number of participants required for within-group measures and interactions in a two-way repeated measures ANOVA was 58 for each group. Using the same method and effect size, the required number of participants for between-subjects measures was 28 for each group. Assuming an attrition rate of 10% at 3 months, the target sample size was set at 128 (64 for each group) to produce the required sample size of 58 for each group.

2.2. Sampling and Randomization

Employees who, according to the results of workplace-provided health checkups required by the Industrial Safety and Health Act, were classified as people whose alcohol intake was at the heavy drinking level (540 ml or more per day) or people who already have a health disorder of γ-GT > 50 U/l were selected for participation. Recruitment was made through the companies by distributing flyers to each individual. After providing informed consent, participants were randomly assigned to the two groups.

2.3. Development of the HAPPY Plus and Training

Referring to the results of a recent field study that used focus group methodology to interview 12 male heavy drinkers [27], the following revisions were made to the HAPPY:

1) A program title was created to improve recruitment. "Learning How to Have a Long-Term Relationship

with Alcohol" was used as the title for the drinking moderation program, because 2 points had become clear. First, there was a strong resistance to reducing drinking (drinking provides an opportunity to socialize and build collegiality, and "being able to hold one's liquor" is tied to the meaning of one's existence, while drinking in moderation is believed to be connected to the disavowal of drinkers' values). Second, there was a lack of foresight regarding long-term health (people do not think about being unable to drink because of health problems; it does not occur to them that their very existence could be threatened if they develop a health problem that makes it physically impossible to drink).

2) Changes were made to amplify participants' perception of the threat to their health in order to increase behavior change rate. The absence of the perception of a threat to health results from a paucity of information and knowledge concerning alcohol-related health problems, with the benefits of drinking emphasized. Therefore, we revised the way in which information was provided, using the Health Belief Model [28] [29], and improved the provision of medical information by instructing the therapist to present the information to participants interactively.

3) Stress management education was added. Because one of the reasons that participants drank alcohol to relieve stress, stress management education was integrated into the program to ensure that participants could learn to cope with stress via alternative means.

4) Measures were added to prevent dropout. We implemented interactive e-mail and telephone follow up between sessions, and integrated motivational interviewing skills into the program presentation, to strengthen communication regarding approval, encouragement, motivation, and sympathy.

5) The self-monitoring method was improved in order for participants to evaluate their drinking behavior objectively. We strengthened participants to set their goals on drinking behaviors and alcohol consumption and to monitor these achievements used a calendar-based diary.

6) Group dynamics were applied. Because customary drinking with work colleagues strengthens collegiality and provides a means via which to be oneself with others, we included group discussions regarding successful drinking (modeling), to increase self-efficacy.

A nurse facilitated this process. To assure the quality of this program, prior to the study, the nurse attended HAPPY training sessions and followed the manual prepared for this program.

2.4. Procedures

As shown in **Figure 1**, participants were assigned to the control (HAPPY) or intervention (HAPPY Plus) group. The trained nurse was assigned as a facilitator for sessions 1 - 3 and follow up for both groups. One group consisted of about six participants. The durations of the sessions and between-session intervals were the same for both groups, with a period of one month between sessions 1 and 2 and two months between sessions 2 and 3 (**Figure 1**).

Session 1 consisted mainly of 1) an explanation regarding the fundamental volume of the workbook, alcohol consumption assessment, and setting moderate-drinking goals; 2) amplification of participants' perception of the threat of alcohol-related health problems; and 3) participants' recording of their alcohol consumption. To amplify the perception of threat, medical information presentation was interactive, and group discussion was included in the intervention group. Session 2 consisted mainly of 1) an explanation regarding the exercise volume of the workbook, alcohol consumption assessment (progress of implementation), and goal resetting; and 2) amplification of participants' perception of the threat of alcohol-related health problems. Session 3 consisted of alcohol consumption assessment (progress of implementation), goal resetting, and a blood test.

2.5. Outcome Evaluation

2.5.1. Primary Endpoint
The primary endpoint was average daily alcohol consumption (number of drinks), which was assessed preintervention and at 1 and 3 months postintervention. Sensible drinking was defined as 2 regular alcohol-free days per week [30]. Sensible drinking recommended by Ministry of Health in Japan includes drinking up to 2 drinks per day for men and 1 drink per day for women [11].

2.5.2. Secondary Endpoints
1) AUDIT scores [19];

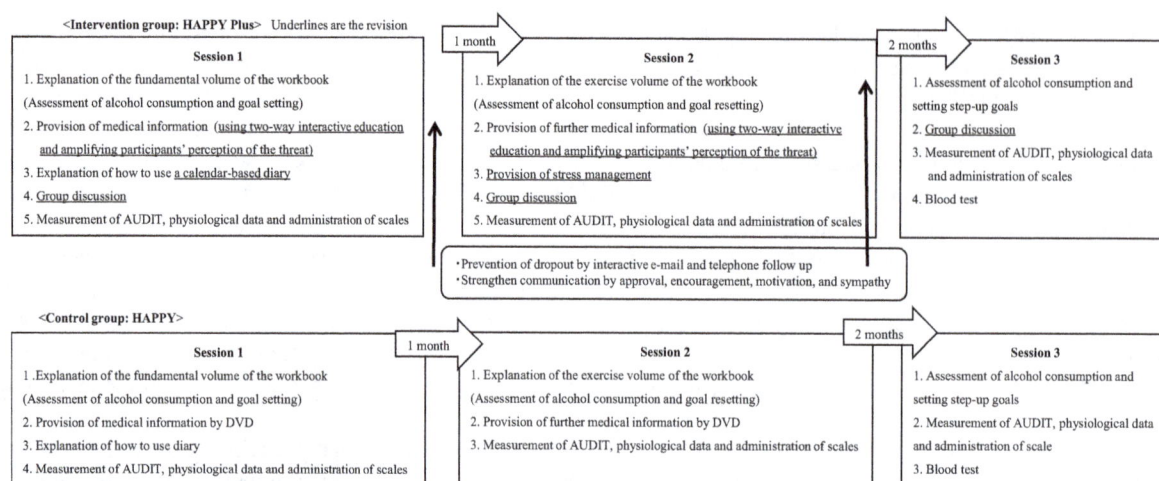

Figure 1. Contents of programs and the process.

2) Physiological indicators: weight, body mass index (BMI), systolic blood pressure, diastolic blood pressure, aspartate transaminase (AST), alanine transaminase (ALT), γ-GT, non-high-density lipoprotein cholesterol (non-HDL), and fasting glucose;

3) Psychological indicators: The General Self-Efficacy [31] [32] and Self-Esteem Scales [33] [34];

4) Achievement of moderate-drinking goals and importance and confidence ratings.

Weight, BMI, and blood pressure were measured by a nurse at each session. Other physiological indicators were measured preintervention and postintervention. The AUDIT and the General Self-Efficacy and Self-Esteem Scales were completed by participants and collected at every session. Blood samples were collected by the nurse at the session site and sent to a laboratory for analysis. Regarding the process indicators, at 1 and 3 months postintervention, participants completed a self-evaluation form concerning goal fulfillment and moderate drinking, with responses chosen from "goal almost achieved", "goal partially achieved", and "goal not achieved". In addition, participants performed self-evaluation during every session, rating the importance of preventing alcohol-related health problems and their confidence in their ability to control alcohol consumption.

The observation period was set at 3 months, because behavioral change could be measured by goal achievement rate and self-efficacy score [35]; we used these measurements as surrogate indicators.

2.6. Statistical Analysis

First, to examine the effects of the HAPPY, a Friedman test was performed to determine the change in overall results over time for both groups, with the items measured at 3 time points for each group. A paired t test was performed to compare items measured at 2 time points (pre- and postintervention). To determine whether the HAPPY Plus yielded superior outcomes, a two-way repeated measures ANOVA or an unpaired t test was performed after determining normality. Participants' achievement of moderate-drinking goals was expressed in terms of proportions of the participant group. A Friedman test was also used to examine changes in importance and confidence ratings over time for each group.

2.7. Study Period

Because the study was performed office by office, participant recruitment and the study procedures were conducted between September 2012 and March 2015.

2.8. Ethical Considerations

Ethical approval for the study was obtained from the Epidemiology Research Ethics Committee at the institution with where the authors were affiliated, and each office of the companies that collaborated in the study. The participants provided written informed consent to participation and the study was performed according to the Declaration of Helsinki.

3. Results

Eighty-eight people agreed to participate in the study. Of these, two withdrew from the study prior to randomization, and three of the control group withdrew prior to initiation of the intervention; all five withdrawals occurred because of business duty burden. Data for 40 participants in the intervention group and 43 in the control group were included in the analysis. Completion rates were 100% and 93.4% for the intervention and control groups, respectively (**Figure 2**).

3.1. Comparison of Demographic and Baseline Data

Participants' mean age was 46.1 ± 8.6 years (range: 25 - 60 years). Their mean alcohol consumption was 5.25 ± 3.23 drinks, and their mean AUDIT score was 14.0 ± 5.53 (**Table 1**). Statistically significant differences were not confirmed for control comparison.

3.2. Effectiveness of the Programs

Table 2 shows the changes in alcohol consumption over time and the physiological and psychological indicators for both groups combined and individually.

Daily alcohol consumption decreased significantly over time in the intervention and control groups and both groups combined (all, $p < 0.001$). However, according to the results of the two-way repeated measures ANOVA, consumption did not differ significantly between groups. Superior outcomes, therefore, were not observed for the HAPPY Plus with respect to the primary endpoint. AUDIT scores decreased significantly over time in the control group ($p < 0.05$) and both groups combined ($p < 0.01$), while scores did not change in the intervention group.

Regarding physiological indicators, BMI decreased significantly in the intervention group ($p < 0.01$) and both groups combined ($p < 0.05$). Systolic blood pressure also decreased significantly in the intervention group and both groups combined (all, $p < 0.05$). However, BMI and systolic blood pressure did not differ significantly between groups.

With respect to liver function, AST and ALT did not change subsequently to the intervention in both groups combined and individually (**Table 3**). However, γ-GT decreased significantly in the control group ($p < 0.05$) and both groups combined ($p < 0.01$), but did not change in the intervention group. In addition, γ-GT did not differ significantly between groups. Non-HDL and fasting glucose decreased very little; therefore, values did not differ significantly between or within groups.

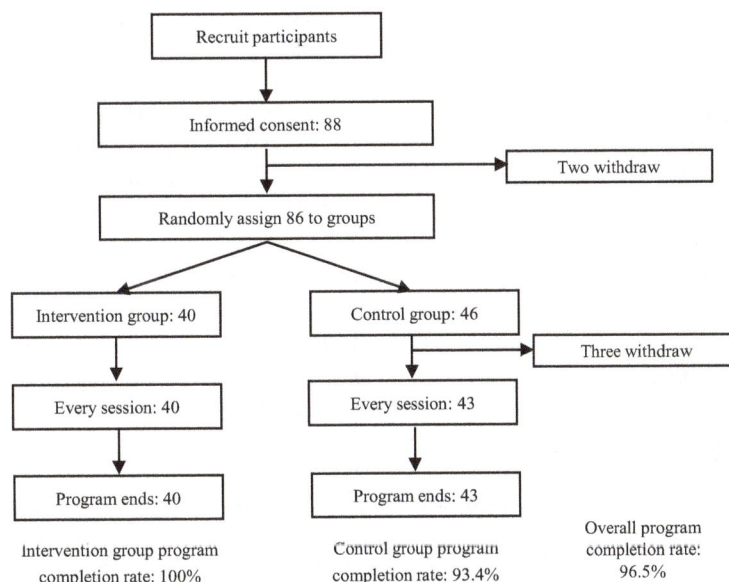

Figure 2. Participation and program completion rates.

Table 1. Baseline characteristics.

Items	Intervention group (n = 40)	Control group (n = 43)	p value
Base characteristics			
Sex (male/female)	30/10	34/9	0.795 n.s.
Age (year), mean ± SD	46.4 ± 9.3	45.7 ± 8.0	0.722 n.s.
Alcohol consumption/day (drinks)	5.27 ± 3.8	5.22 ± 2.7	0.951 n.s.
AUDIT score	13.3 ± 5.9	14.7 ± 5.1	0.244 n.s.
Physiological indicators (mean ± SD)			
Weight (kg)	68.9 ± 13.1	68.7 ± 13.3	0.959 n.s.
Body mass index	23.9 ± 3.5	24.2 ± 3.5	0.697 n.s.
Systolic blood pressure (mmHg)	132.1 ± 19.6	130.5 ± 18.8	0.707 n.s.
Diastolic blood pressure (mmHg)	85.4 ± 15.3	82.9 ± 13.6	0.423 n.s.
AST (U/l)	25.6 ± 9.8	27.4 ± 14.7	0.512 n.s.
ALT (U/l)	28.4 ± 19.0	28.4 ± 21.7	0.997 n.s.
γ-GT (U/l)	68.5 ± 75.4	90.1 ± 109.7	0.304 n.s.
Non-HDL (mg/dl)	135.4 ± 41.1	141.7 ± 41.6	0.626 n.s.
Fasting glucose (mg/dl)	99.8 ± 13.2	96.1 ± 16.5	0.266 n.s.
Psychological indicators			
Self-efficacy score	9.9 ± 4.1	9.1 ± 4.3	0.450 n.s.
Self-esteem score	22.7 ± 3.7	22.3 ± 3.3	0.583 n.s.

Sex: chi-squared test; Psychological indicators: Mann-Whitney U test; Other: unpaired t test Abbreviations: γ-GT: γ-glutamyltranspeptidase; ALT: alanine transaminase; AST: aspartate transaminase; AUDIT: Alcohol Use Disorders Identification Test; non-HDL: non-high-density lipoprotein cholesterol; SD: standard deviation; n.s.: No Significant

Regarding γ-GT, a pre/postintervention comparison was performed for participants with baseline values exceeding the reference value (>50 U/l; **Table 4**). Large reductions, all of which were statistically significant, were observed in the intervention and control groups (all, $p < 0.05$) and both groups combined ($p < 0.01$). However, no significant difference was observed between groups.

Self-efficacy increased significantly in the control group ($p < 0.05$) and both groups combined ($p < 0.01$). However, scores in the intervention group did not change and did not differ significantly between groups. Scores in self-esteem were observed unchanged in both groups combined and individually (**Table 2**).

Participants' goal achievement levels are shown in **Table 5**, and changes in their confidence levels over time and ratings for perception of the importance of preventing alcohol-related health problems are shown in **Table 6**. At both 1 and 3 months postintervention, relative to that of the control group, a higher proportion (60%) of participants in the intervention group had chosen the "goal almost achieved" response. Preintervention perception of the importance of preventing alcohol-related health problems was high in both groups, but no postintervention increases were observed. Confidence levels increased significantly in the intervention and control groups (all, $p < 0.05$). In addition, slight changes in goal achievement levels were observed in the intervention and control groups over time.

3.3. Participant Evaluations of Program Improvements

Table 7 shows the results of participants' evaluations of the programs. The HAPPY Plus evaluation included the improvements applied to address the weak points of the HAPPY. Approximately 80% of participants rated the improvements as good or very good. In contrast, 32.5% rated the provision of information concerning stress

Table 2. Changes in alcohol consumption and physiological and psychological indicators over time.

	Both Groups (n = 83)				Intervention Group (n = 40)				Control Group (n = 43)				Two-way repeated measures ANOVA (upper: F value; lower: p value)		
	Preintervention	After 1 month	After 3 months	p value	Preintervention	After 1 month	After 3 months	p value	Preintervention	After 1 month	After 3 months	p value	Interaction	Between groups	Within groups
Alcohol consumption day	5.25 ± 3.23	4.10 ± 2.71	3.76 ± 2.65	<0.001	5.27 ± 3.77	4.25 ± 3.12	3.82 ± 2.87	<0.001	5.22 ± 2.68	3.96 ± 2.30	3.70 ± 2.46	<0.001	0.272	0.062	41.931
													0.687	0.804	<0.001
AUDIT score	14.0 ± 5.53	12.9 ± 5.39	12.5 ± 5.51	0.004	13.3 ± 5.92	12.4 ± 5.65	12.2 ± 5.45	0.136	14.7 ± 5.12	13.4 ± 5.16	12.7 ± 5.63	0.022	0.689	0.744	8.025
													0.503	0.391	<0.001
Weight (kg)	68.8 ± 13.1	68.8 ± 13.0	68.5 ± 12.9	0.151	68.9 ± 13.1	68.9 ± 13.1	68.5 ± 13.1	0.015	68.7 ± 13.0	68.7 ± 13.0	68.5 ± 12.8	0.925	0.171	0.002	1.205
													0.793	0.964	0.296
Body Mass Index	24.1 ± 3.5	23.9 ± 3.5	23.8 ± 3.4	0.048	23.9 ± 3.5	23.6 ± 3.5	23.5 ± 3.5	0.005	24.2 ± 3.5	24.1 ± 3.4	24.0 ± 3.4	0.974	0.557	0.322	3.562
													0.489	0.572	0.054
Systolic blood pressure (mmHg)	131.3 ± 19.1	128.5 ± 16.2	127.1 ± 18.1	0.032	132.1 ± 19.6	126.9 ± 16.9	125.9 ± 20.8	0.019	130.5 ± 18.8	129.9 ± 15.5	128.3 ± 15.3	0.572	1.710	0.116	5.302
													0.184	0.734	0.006
Diastolic blood pressure (mmHg)	84.1 ± 14.5	84.8 ± 13.0	82.6 ± 15.2	0.818	85.4 ± 15.3	85.3 ± 13.5	81.5 ± 17.6	0.337	82.9 ± 13.6	84.3 ± 12.8	83.6 ± 12.7	0.742	1.949	0.027	1.835
													0.146	0.870	0.163
Self-efficacy	9.5 ± 4.2	10.0 ± 4.5	10.4 ± 4.5	0.002	9.9 ± 4.1	10.5 ± 4.3	10.9 ± 4.4	0.055	9.1 ± 4.3	9.5 ± 4.7	9.9 ± 4.6	0.040	0.250	0.908	11.493
													0.735	0.343	<0.001
Self-esteem	22.5 ± 3.5	22.7 ± 3.8	23.3 ± 4.0	0.055	22.7 ± 3.7	23.0 ± 4.0	23.6 ± 4.3	0.129	22.3 ± 3.3	22.5 ± 3.6	23.0 ± 3.6	0.333	0.136	0.435	6.762
													0.854	0.511	0.002

Abbreviations: AUDIT: Alcohol Use Disorders Identification Test.

Table 3. Changes in blood test data over time.

	Both Groups (n = 83)			Intervention Group (n = 43)			Control Group (n = 43)			Unpaired t test p value	
	Preintervention	Postintervention	p value	Preintervention	Postintervention	p value	Preintervention	Postintervention	p value	Preintervention	Postintervention
AST (U/l)	26.6 ± 12.7	24.5 ± 9.4	0.060	25.6 ± 9.8	25.0 ± 10.7	0.647	27.7 ± 15.0	24.0 ± 7.9	0.055	0.512	0.627
ALT (U/l)	28.5 ± 20.5	27.1 ± 16.6	0.331	28.4 ± 19.0	27.6 ± 19.1	0.663	28.5 ± 22.2	26.5 ± 13.8	0.377	0.997	0.769
γ-GT (U/l)	80.5 ± 95.6	64.3 ± 65.2	0.009	68.5 ± 75.4	59.7 ± 70.2	0.114	92.6 ± 111.8	69.0 ± 60.3	0.033	0.304	0.529
Non-HDL (mg/dl)	138.3 ± 41.0	141.6 ± 41.9	0.400	135.4 ± 41.1	138.8 ± 45.7	0.486	141.7 ± 41.6	144.9 ± 37.6	0.629	0.626	0.631
Fasting glucose (mg/dl)	98.1 ± 15.1	98.9 ± 20.5	0.647	99.8 ± 13.2	98.5 ± 14.0	0.644	96.2 ± 16.8	99.3 ± 25.8	0.179	0.266	0.828

Abbreviations: γ-GT: γ-glutamyltranspeptidase; ALT: alanine transaminase; AST: aspartate transaminase; non-HDL: non-high-density lipoprotein cholesterol.

Table 4. Participants' γ-GT values exceeding the reference value.

		Wilcoxon rank sum test			Mann-Whitney U test p value	
	n	Preintervention	Postintervention	p value	Preintervention	Postintervention
Both groups	32	151.8 ± 118.9	108.1 ± 81.5	0.001	0.459	0.352
Intervention group	14	132.6 ± 98.6	103.0 ± 100.3	0.041		
Control group	18	166.8 ± 133.4	112.0 ± 66.2	0.014		

Abbreviations: γ-GT: γ-glutamyltranspeptidase.

Table 5. Change in participants' goal achievement over time.

	Intervention group (n = 40)		Control group (n = 43)	
	After 1 month	After 3 months	After 1 month	After 3 months
Goal almost achieved, n (%)	24 (60.0)	24 (60.0)	16 (37.2)	18 (41.9)
Goal partially achieved, n (%)	14 (35.0)	13 (32.5)	17 (39.5)	18 (41.9)
Goal not achieved, n (%)	2 (5.0)	3 (7.5)	10 (23.3)	7 (16.3)
Total	40 (100.0)	40 (100.0)	43 (100.0)	43 (100.0)

Table 6. Changes in ratings for importance and confidence related to drinking in moderation over time.

	Intervention Group (n = 40)				Control group (n = 43)			
	Preintervention	After 1 month	After 3 months	p value	Preintervention	After 1 month	After 3 months	p value
Importance rating	7.15 ± 2.21	7.33 ± 1.73	7.53 ± 2.00	0.911	7.14 ± 2.57	7.26 ± 2.28	7.28 ± 2.15	0.940
Confidence rating	5.43 ± 2.07	5.78 ± 2.28	6.23 ± 1.90	0.020	5.05 ± 1.98	5.81 ± 1.93	5.93 ± 2.28	0.041

Table 7. Overall program evaluations.

	n	Very good (Long)	Good (A little long)	Neither	Bad (A little short)	Very bad (Short)	No response
HAPPY Plus							
Alcohol-related health problem slides	40	8 (20.0%)	25 (62.5%)	6 (15.0%)	0 (0.0%)	0 (0.0%)	1
Alcohol-related health problem explanations	40	9 (22.5%)	26 (65.0%)	4 (10.0%)	0 (0.0%)	0 (0.0%)	1
Support via telephone and e-mail	40	8 (20.0%)	22 (55.0%)	9 (22.5%)	0 (0.0%)	0 (0.0%)	1
Group discussions	40	9 (22.5%)	23 (57.5%)	7 (17.5%)	0 (0.0%)	0 (0.0%)	1
Learning materials for stress management	40	6 (15.0%)	20 (50.0%)	13 (32.5%)	0 (0.0%)	0 (0.0%)	1
Alcohol consumption diary: frequency of use	40	29 (72.5%)	6 (15.0%)	4 (10.0%)	1 (2.5%)	0 (0.0%)	0
Alcohol consumption diary: ease of use	40	7 (17.5%)	21 (52.5%)	11 (27.5%)	1 (2.5%)	0 (0.0%)	0
Information included with the alcohol consumption diary	40	7 (17.5%)	30 (75.0%)	3 (7.5%)	0 (0.0%)	0 (0.0%)	0
HAPPY							
Alcohol consumption diary: frequency of use	43	21 (48.8%)	14 (32.6%)	4 (9.3%)	2 (4.7%)	1 (2.3%)	1
Alcohol consumption diary: ease of use	43	3 (7.0%)	24 (55.8%)	10 (23.3%)	5 (11.6%)	0 (0.0%)	1
Information included with the alcohol consumption diary	43	1 (2.3%)	36 (83.7%)	5 (11.6%)	0 (0.0%)	0 (0.0%)	1

management as "neither". The HAPPY Plus revised alcohol consumption diary received a number of positive reviews.

4. Discussion

4.1. Study Participation

As the participants' baseline daily alcohol consumption and AUDIT scores indicated harmful use but did not fall within the alcohol dependence range; in addition, almost 40% of the participants already caused alcoholic liver disease, the study appears to have been successful in recruiting a sample in need of lifestyle modification. Collaborating with companies and the change in the program title facilitated the engagement process. These improvements appeared effective. In addition, the efforts to retain participants by e-mail and telephone follow up in the HAPPY Plus appeared successful, as 100% of the participants completed the study.

4.2. Effects of the HAPPY and HAPPY Plus

Since HAPPY Plus is a revision of the HAPPY, we examined effectiveness of both groups combined first. While significant changes occurred in the primary endpoint, average daily alcohol consumption, and secondary endpoints, AUDIT scores, BMI, systolic blood pressure, and γ-GT, were observed with both programs. The HAPPY, which provides feedback via the use of AUDIT scores to give participants with a clear understanding of their current alcohol use, relevant medical knowledge, and a tool of self-monitoring their consumption using diaries, exerted a direct effect on the reduction of alcohol consumption, showed the similar effect to that exerted by the BI [36]. As a secondary effect, the results confirmed a decrease in blood pressure, which was also suggested in the positive relationships between alcohol intake and hypertension shown in other studies [37]-[39].

On the other hand, although alcohol intake is related to risk of glucose intolerance [40] and elevated fatty acid levels [41], there were no improvements in these indicators. This may have occurred because there were only three participants whose results exceeded the reference values for diabetes. More important reason is that the program did not include diet and exercise education. This is explained in comparison with disease management programs which include comprehensive health risk behavior modification [35] and the metabolic syndrome life-style change education [42], which proved improvement in indicators for not only alcohol consumption but also blood glucose, blood pressure, and lipids. Especially, Iyatomi *et al.* showed significant improvement for targeting high-risk drinkers whose AUDIT scores of at least 10 or consumed at least 21 drinks per week [42]. Therefore, we need to improve the programs; once the effects of moderate alcohol consumption have increased, the next step is to guide participants into programs including disease prevention programs that provide good dietary and exercise guidance or those that aim to improve overall health behavior.

In addition, scores for self-efficacy and self-esteem improved over time. This suggests that the intervention elements included in the HAPPY, such as empathy, goal setting and evaluation, could have been effective in providing a successful experience in drinking moderation.

4.3. Effects of the HAPPY Plus vs. the HAPPY

Goal achievement was considerably higher in the HAPPY Plus, as further information concerning alcohol-related health problems was provided, presentation was interactive, group dynamics were introduced, and telephone and e-mail follow up were added. Aside from this finding, the HAPPY Plus was not shown to be superior to the HAPPY.

A considerable reason is that there were control group participants whose data values were extreme, and improvements in these participants' data exerted a strong influence on the results. Moreover, even in the HAPPY Plus, with behavior modification enhancement, the goal achievement rate was only 60%; notwithstanding the finding that there was a significant decrease in AUDIT scores in both groups combined. The average score did not fall below the dangerous consumption level. Further, despite a large and statistically significant reduction in γ-GT values in both groups combined, the average value did not decrease sufficiently to reach the normal range.

Another explanation for this could be that, even though the medium and method were altered, feedback, advice, goal setting, self-monitoring, and acquisition of medical knowledge were included in both programs. Moreover, as company employees, participants could be assumed to possess sufficient cognitive ability to adapt an approach to suit their needs and use the Internet and other resources to obtain information as required. In fact, some participants stated that the alcohol consumption diary required improvement and created their own spreadsheet programs. However, the diary used in the HAPPY Plus demonstrated some strengths. The calendar style exerted a self-monitoring effect, as participants were able to grasp the relationship between changes in their behavior and alcohol consumption, such as "the relationship between weekend dinner parties and alcohol consumption" and "setting alcohol-free days and its effects", at a glance. While the introduction of a drinking diary was not shown to exert a significant effect in one study [43], Hara *et al.* [44] described the effectiveness of moderate-drinking goals and a drinking diary. Nevertheless, with the finding that levels of achievement of behavioral goals were high in the HAPPY Plus, using a longer measurement period, it is conceivable that results could be reflected in improved physiological indicators and AUDIT scores.

In addition, participants' evaluations of the stress management section of the program were low, and it did not exert a direct effect on controlling drinking behavior. Although entirely within the realm of conjecture, because this was a group intervention implemented in the workplace, it is possible that participants felt unable to discuss stress. Even though some studies have indicated that drinking behavior was associated with stress coping in men [45], rather than drinking serving as a means of relieving stress, it could simply reflect a daily habit, as some participants value drinking for its own sake, and their drinking is not related to stress relief [27]. Therefore, stress management could be deleted for the group intervention.

Regarding the use of group interventions in the workplace, in recent years, Internet-based programs designed to assist individuals in reducing their drinking have multiplied in other countries, and there is evidence to support their effectiveness [46]. In particular, because such programs are easily accessible, they are useful for minors engaging in drinking illegally [47]. However, given that the development of web-based programs to reduce drinking has just begun in Japan, the use of group interventions should not be underestimated for several reasons. The biggest reason is that in Japan, drinking is often work related, and peer effect should not be underestimated.

The results of this study suggested that convincing heavy drinkers to participate in and complete such programs requires an enforcement mechanism.

4.4. Summary and Future Improvements

Both the HAPPY and HAPPY Plus were found to reduce daily alcohol consumption. In addition, to support participants with metabolic syndrome and respect to their dietary problems, the revised version of HAPPY that includes improvement of overall health behaviors is required. To improve program participation and completion rates, it was important to direct appeal for participation to companies, establish work-based groups, and conduct e-mail and telephone follow-up between sessions. Finally, since goal achievement rate was high in HAPPY Plus, it might be necessary to observe changes in drinking behavior over a period of at least a year rather than relying on surrogate indicators.

Conflicts of Interest

The authors declare that there are no conflicts of interest associated with this manuscript.

Funding

No funding was received for this study.

Access to Study Data

All authors had access to the study data.

References

[1] World Health Organization (2010) The Global Strategy to Reduce the Harmful use of Alcohol. World Health Organization, Geneva. http://www.who.int/substance_abuse/msbalcstragegy.pdf

[2] World Health Organization (1992) The ICD-10 Classification of Mental and Behavioral Disorders: Clinical Descriptions and Diagnostic Guidelines. World Health Organization, Geneva. http://www.who.int/classifications/icd/en/bluebook.pdf

[3] Ikeda, N., Saito, E., Kondo, N., Inoue, M., Ikeda, S., Satoh, T., et al. (2011) What Has Made the Population of Japan Healthy? The Lancet, 378, 1094-1105. http://dx.doi.org/10.1016/S0140-6736(11)61055-6

[4] World Health Organization (2009) Global Health Risks: Mortality and Burden of Disease Attributable to Selected Major Risks. World Health Organization, Geneva.

[5] Tsugane, S., Michael T.F., Sasaki, S. and Baba, S. (1999) Alcohol Consumption and All-Cause and Cancer Mortality Among Middle-Aged Japanese Men: Seven Year Follow-Up of the JPHC Study Cohort I. American Journal of Epidemiology, 150, 1201-1207. http://aje.oxfordjournals.org/content/150/11/1201.full.pdf http://dx.doi.org/10.1093/oxfordjournals.aje.a009946

[6] Matsushita, S. and Higuchi, S. (2009) Alcohol-Related Disorders and Suicide. Psychiatria et Neurologia Japonica, 111, 1191-1202.

[7] Ministry of Health, Labour and Welfare (2015) "Drinking and Accidents". Health Information Website for the Prevention of Lifestyle Diseases [Seikatsushūkanbyō-yobō no tame no kenkōjōhōsaito "Inshu to jiko"]. Ministry of Health, Labour and Welfare, Tokyo. http://www.e-healthnet.mhlw.go.jp/information/alcohol/a-06-004.html

[8] Health Insurance Association of Tokio Marine Nichido (2015) Visualizing Health Issues through Collaboration between Insurers and Business Owners Based on the "Health Cost Management" Framework ["Kenkōkeiei" no wakugu-minimotozuitahokensha/jigyōnushi no korabo-herusuniyorukenkō-kadai no kashika]. Health Insurance Association of Tokyo Marine Nichido, Tokyo. http://www.mhlw.go.jp/file/06-Seisakujouhou-12400000-Hokenkyoku/houkoku12.pdf

[9] Health, Labour and Welfare Statistics Association (2004) Welfare Indicators 2004 Special Edition: National Health Trend [Kokumin-eisei no dōkō "Kōsei no shihyō" rinji-zōkan 2004]. Health, Labour and Welfare Statistics Association, Tokyo.

[10] Higuchi, S. (2004) Research on the Prevention of Problems Related to Drinking in Adults: 2003 Annual Report [Kōseirōdōkagakukenkyūhihojokin, Seijin no inshujittai to kanrenmondai no yobōnikansurukenkyū]. Health and Labor Sciences Research Grant.

[11] Health Japan 21 (2012) Reference Data Relating to the Promotion of Health Japan 21 (The Second Term) (Kenkō

Nippon 21 (dai 2 ji) no suishinnikansurusankōshiryō). Nutrition Committee for Regional Health Services and the Promotion of Health, Health and Science Council.

[12] Babor, T.F. and Higgins-Biddle, J.C. (2001) Brief Intervention for Hazardous and Harmful Drinking: A Manual for Use in Primary Care. World Health Organization, Department of Mental Health and Substance Abuse, Geneva.

[13] Wilk, A., Jensen, N. and Havighurst, T. (1997) Meta-Analysis of Randomized Control Trials Addressing Brief Interventions in Heavy Alcohol Drinkers. *Journal of General Internal Medicine*, **12**, 274-283. http://dx.doi.org/10.1007/s11606-006-5063-z

[14] National Guideline Clearinghouse (2011) Guideline Title: Problem Drinking, Agency for Healthcare Research and Quality. http://www.guideline.gov/content.aspx?id=38894&search=problem+drinking

[15] National Institute for Health and Clinical Excellence (2010) Alcohol-Use Disorders: Preventing Harmful Drinking. Public Health Guidance 24. National Institute for Health and Clinical Excellence, National Health Service, UK. http://www.nice.org.uk/guidance/ph24

[16] Scottish Intercollegiate Guidelines Network (2003) The Management of Harmful Drinking and Alcohol Dependence in Primary Care. Publication No.74. http://www.sign.ac.uk/pdf/sign74.pdf

[17] McQueen, J., Howe, T.E., Allan, L., Mains, D. and Hardy, V. (2011) Brief Interventions for Heavy Alcohol Users Admitted to General Hospital Wards. *Cochrane Database of Systematic Reviews*, **8**, Article ID: CD005191. http://dx.doi.org/10.1002/14651858.cd005191.pub3

[18] Yuzuriha, T. (2010) User Manual for the HAPPY Program of Early Intervention Strategies for Alcohol Problems, 2nd Edition (Arukōrumondaisōkikainyū no sutoratejī HAPPY puroguramushiyōmanuarudai 2 ban). National Hospital Organization, Hizen Psychiatric Center, 35-47.

[19] Hiro, H. and Shima, S. (1996) Availability of the Alcohol Use Disorders Identification Test (AUDIT) for a Complete Health Examination in Japan. *Nihon Arukoru Yakubutsu Igakkai Zasshi*, **31**, 437-450.

[20] Sunami, T. and Yuzuriha, T. (2012) The Importance of Early Intervention with Heavy Drinkers: The Practice of Brief Interventions (Taryōinshushani tai surusōki-kainyū no jūyōsei: Burīfuintābenshyon no jissenkara). *The Journal of Public Health Practice*, **76**, 195-199.

[21] Hara, T., Muto, T., Yoshimori, C., Ishido, K., Higuchi, S. and Yuzuriha, T. (2009) The Effectiveness of a Group Intervention Program for Heavy Drinkers in the Workplace. *Japanese Journal of Alcohol Studies & Drug Dependence*, **44**, 290-291.

[22] Yoshioka, K. (2009) Empirical Testing of the Effectiveness of Interventions of the HAPPY Alcohol Dependence Prevention Program in Workers with Alcohol-Related Problems (Arukōruizonshōyobōpuroguramu (HAPPY) kainyū no kōkakenshō, arukōrikanrenmondai o motsushūrōsha o taishōni shite). *The Journal of the Japanese Society of Alcohol-Related Problems*, **11**, 117-121.

[23] Ministry of Health, Labour and Welfare (2014) 2012 Implementation Status for Lifestyle Disease Checkups and Counseling (Heisei 24 nendotokuteikenkōshinsa—Tokuteihokenshidō no jisshijōkyō). Ministry of Health, Labour and Welfare, Tokyo.

[24] Ames, G.M. and Bennett, J.B. (2011) Prevention Interventions of Alcohol Problems in the Workplace: A Review and Guiding Framework. *Alcohol Research & Health*, **34**, 175-187. http://pubs.niaaa.nih.gov/publications/arh342/175-187.htm

[25] McPherson, T.L., Goplerud, E., Olufokunbi-Sam, D., Jacobus-Kantor, L., Lusby-Treber, K. and Walsh, T. (2009) Workplace Alcohol Screening, Brief Intervention, and Referral to Treatment (SBIRT): A Survey of Employer and Vendor Practices. *Journal of Workplace Behavioral Health*, **24**, 285-306. http://dx.doi.org/10.1080/15555240903188372

[26] Fleming, M.F., Barry, K.L., Manwell, L.B., Johnson, K. and London, R. (1997) Brief Physician Advice for Problem Alcohol Drinkers: A Randomized Controlled Trial in Community-Based Primary Care Practices. *The Journal of the American Medical Association*, **277**, 1039-1045. http://www.ncbi.nlm.nih.gov/pubmed/9091691 http://dx.doi.org/10.1001/jama.1997.03540370029032

[27] Harada, K. and Moriyama, M. (2013). Drinkers' Life Value and Their Resistance to Moderation in Drinking. *Japan Academy of Psychiatric and Mental Health Nursing*, **22**, 31-39.

[28] Rosenstock, I.M. (1974) Historical Origins of the Health Belief Model. *Health Education Monographs*, **2**, 328-335. http://dx.doi.org/10.1177/109019817400200403

[29] Becker, M.H. (1974) The Health Belief Model and Personal Health Behavior. *Health Education Monographs*, **2**, 324-508. http://dx.doi.org/10.1177/109019817400200407

[30] Health and Medicine Alcohol Association (2008) The 10 Articles of Sensible Drinking (Tekiseiinshu no 10 kajō). Health and Medicine Alcohol Association, Tokyo. http://arukenkyo.or.jp/health/proper/index.html

[31] Bandura, A. (1977) Self-Efficacy: Toward a Unifying Theory of Behavioral Change. *Psychological Review*, **84**, 191-215. http://archive2.cra.org/Activities/craw_archive/dmp/awards/2007/Tolbert/self-efficacy.pdf http://dx.doi.org/10.1037/0033-295X.84.2.191

[32] Sakano, Y. and Tojo, M. (1986) General Self-Efficacy Scale (Ippanseijikokouryokukan Syakudo no sakuseinokokoromi). *Kodoryohokenkyu*, **12**, 73-82.

[33] Rosenberg, M. (1965) Society and the Adolescent Self-Image. Princeton University Press, Princeton.

[34] Mimura, C. and Griffiths, P. (2007) A Japanese Version of the Rosenberg Self-Esteem Scale: Translation and Equivalence Assessment. *Journal of Psychosomatic Research*, **62**, 589-594. http://dx.doi.org/10.1016/j.jpsychores.2006.11.004

[35] Kazawa, K. and Moriyama, M. (2013) Effects of a Self-Management Skills-Acquisition Program on Pre-Dialysis Patients with Diabetic Nephropathy. *Nephrology Nursing Journal*, **40**, 141-149.

[36] Gail, D.O., Michael, V.P., Linda, C.D., David, A.F., Susan, H.B., Marek, C.C., *et al.* (2012) A Brief Intervention Reduces Hazardous and Harmful Drinking in Emergency Department Patients. *Annals of Emergency Medicine*, **51**, 742-750.

[37] McMahon, S. (1987) Alcohol Consumption and Hypertension. *Hypertension*, **9**, 111-121. http://dx.doi.org/10.1161/01.HYP.9.2.111

[38] Marmot, M.G., Elliott, P., Shipley, M.J., Dyer, A.R., Ueshima, H., Beevers, D.G., *et al.* (1994) Alcohol and Blood Pressure: The INTERSALT Study. *British Medical Journal*, **308**, 1263-1267. http://dx.doi.org/10.1136/bmj.308.6939.1263

[39] Okamura, T., Tanaka, T., Yoshita, K., Chiba, N., Takebayashi, T., Kikuchi, Y., *et al.*, HIPOP-OHP Research Group (2004) Specific Alcoholic Beverage and Blood Pressure in a Middle-Aged Japanese Population: The High-Risk and Population Strategy for Occupational Health Promotion (HIPOP-OHP) Study. *Journal of Human Hypertension*, **18**, 9-16. http://dx.doi.org/10.1038/sj.jhh.1001627

[40] Kiyohara, Y., Shinohara, A., Kato, I., Shirota, T., Kubo, M., Tanizaki, Y., *et al.* (2003) Dietary Factors and Development of Impaired Glucose Tolerance and Diabetes in a General Japanese Population: Hisayama Study. *Journal of Epidemiology*, **13**, 251-258. http://dx.doi.org/10.2188/jea.13.251

[41] Ben, G., Gnudi, L., Maran, A., Gigante, A., Duner, E., Iori, E., *et al.* (1991) Effects of Chronic Alcohol Intake on Carbohydrate and Lipid Metabolism in Subjects with Type II (Non-Insulin-Dependent) Diabetes. *The American Journal of Medicine*, **90**, 70-76. http://dx.doi.org/10.1016/0002-9343(91)90508-U

[42] Iyadomi, M., Endo, K., Hara, T., Yuzuriha, T., Ichiba, M. and Tsutsumi, A. (2013) Effects of a Group Alcohol Intervention (S-HAPPY Program) at the Workplace for High Risk Alcohol Drinkers Using the Framework of the Specific Health Examination and Health Guidance System of the Metabolic Syndrome [Tokutei Hoken Shido no Wakugumi wo Riyoushita Hai-RisukuInshushani Taisuru Shokuikini Okeru Shudan Sesshu Shido (S-HAPPY Puroguramu) no Kouka]. *The Journal of Science of Labour*, **89**, 155-165.

[43] Ito, C., Yuzuriha, T., Noda, T., Ojima, T., Hiro, H. and Higuchi, S. (2015) Brief Intervention in the Workplace for Heavy Drinkers: A Randomized Clinical Trial in Japan. *Alcohol and Alcoholism*, **50**, 157-163. http://dx.doi.org/10.1093/alcalc/agu090

[44] Hara, T., Muto, T., Yoshimori, C., Ishido, K., Sunami, T., Endo, K. and Yuzuriha, T. (2011) Effectiveness of Drinking Plan and Drinking Diary in Intervention Program (HAPPY Program) for Heavy Drinkers [Taryou Inshusha Kainyu Puroguramu (HAPPY Program) ni Okeru Inshumokuhyou to Inshunikki no Yukouseinitsuite]. *Japanese Journal of Alcohol Studies & Drug Dependence*, **46**, 347-356.

[45] Urakawa, K. and Hagi, N. (2008) Relationships between Worker Stress Coping Behaviors and Occupational Stress (Kinrōsha no sutoresutaishokōdō to shokugyōseisutoresu to no kanren). *Mie Nursing Journal*, **10**, 89-92.

[46] Hester, R.K., Delaney, H.D. and Campbell, W. (2011) ModerateDrinking.com and Moderation Management: Outcomes of a Randomized Clinical Trial with Non-Dependent Problem Drinkers. *Journal of Consulting and Clinical Psychology*, **79**, 215-224. http://www.ncbi.nlm.nih.gov/pmc/articles/PMC3066281/pdf/nihms271551.pdf http://dx.doi.org/10.1037/a0022487

[47] Spijkerman, R., Roek, M.A., Vermulst, A., Lemmers, L., Huiberts, A. and Engels, R.C. (2010) Effectiveness of a Web-Based Brief Alcohol Intervention and Added Value of Normative Feedback in Reducing Underage Drinking: A Randomized Controlled Trial. *Journal of Medical Internet Research*, **12**, e65. http://dx.doi.org/10.2196/jmir.1465 http://www.ncbi.nlm.nih.gov/pubmed/21169172

7

Comparison of Survey Sampling Methods for Estimation of Vaccination Coverage in an Urban Setup of Assam, India

Dilip C. Nath*, Bhushita Patowari

Department of Statistics, Gauhati University, Guwahati, India
Email: *dilipc.nath@gmail.com, pbhushita@yahoo.com

Abstract

Background: Immunization averts a large number of children in each year. The burden of vaccine preventable diseases remains high in developing countries compared to developed countries. To overcome from this burden different types of immunization programs have been implemented. For better immunization coverage in developing countries, considerable progress is to be made to improve the knowledge and awareness regarding importance of vaccines. In this study a comparative study of immunization coverage under two sampling methods has been performed. Methods: In this study variance and design effect of proportion of children vaccinated against different types of vaccines (BCG, OPV, DPT, Hepatitis B, Hib, Measles and MMR) are estimated under two stage (30 × 30) cluster and systematic sampling for comparison of these two survey sampling methods. Also the homogeneity of clusters has been tested by using chi-square test. Results: It is observed that BCG, OPV and DPT vaccination coverage is more than 90% whereas Hepatitis B, Measles, Hib and MMR vaccination coverage is between 50% - 64% only. Here systematic random sampling is more complicated than two stage (30 × 30) cluster sampling. Also the result shows that the clusters are homogeneous with respect to proportion of children vaccinated. Conclusion: There is no significant difference between the two survey methodologies regarding the point estimation of vaccination coverage but estimation of variances of vaccination coverage is less in two stage (30 × 30) cluster sampling than that of the systematic sampling. Also the clusters are homogeneous. Very less improvement has been observed in case of fully vaccination coverage than the previous study. From the study it can be said that two stage (30 × 30) cluster sampling will be preferred to systematic sampling and simple random sampling method.

Keywords

Vaccine Coverage, Cluster Sampling, Systematic Sampling, Design Effect, Marascuilo Procedure

*Corresponding author.

1. Introduction

World Health Organization (WHO) recommends that all children should receive one dose of Bacillis Calmette-Guerin Vaccine (BCG), three doses of diphtheria-tetanus-pertusis vaccine (DPT), three doses of either oral polio vaccine (OPV) or inactivated polio vaccine (IPV), three doses of hepatitis B vaccine, and one dose of a measles virus-containing vaccine (MVCV), either anti-measles alone or in combination with other antigens. It also recommends three doses of vaccine against infection with Haemophilus influenza type b (Hib). To boost immunity at older ages, additional immunizations are recommended for healthcare workers, travelers, high-risk groups and people in areas where the risk of specific vaccine-preventable diseases is high [1]. The important role played by the WHO's EPI (Expanded Programme on Immunization) Cluster Survey in the success of national immunization programme efforts in many countries is widely recognized. The programme monitoring capability provided through the conduct of periodic cluster surveys has been especially important in developing country settings, where administrative records are often incomplete [2]. Together with EPI sampling other survey sampling has been compared in different studies [3]-[5]. According to WHO coverage of BCG vaccine is 87%, DPT3 vaccine is 72% and OPV3 vaccine is 70% in 2011 [6]. In a study Phukan *et al.* reported that the children of Assam in the North-East Region of India have consistently evidenced low rates for routine childhood immunizations. About 62.2% of the children were fully immunized [7]. Children are considered fully immunized if they receive one dose of BCG, three doses of OPV and DPT each and one dose of measles vaccine before reaching one year of age.

In this study estimates of vaccination coverage have been compared using design effect and variance of estimated proportion of children vaccinated against BCG, OPV, DPT, Hepatitis B, Hib, Measles and MMR (measles mumps rubella) vaccines under two stage (30 × 30) cluster sampling and systematic random sampling.

2. Methods

The data that has been used in this study is taken from a survey "Comparison of Two Survey Methodologies to Estimate Total Vaccination Coverage" sponsored by Indian Council of Medical Research (ICMR), New Delhi. It has been collected during the period from January to October, 2011 using following sampling techniques.

Two stage (30 × 30) cluster sampling: In this method the population needs to be divided into a complete set of non-overlapping subpopulations, usually defined by geographic or political boundaries. These subpopulations are called clusters. In the first stage, 30 of these clusters are sampled with probability proportionate to the size (PPS) of the population in the cluster. Sampling with probability proportionate to size allows the larger clusters to have a greater chance of being selected. The clusters are sampled without replacement. In the second stage of sampling, thirty subjects are selected within each cluster. Although the sampling unit is the individual subject, the sampling is conducted on the household level. Cluster sampling is often a practical approach to surveys because it samples by groups (clusters) of elements rather than by individual elements. It simplifies the task of constructing sampling frames, and it reduces the survey costs [8]. The advantages of two stage (30 × 30) cluster sampling over other designs are same as cluster sampling. A sampling frame listing all elements in the population may be impossible or costly to obtain, whereas to obtain a list of all clusters may be easy. Also the cost of obtaining data may be inflated by travel cost if the sampled elements are spread over a large geographic area.

Systematic random sampling: Systematic sampling is a random method of sampling in which only the first unit is selected with the help of random numbers and the rest get selected automatically according to some pre-designed pattern. If the population size $N = nk$, where n is the sample size and k is an integer, and a random number less than or equal to k be selected and every k^{th} unit thereafter. This procedure is linear systematic sampling. When $N \neq nk$ then every k^{th} unit be included in a circular manner till the whole list is exhausted, it is called circular systematic sampling. Systematic sampling is commonly used as an alternative to simple random sampling (SRS) because of its simplicity. It selects every k^{th} element after a random start (between 1 and k). Its procedural tasks are simple, and the process can easily be checked, whereas it is difficult to verify SRS by examining the results. It is often used in the final stage of multistage sampling when the fieldworker is instructed to select a predetermined proportion of units from the listing of dwellings in a street block. The systematic sampling procedure assigns each element in a population the same probability of being selected [8].

With the two stage (30 × 30) cluster sampling method in the first stage 30 wards are selected and in the second stage 30 units from each ward are selected. For the selection of second stage units in a selected ward only the first household is randomly selected. After the first household is visited, the surveyor moves to the "next" household, which is defined as the one whose front door is closest to the one just visited. Where there are bylane in a particular lane survey procedure is carried out in that place according to the serial household number in that bylane. This process continues until all 30 eligible subjects are found. The subjects are chosen by selecting a household and for more than one eligible subject (children from 6 months to 5 years of age) in a household all are selected.

After completing the 1st sampling method (that is two stage (30 × 30) cluster sampling) in a ward, 2nd sampling method (systematic random sampling) is carried out in same ward. In this sampling technique a random number is selected from random number table on the basis of the number of household in a lane where the survey was carried out in case of two stage (30 × 30) cluster sampling and this became the first sampling unit (household) of the systematic random sampling. After that each household is selected at an interval of 10 household and continuing the process until the 30 sampling units are not completed. Here the interval of household is taken as 10 so that the interval is neither too small nor too large. If we take the interval too small then we should get so many repetitions of the samples from two stage (30 × 30) cluster sampling which results same sampling unit in the 2nd sampling method (systematic sampling) and if we take the interval too large then there should not be any similarity between the two sampling methodologies as the larger interval will cover larger area and both the sampling techniques would take different places.

3. Statistical Analysis

Analysis has been carried out in the following two sections.

3.1. Section A

Here, variance of proportion of vaccination coverage and design effect of the same has been estimated.

Let, P = proportion of children who are vaccinated

Since same number of children has sampled per cluster, estimate of P $\left(\hat{P}\right)$ is given by

$$\hat{P} = \sum_{i=1}^{n=30} \frac{p_i}{n} \tag{1}$$

where p_i = the proportion of surveyed children in i^{th} cluster

n = the number of clusters

Then approximate estimated variance of $\hat{P}_c$ under cluster sampling [4] is given by

$$\hat{v}\left(\hat{P}_c\right) = \sum_{i=1}^{n}\left(p_i - \hat{P}\right)^2 \Big/ \left[n(n-1)\right] \tag{2}$$

Again the estimated variance of $\hat{P}_{sy}$ under systematic sampling [9] is

$$\hat{v}\left(\hat{P}_{sy}\right) = \left(\frac{N-n}{N}\right)\frac{\hat{p}(1-\hat{p})}{n-1} \tag{3}$$

An approximate 95% confidence interval on P can be obtained by using

$$\hat{P} \pm 1.96\sqrt{v\left(\hat{P}\right)} \tag{4}$$

The design effect may be estimated as

$$deff = \frac{\hat{v}(\text{esimated proportion under specified sampling})}{\hat{v}\left(\hat{P}_s\right)} \tag{5}$$

where

$$\hat{v}\left(\hat{P}_s\right) = \hat{P}(1-\hat{P}) \Big/ \left[\left(\sum_{i=1}^{n=30} n_i\right) - 1\right] \tag{6}$$

is the estimated variance under simple random sampling [4].

Also the design effect for cluster sampling vs systematic sampling is obtained as

$$deff = \frac{\hat{v}\left(\hat{P}_c\right)}{\hat{v}\left(\hat{P}_{sy}\right)} \tag{7}$$

3.2. Section B

In this section homogeneity of clusters have been tested by using chi-square test. That is to test equality of proportion of children vaccinated in each clusters. The test procedure is carried out taking Hepatitis B (at birth) vaccine (two stage (30 × 30) cluster sampling).

The null hypothesis is that there are no significant differences among the proportions of children vaccinated against Hepatitis B (at birth) in each clusters.

H_0: $P_1 = P_2 = \cdots = P_{30}$

Against the alternative that all the proportions are not equal.

H_1: Not all P_j's are equal (where $j = 1, 2, \cdots, 30$)

The test statistic is

$$\chi^2 = \sum \frac{\left(f_o - f_e\right)^2}{f_e} \tag{8}$$

where

f_o = observed frequency in a particular cell of a 2 × 30 contingency table

f_e = expected frequency in a particular cell if the null hypothesis is true

If the null hypothesis is true the proportions are all equal across the population. And rejecting the null hypothesis only allows to reach the conclusion that all proportions are not equal. But the test statistics does not give any information about proportions that differ. To identify the differences between proportions we will rely on a multiple comparison procedure. The Marascuilo procedure [10] enables us to make comparisons between all pairs of groups. In this procedure the absolute value of the pairwise difference between sample proportions has to be computed. The absolute values of these differences are the test statistics. For each pairwise comparison a critical value is computed as follows:

$$CV_{ij} = \sqrt{\chi^2_{\alpha,k-1}} \sqrt{\frac{\overline{p}_i\left(1 - \overline{p}_i\right)}{n_i} + \frac{\overline{p}_j\left(1 - \overline{p}_j\right)}{n_j}} \tag{9}$$

where α = level of significance, k = number of clusters

To compare each of test statistics with the corresponding critical value a specific pair is significantly different if the absolute difference in the sample proportion $\left|p_i - p_j\right|$ is greater than its critical range.

4. Results

Table 1 gives estimated coverage of BCG (at birth), OPV (OPV1 at birth, OPV2 at 6 weeks, OPV3 at 10 weeks, OPV4 at 14 weeks, OPV5 at 15 - 18 months and OPV6 at 5 years), DPT (DPT1 at 6 weeks, DPT2 at 10 weeks, DPT3 at 14 weeks, DPT4 at 15 - 18 months and DPT5 at 5 years), Hepatitis B (HepB1 at birth and HepB2 at 6 weeks), Hib (Hib1 at 6 weeks, Hib2 at 10 weeks and Hib3 at 14 weeks), Measles (at 9 months) and MMR (at 15 - 18 months) vaccine with 95% confidence intervals under two stage cluster and systematic sampling. Coverage of BCG vaccine is 99%, OPV and DPT vaccine coverage is more than 90% except for OPV6 and DPT5. But coverage of Hepatitis B, Hib, Measles and MMR vaccines are only between 50% - 64%. Though the individual vaccination coverage is high for BCG, OPV and DPT vaccine but fully vaccination coverage is only 63.52%. Both the survey methods have given point estimates of vaccination coverage with less difference.

Estimated variance of proportion of vaccination coverage is given in **Table 2**. It is seen that variances are less in case of two stage cluster sampling than the systematic sampling for all the vaccines namely BCG, OPV, DPT, Hepatitis B, Hib, Measles and MMR that are considered in the study. So the interval estimation of vaccination coverage has given better estimate in case of two stage (30 × 30) cluster sampling than the systematic sampling with less standard error (SE).

Table 1. Estimated coverage of vaccines under two stage cluster (30 × 30) and systematic sampling.

Vaccine		Two stage cluster (30 × 30)		Systematic sampling	
		Coverage estimate	95% CI	Coverage estimate	95% CI
BCG		0.99	(0.98, 0.99)	0.99	(0.98, 0.99)
OPV	OPV1	0.99	(0.98, 0.99)	0.99	(0.98,0.99)
	OPV2	0.98	(0.97, 0.98)	0.99	(0.98,0.99)
	OPV3	0.98	(0.97, 0.98)	0.99	(0.98,0.99)
	OPV4	0.97	(0.96, 0.97)	0.99	(0.98,0.99)
	OPV5	0.90	(0.89, 0.90)	0.89	(0.86,0.91)
	OPV6	0.54	(0.53, 0.54)	0.54	(0.50,0.57)
DPT	DPT1	0.98	(0.97, 0.98)	0.99	(0.98,0.99)
	DPT2	0.98	(0.97, 0.98)	0.99	(0.98,0.99)
	DPT3	0.97	(0.96, 0.97)	0.98	(0.98,0.99)
	DPT4	0.90	(0.89, 0.90)	0.90	(0.88,0.91)
	DPT5	0.52	(0.51, 0.52)	0.51	(0.47,0.54)
Hepatitis B	HepB1	0.58	(0.57, 0.58)	0.56	(0.52,0.59)
	HepB2	0.59	(0.58, 0.59)	0.56	(0.52,0.59)
Hib	Hib1	0.57	(0.56, 0.57)	0.55	(0.51,0.58)
	Hib2	0.57	(0.56, 0.57)	0.55	(0.51,0.58)
	Hib3	0.57	(0.50, 0.64)	0.55	(0.51,0.58)
Measles		0.64	(0.63, 0.64)	0.64	(0.60, 0.67)
MMR		0.52	(0.51, 0.52)	0.50	(0.46, 0.53)

Table 2. Estimated variance of proportion of vaccination coverage $\left(\hat{P} \right)$.

Vaccines		Methodology	
		Two stage cluster (30 × 30)	Systematic sampling
BCG		9.2009×10^{-09}	2.44173×10^{-06}
OPV	OPV1	1.1947×10^{-08}	4.87257×10^{-06}
	OPV2	3.2958×10^{-08}	9.70164×10^{-06}
	OPV3	3.2134×10^{-08}	1.32949×10^{-05}
	OPV4	1.2785×10^{-07}	1.56768×10^{-05}
	OPV5	5.4684×10^{-06}	2.29435×10^{-04}
	OPV6	6.0007×10^{-07}	1.06516×10^{-04}
	OPV7	9.5874×10^{-07}	2.73425×10^{-04}
DPT	DPT1	3.2958×10^{-08}	9.70164×10^{-06}
	DPT2	6.4818×10^{-08}	1.20999×10^{-05}
	DPT3	9.4344×10^{-08}	1.32949×10^{-05}
	DPT4	6.4134×10^{-07}	1.03118×10^{-04}
	DPT5	9.8328×10^{-07}	2.75069×10^{-04}
Hepatitis B	HepB1	1.1741×10^{-06}	2.7177×10^{-04}
	HepB2	1.1741×10^{-06}	2.71907×10^{-04}
Hib	Hib1	1.2841×10^{-06}	2.72553×10^{-04}
	Hib2	1.2814×10^{-06}	2.72303×10^{-04}
	Hib3	1.305×10^{-06}	2.72429×10^{-04}
Measles		1.6381×10^{-06}	2.53068×10^{-04}
MMR		1.702×10^{-06}	2.75305×10^{-04}

Table 3 represents estimates of design effect of proportion of children vaccinated against different types of vaccines. Design effect estimates are calculated for two stage cluster sampling vs simple random sampling, systematic sampling vs simple random sampling and cluster sampling vs systematic sampling. It is seen that design effect estimates are high in systematic sampling vs simple random sampling rather than the two stage cluster sampling vs simple random sampling and cluster sampling vs systematic sampling for all the vaccines considered here.

To study the homogeneity of clusters chi-square test has been performed. Here calculated value of χ^2 is 116.68 with 29 d.f. and p value is 0.00 that is the test statistic is significant and we reject the null hypothesis and concluded that the proportions of children vaccinated against Hepatitis B (at birth) are not equal. Let us start with computing all the proportions of children vaccinated against Hepatitis B (at birth) (given in **Table 4**).

Table 3. Estimates of design effect of proportion of children vaccinated.

Vaccine		Design effect		
		Cluster vs SRS	Systematic vs SRS	Cluster vs systematic
BCG		0.000835516	0.221728395	0.003768
OPV	OPV1	0.001084923	0.442469136	0.002452
	OPV2	0.001511716	0.880987654	0.003397
	OPV3	0.0014739	1.207284	0.002417
	OPV4	0.003949769	1.423580247	0.008155
	OPV5	0.022256	0.933037	0.023834
	OPV6	0.005094	0.831239	0.005634
	OPV7	0.001308	0.411678	0.003506
DPT	DPT1	0.001511716	0.880987654	0.003397
	DPT2	0.002973041	1.098765432	0.005357
	DPT3	0.002914598	1.207283951	0.007096
	DPT4	0.0054443	0.87535464	0.00622
	DPT5	0.00133547	0.41166791	0.003575
Hepatitis B	HepB1	0.004333	0.991563	0.00432
	HepB2	0.004364	0.992063	0.004318
Hib	Hib1	0.004710096	0.99	0.004712
	Hib2	0.0047	0.989091	0.004706
	Hib3	0.0047867	0.9895506	0.00479
Measles		0.0059581	0.9380207	0.006473
MMR		0.0052098	0.8413334	0.006182

Table 4. Estimated proportions of children vaccinated against Hepatitis B (at birth).

Sl. No.	Ward No.	Estimated proportions	
1	2	p_1	0.17
2	4	p_2	0.70
3	5	p_3	0.23
4	11	p_4	0.93
5	12	p_5	0.53
6	15	p_6	0.60
7	17	p_7	0.47
8	18	p_8	0.70
9	24	p_9	0.17

Continued

10	25	p_{10}	0.67
11	26	p_{11}	0.63
12	33	p_{12}	0.73
13	35	p_{13}	0.40
14	36	p_{14}	0.63
15	37	p_{15}	0.63
16	38	p_{16}	0.43
17	40	p_{17}	0.53
18	42	p_{18}	0.73
19	43	p_{19}	0.67
20	46	p_{20}	0.53
21	47	p_{21}	0.57
22	48	p_{22}	0.60
23	50	p_{23}	0.80
24	51	p_{24}	0.63
25	53	p_{25}	0.67
26	54	p_{26}	0.63
27	55	p_{27}	0.37
28	57	p_{28}	0.70
29	59	p_{29}	0.57
30	60	p_{30}	0.83

It is seen that Hepatitis B (at birth) vaccine coverage is higher for ward number 11 ($p_4 = 0.93$) than all other wards. After that $|p_i - p_j|$ and CV_{ij} are computed and compared each of test statistics with the corresponding critical value CV_{ij} (given in **Table 5**).

Results are significant only for proportion of Hepatitis B (at birth) vaccine coverage for ward number 1 vs ward number 4 (p_1 vs p_4), ward number 1 vs ward number 30 (p_1 vs p_{30}), ward number 3 vs ward number 4 (p_3 vs p_4), ward number 4 vs ward number 9 (p_4 vs p_9) and ward number 9 vs ward number 30 (p_9 vs p_{30}). That is these proportions are not equal. Out of 435 pairs of proportions of vaccination coverage only 5 pairs of proportions are unequal.

5. Discussion

Estimates of variances and design effect have been used by Milligan *et al.* [4] to compare two cluster sampling methods for health surveys in developing countries. Both the methods gave very similar point estimates of vaccination coverage. The estimates of the proportion fully vaccinated were 0.56 (EPI) and 0.54 (segmented method) and suggest that EPI method can give accurate and precise results. On the basis of this previous study the current study tries to estimate the design effect of vaccination coverage of the considered study population. In a study of comparison of survey methodologies relative feasibility of the sampling methodologies was assessed by Luman *et al.* [3]. Coverage with routine vaccinations among children aged 12 - 23 months was much lower than coverage achieved through the measles SIA (supplemental immunization activities). Also Katz *et al.* studied bias estimate and design effects associated with the EPI sampling design [11]. Brogan *et al.* suggested techniques for improving the accuracy of the EPI cluster survey method [12]. In Bangladesh overall only 64.1% of children received the measles vaccine, polio1 has the highest coverage rate in both urban and rural areas. The study also reported that percentage of receiving DPT and polio vaccine decreases when higher doses are given [13]. Chhabra *et al.* studied the factors affecting the vaccination coverage in two urbanized villages of East Delhi. The coverage levels were highest for BCG (82.7%) and DPT/OPV1 (81.5%) and lowest for HBV3 (24.3%). About 65.3% had received primary immunization while only 41.6% of children had received MMR vaccine [14].

Table 5. Pairwise Comparison of test statistics ($|p_i - p_j|$) and critical values (CV_{ij}).

Sl No.	$|p_i - p_j|$		CV_{ij}	Sl No.	$|p_i - p_j|$		CV_{ij}	Sl No.	$|p_i - p_j|$		CV_{ij}
1	$p_1 - p_2$	0.53	0.71	146	$p_6 - p_{17}$	0.07	0.83	291	$p_{13} - p_{22}$	0.20	0.83
2	$p_1 - p_3$	0.06	0.67	147	$p_6 - p_{18}$	0.13	0.79	292	$p_{13} - p_{23}$	0.40	0.75
3	$p_1 - p_4^*$	**0.76**	**0.54**	148	$p_6 - p_{19}$	0.07	0.81	293	$p_{13} - p_{24}$	0.23	0.82
4	$p_1 - p_5$	0.36	0.74	149	$p_6 - p_{20}$	0.07	0.83	294	$p_{13} - p_{25}$	0.27	0.81
5	$p_1 - p_6$	0.43	0.74	150	$p_6 - p_{21}$	0.03	0.83	295	$p_{13} - p_{26}$	0.23	0.82
6	$p_1 - p_7$	0.30	0.74	151	$p_6 - p_{22}$	0.00	0.83	296	$p_{13} - p_{27}$	0.03	0.82
7	$p_1 - p_8$	0.53	0.71	152	$p_6 - p_{23}$	0.20	0.75	297	$p_{13} - p_{28}$	0.30	0.80
8	$p_1 - p_9$	0.00	0.63	153	$p_6 - p_{24}$	0.03	0.82	298	$p_{13} - p_{29}$	0.17	0.83
9	$p_1 - p_{10}$	0.50	0.72	154	$p_6 - p_{25}$	0.07	0.81	299	$p_{13} - p_{30}$	0.43	0.74
10	$p_1 - p_{11}$	0.46	0.73	155	$p_6 - p_{26}$	0.03	0.82	300	$p_{14} - p_{15}$	0.00	0.81
11	$p_1 - p_{12}$	0.56	0.69	156	$p_6 - p_{27}$	0.23	0.82	301	$p_{14} - p_{16}$	0.20	0.82
12	$p_1 - p_{13}$	0.23	0.74	157	$p_6 - p_{28}$	0.10	0.80	302	$p_{14} - p_{17}$	0.10	0.83
13	$p_1 - p_{14}$	0.46	0.73	158	$p_6 - p_{29}$	0.03	0.83	303	$p_{14} - p_{18}$	0.10	0.78
14	$p_1 - p_{15}$	0.46	0.73	159	$p_6 - p_{30}$	0.23	0.74	304	$p_{14} - p_{19}$	0.04	0.80
15	$p_1 - p_{16}$	0.26	0.74	160	$p_7 - p_8$	0.23	0.81	305	$p_{14} - p_{20}$	0.10	0.83
16	$p_1 - p_{17}$	0.36	0.74	161	$p_7 - p_9$	0.30	0.74	306	$p_{14} - p_{21}$	0.06	0.82
17	$p_1 - p_{18}$	0.56	0.69	162	$p_7 - p_{10}$	0.20	0.82	307	$p_{14} - p_{22}$	0.03	0.82
18	$p_1 - p_{19}$	0.50	0.72	163	$p_7 - p_{11}$	0.16	0.83	308	$p_{14} - p_{23}$	0.17	0.75
19	$p_1 - p_{20}$	0.36	0.74	164	$p_7 - p_{12}$	0.26	0.80	309	$p_{14} - p_{24}$	0.00	0.81
20	$p_1 - p_{21}$	0.40	0.74	165	$p_7 - p_{13}$	0.07	0.83	310	$p_{14} - p_{25}$	0.04	0.80
21	$p_1 - p_{22}$	0.43	0.74	166	$p_7 - p_{14}$	0.16	0.83	311	$p_{14} - p_{26}$	0.00	0.81
22	$p_1 - p_{23}$	0.63	0.65	167	$p_7 - p_{15}$	0.16	0.83	312	$p_{14} - p_{27}$	0.26	0.81
23	$p_1 - p_{24}$	0.46	0.73	168	$p_7 - p_{16}$	0.04	0.84	313	$p_{14} - p_{28}$	0.07	0.79
24	$p_1 - p_{25}$	0.50	0.72	169	$p_7 - p_{17}$	0.06	0.84	314	$p_{14} - p_{29}$	0.06	0.82
25	$p_1 - p_{26}$	0.46	0.73	170	$p_7 - p_{18}$	0.26	0.80	315	$p_{14} - p_{30}$	0.20	0.73
26	$p_1 - p_{27}$	0.20	0.73	171	$p_7 - p_{19}$	0.20	0.82	316	$p_{15} - p_{16}$	0.20	0.82
27	$p_1 - p_{28}$	0.53	0.71	172	$p_7 - p_{20}$	0.06	0.84	317	$p_{15} - p_{17}$	0.10	0.83
28	$p_1 - p_{29}$	0.40	0.74	173	$p_7 - p_{21}$	0.10	0.84	318	$p_{15} - p_{18}$	0.10	0.78
29	$p_1 - p_{30}^*$	**0.66**	**0.63**	174	$p_7 - p_{22}$	0.13	0.83	319	$p_{15} - p_{19}$	0.04	0.80
30	$p_2 - p_3$	0.47	0.74	175	$p_7 - p_{23}$	0.33	0.76	320	$p_{15} - p_{20}$	0.10	0.83
31	$p_2 - p_4$	0.23	0.62	176	$p_7 - p_{24}$	0.16	0.83	321	$p_{15} - p_{21}$	0.06	0.82
32	$p_2 - p_5$	0.17	0.81	177	$p_7 - p_{25}$	0.20	0.82	322	$p_{15} - p_{22}$	0.03	0.82
33	$p_2 - p_6$	0.10	0.80	178	$p_7 - p_{26}$	0.16	0.83	323	$p_{15} - p_{23}$	0.17	0.75
34	$p_2 - p_7$	0.23	0.81	179	$p_7 - p_{27}$	0.10	0.83	324	$p_{15} - p_{24}$	0.00	0.81
35	$p_2 - p_8$	0.00	0.77	180	$p_7 - p_{28}$	0.23	0.81	325	$p_{15} - p_{25}$	0.04	0.80
36	$p_2 - p_9$	0.53	0.71	181	$p_7 - p_{29}$	0.10	0.84	326	$p_{15} - p_{26}$	0.00	0.81
37	$p_2 - p_{10}$	0.03	0.78	182	$p_7 - p_{30}$	0.36	0.74	327	$p_{15} - p_{27}$	0.26	0.81
38	$p_2 - p_{11}$	0.07	0.79	183	$p_8 - p_9$	0.53	0.71	328	$p_{15} - p_{28}$	0.07	0.79
39	$p_2 - p_{12}$	0.03	0.76	184	$p_8 - p_{10}$	0.03	0.78	329	$p_{15} - p_{29}$	0.06	0.82
40	$p_2 - p_{13}$	0.30	0.80	185	$p_8 - p_{11}$	0.07	0.79	330	$p_{15} - p_{30}$	0.20	0.73
41	$p_2 - p_{14}$	0.07	0.79	186	$p_8 - p_{12}$	0.03	0.76	331	$p_{16} - p_{17}$	0.10	0.84
42	$p_2 - p_{15}$	0.07	0.79	187	$p_8 - p_{13}$	0.30	0.80	332	$p_{16} - p_{18}$	0.30	0.79
43	$p_2 - p_{16}$	0.27	0.80	188	$p_8 - p_{14}$	0.07	0.79	333	$p_{16} - p_{19}$	0.24	0.81

Continued

44	$p_2 - p_{17}$	0.17	0.81	189	$p_8 - p_{15}$	0.07	0.79	334	$p_{16} - p_{20}$	0.10	0.84
45	$p_2 - p_{18}$	0.03	0.76	190	$p_8 - p_{16}$	0.27	0.80	335	$p_{16} - p_{21}$	0.14	0.83
46	$p_2 - p_{19}$	0.03	0.78	191	$p_8 - p_{17}$	0.17	0.81	336	$p_{16} - p_{22}$	0.17	0.83
47	$p_2 - p_{20}$	0.17	0.81	192	$p_8 - p_{18}$	0.03	0.76	337	$p_{16} - p_{23}$	0.37	0.76
48	$p_2 - p_{21}$	0.13	0.80	193	$p_8 - p_{19}$	0.03	0.78	338	$p_{16} - p_{24}$	0.20	0.82
49	$p_2 - p_{22}$	0.10	0.80	194	$p_8 - p_{20}$	0.17	0.81	339	$p_{16} - p_{25}$	0.24	0.81
50	$p_2 - p_{23}$	0.10	0.72	195	$p_8 - p_{21}$	0.13	0.80	340	$p_{16} - p_{26}$	0.20	0.82
51	$p_2 - p_{24}$	0.07	0.79	196	$p_8 - p_{22}$	0.10	0.80	341	$p_{16} - p_{27}$	0.06	0.82
52	$p_2 - p_{25}$	0.03	0.78	197	$p_8 - p_{23}$	0.10	0.72	342	$p_{16} - p_{28}$	0.27	0.80
53	$p_2 - p_{26}$	0.07	0.79	198	$p_8 - p_{24}$	0.07	0.79	343	$p_{16} - p_{29}$	0.14	0.83
54	$p_2 - p_{27}$	0.33	0.79	199	$p_8 - p_{25}$	0.03	0.78	344	$p_{16} - p_{30}$	0.40	0.74
55	$p_2 - p_{28}$	0.00	0.77	200	$p_8 - p_{26}$	0.07	0.79	345	$p_{17} - p_{18}$	0.20	0.80
56	$p_2 - p_{29}$	0.13	0.80	201	$p_8 - p_{27}$	0.33	0.79	346	$p_{17} - p_{19}$	0.14	0.82
57	$p_2 - p_{30}$	0.13	0.71	202	$p_8 - p_{28}$	0.00	0.77	347	$p_{17} - p_{20}$	0.00	0.84
58	$\boldsymbol{p_3 - p_4}^*$	**0.70**	**0.59**	203	$p_8 - p_{29}$	0.13	0.80	348	$p_{17} - p_{21}$	0.04	0.84
59	$p_3 - p_5$	0.30	0.78	204	$p_8 - p_{30}$	0.13	0.71	349	$p_{17} - p_{22}$	0.07	0.83
60	$p_3 - p_6$	0.37	0.77	205	$p_9 - p_{10}$	0.50	0.72	350	$p_{17} - p_{23}$	0.27	0.76
61	$p_3 - p_7$	0.24	0.78	206	$p_9 - p_{11}$	0.46	0.73	351	$p_{17} - p_{24}$	0.10	0.83
62	$p_3 - p_8$	0.47	0.74	207	$p_9 - p_{12}$	0.56	0.69	352	$p_{17} - p_{25}$	0.14	0.82
63	$p_3 - p_9$	0.06	0.67	208	$p_9 - p_{13}$	0.23	0.74	353	$p_{17} - p_{26}$	0.10	0.83
64	$p_3 - p_{10}$	0.44	0.75	209	$p_9 - p_{14}$	0.46	0.73	354	$p_{17} - p_{27}$	0.16	0.83
65	$p_3 - p_{11}$	0.40	0.76	210	$p_9 - p_{15}$	0.46	0.73	355	$p_{17} - p_{28}$	0.17	0.81
66	$p_3 - p_{12}$	0.50	0.73	211	$p_9 - p_{16}$	0.26	0.74	356	$p_{17} - p_{29}$	0.04	0.84
67	$p_3 - p_{13}$	0.17	0.77	212	$p_9 - p_{17}$	0.36	0.74	357	$p_{17} - p_{30}$	0.30	0.74
68	$p_3 - p_{14}$	0.40	0.76	213	$p_9 - p_{18}$	0.56	0.69	358	$p_{18} - p_{19}$	0.06	0.77
69	$p_3 - p_{15}$	0.40	0.76	214	$p_9 - p_{19}$	0.50	0.72	359	$p_{18} - p_{20}$	0.20	0.80
70	$p_3 - p_{16}$	0.20	0.77	215	$p_9 - p_{20}$	0.36	0.74	360	$p_{18} - p_{21}$	0.16	0.79
71	$p_3 - p_{17}$	0.30	0.78	216	$p_9 - p_{21}$	0.40	0.74	361	$p_{18} - p_{22}$	0.13	0.79
72	$p_3 - p_{18}$	0.50	0.73	217	$p_9 - p_{22}$	0.43	0.74	362	$p_{18} - p_{23}$	0.07	0.71
73	$p_3 - p_{19}$	0.44	0.75	218	$p_9 - p_{23}$	0.63	0.65	363	$p_{18} - p_{24}$	0.10	0.78
74	$p_3 - p_{20}$	0.30	0.78	219	$p_9 - p_{24}$	0.46	0.73	364	$p_{18} - p_{25}$	0.06	0.77
75	$p_3 - p_{21}$	0.34	0.77	220	$p_9 - p_{25}$	0.50	0.72	365	$p_{18} - p_{26}$	0.10	0.78
76	$p_3 - p_{22}$	0.37	0.77	221	$p_9 - p_{26}$	0.46	0.73	366	$p_{18} - p_{27}$	0.36	0.78
77	$p_3 - p_{23}$	0.57	0.69	222	$p_9 - p_{27}$	0.20	0.73	367	$p_{18} - p_{28}$	0.03	0.76
78	$p_3 - p_{24}$	0.40	0.76	223	$p_9 - p_{28}$	0.53	0.71	368	$p_{18} - p_{29}$	0.16	0.79
79	$p_3 - p_{25}$	0.44	0.75	224	$p_9 - p_{29}$	0.40	0.74	369	$p_{18} - p_{30}$	0.10	0.69
80	$p_3 - p_{26}$	0.40	0.76	225	$\boldsymbol{p_9 - p_{30}}^*$	**0.66**	**0.63**	370	$p_{19} - p_{20}$	0.14	0.82
81	$p_3 - p_{27}$	0.14	0.76	226	$p_{10} - p_{11}$	0.04	0.80	371	$p_{19} - p_{21}$	0.10	0.81
82	$p_3 - p_{28}$	0.47	0.74	227	$p_{10} - p_{12}$	0.06	0.77	372	$p_{19} - p_{22}$	0.07	0.81
83	$p_3 - p_{29}$	0.34	0.77	228	$p_{10} - p_{13}$	0.27	0.81	373	$p_{19} - p_{23}$	0.13	0.74
84	$p_3 - p_{30}$	0.60	0.67	229	$p_{10} - p_{14}$	0.04	0.80	374	$p_{19} - p_{24}$	0.04	0.80
85	$p_4 - P_p$	0.40	0.67	230	$p_{10} - p_{15}$	0.04	0.80	375	$p_{19} - p_{25}$	0.00	0.79
86	$p_4 - p_6$	0.33	0.66	231	$p_{10} - p_{16}$	0.24	0.81	376	$p_{19} - p_{26}$	0.04	0.80
87	$p_4 - p_7$	0.46	0.67	232	$p_{10} - p_{17}$	0.14	0.82	377	$p_{19} - p_{27}$	0.30	0.80

Continued

#	Pair			#	Pair			#	Pair		
88	$p_4 - p_8$	0.23	0.62	233	$p_{10} - p_{18}$	0.06	0.77	378	$p_{19} - p_{28}$	0.03	0.78
89	$p_4 - p_9^*$	**0.76**	**0.54**	234	$p_{10} - p_{19}$	0.00	0.79	379	$p_{19} - p_{29}$	0.10	0.81
90	$p_4 - p_{10}$	0.26	0.64	235	$p_{10} - p_{20}$	0.14	0.82	380	$p_{19} - p_{30}$	0.16	0.72
91	$p_4 - p_{11}$	0.30	0.65	236	$p_{10} - p_{21}$	0.10	0.81	381	$p_{20} - p_{21}$	0.04	0.84
92	$p_4 - p_{12}$	0.20	0.61	237	$p_{10} - p_{22}$	0.07	0.81	382	$p_{20} - p_{22}$	0.07	0.83
93	$p_4 - p_{13}$	0.53	0.66	238	$p_{10} - p_{23}$	0.13	0.74	383	$p_{20} - p_{23}$	0.27	0.76
94	$p_4 - p_{14}$	0.30	0.65	239	$p_{10} - p_{24}$	0.04	0.80	384	$p_{20} - p_{24}$	0.10	0.83
95	$p_4 - p_{15}$	0.30	0.65	240	$p_{10} - p_{25}$	0.00	0.79	385	$p_{20} - p_{25}$	0.14	0.82
96	$p_4 - p_{16}$	0.50	0.66	241	$p_{10} - p_{26}$	0.04	0.80	386	$p_{20} - p_{26}$	0.10	0.83
97	$p_4 - p_{17}$	0.40	0.67	242	$p_{10} - p_{27}$	0.30	0.80	387	$p_{20} - p_{27}$	0.16	0.83
98	$p_4 - p_{18}$	0.20	0.61	243	$p_{10} - p_{28}$	0.03	0.78	388	$p_{20} - p_{28}$	0.17	0.81
99	$p_4 - p_{19}$	0.26	0.64	244	$p_{10} - p_{29}$	0.10	0.81	389	$p_{20} - p_{29}$	0.04	0.84
100	$p_4 - p_{20}$	0.40	0.67	245	$p_{10} - p_{30}$	0.16	0.72	390	$p_{20} - p_{30}$	0.30	0.74
101	$p_4 - p_{21}$	0.36	0.66	246	$p_{11} - p_{12}$	0.10	0.78	391	$p_{21} - p_{22}$	0.03	0.83
102	$p_4 - p_{22}$	0.33	0.66	247	$p_{11} - p_{13}$	0.23	0.82	392	$p_{21} - p_{23}$	0.23	0.76
103	$p_4 - p_{23}$	0.13	0.57	248	$p_{11} - p_{14}$	0.00	0.81	393	$p_{21} - p_{24}$	0.06	0.82
104	$p_4 - p_{24}$	0.30	0.65	249	$p_{11} - p_{15}$	0.00	0.81	394	$p_{21} - p_{25}$	0.10	0.81
105	$p_4 - p_{25}$	0.26	0.64	250	$p_{11} - p_{16}$	0.20	0.82	395	$p_{21} - p_{26}$	0.06	0.82
106	$p_4 - p_{26}$	0.30	0.65	251	$p_{11} - p_{17}$	0.10	0.83	396	$p_{21} - p_{27}$	0.20	0.82
107	$p_4 - p_{27}$	0.56	0.65	252	$p_{11} - p_{18}$	0.10	0.78	397	$p_{21} - p_{28}$	0.13	0.80
108	$p_4 - p_{28}$	0.23	0.62	253	$p_{11} - p_{19}$	0.04	0.80	398	$p_{21} - p_{29}$	0.00	0.83
109	$p_4 - p_{29}$	0.36	0.66	254	$p_{11} - p_{20}$	0.10	0.83	399	$p_{21} - p_{30}$	0.26	0.74
110	$p_4 - p_{30}$	0.10	0.54	255	$p_{11} - p_{21}$	0.06	0.82	400	$p_{22} - p_{23}$	0.20	0.75
111	$p_5 - p_6$	0.07	0.83	256	$p_{11} - p_{22}$	0.03	0.82	401	$p_{22} - p_{24}$	0.03	0.82
112	$p_5 - p_7$	0.06	0.84	257	$p_{11} - p_{23}$	0.17	0.75	402	$p_{22} - p_{25}$	0.07	0.81
113	$p_5 - p_8$	0.17	0.81	258	$p_{11} - p_{24}$	0.00	0.81	403	$p_{22} - p_{26}$	0.03	0.82
114	$p_5 - p_9$	0.36	0.74	259	$p_{11} - p_{25}$	0.04	0.80	404	$p_{22} - p_{27}$	0.23	0.82
115	$p_5 - p_{10}$	0.14	0.82	260	$p_{11} - p_{26}$	0.00	0.81	405	$p_{22} - p_{28}$	0.10	0.80
116	$p_5 - p_{11}$	0.10	0.83	261	$p_{11} - p_{27}$	0.26	0.81	406	$p_{22} - p_{29}$	0.03	0.83
117	$p_5 - p_{12}$	0.20	0.80	262	$p_{11} - p_{28}$	0.07	0.79	407	$p_{22} - p_{30}$	0.23	0.74
118	$p_5 - p_{13}$	0.13	0.83	263	$p_{11} - p_{29}$	0.06	0.82	408	$p_{23} - p_{24}$	0.17	0.75
119	$p_5 - p_{14}$	0.10	0.83	264	$p_{11} - p_{30}$	0.20	0.73	409	$p_{23} - p_{25}$	0.13	0.74
120	$p_5 - p_{15}$	0.10	0.83	265	$p_{12} - p_{13}$	0.33	0.79	410	$p_{23} - p_{26}$	0.17	0.75
121	$p_5 - p_{16}$	0.10	0.84	266	$p_{12} - p_{14}$	0.10	0.78	411	$p_{23} - p_{27}$	0.43	0.75
122	$p_5 - p_{17}$	0.00	0.84	267	$p_{12} - p_{15}$	0.10	0.78	412	$p_{23} - p_{28}$	0.10	0.72
123	$p_5 - p_{18}$	0.20	0.80	268	$p_{12} - p_{16}$	0.30	0.79	413	$p_{23} - p_{29}$	0.23	0.76
124	$p_5 - p_{19}$	0.14	0.82	269	$p_{12} - p_{17}$	0.20	0.80	414	$p_{23} - p_{30}$	0.03	0.65
125	$p_5 - p_{20}$	0.00	0.84	270	$p_{12} - p_{18}$	0.00	0.75	415	$p_{24} - p_{25}$	0.04	0.80
126	$p_5 - p_{21}$	0.04	0.84	271	$p_{12} - p_{19}$	0.06	0.77	416	$p_{24} - p_{26}$	0.00	0.81
127	$p_5 - p_{22}$	0.07	0.83	272	$p_{12} - p_{20}$	0.20	0.80	417	$p_{24} - p_{27}$	0.26	0.81
128	$p_5 - p_{23}$	0.27	0.76	273	$p_{12} - p_{21}$	0.16	0.79	418	$p_{24} - p_{28}$	0.07	0.79
129	$p_5 - p_{24}$	0.10	0.83	274	$p_{12} - p_{22}$	0.13	0.79	419	$p_{24} - p_{29}$	0.06	0.82
130	$p_5 - p_{25}$	0.14	0.82	275	$p_{12} - p_{23}$	0.07	0.71	420	$p_{24} - p_{30}$	0.20	0.73
131	$p_5 - p_{26}$	0.10	0.83	276	$p_{12} - p_{24}$	0.10	0.78	421	$p_{25} - p_{26}$	0.04	0.80

Continued

132	$p_5 - p_{27}$	0.16	0.83	277	$p_{12} - p_{25}$	0.06	0.77	422	$p_{25} - p_{27}$	0.30	0.80
133	$p_5 - p_{28}$	0.17	0.81	278	$p_{12} - p_{26}$	0.10	0.78	423	$p_{25} - p_{28}$	0.03	0.78
134	$p_5 - p_{29}$	0.04	0.84	279	$p_{12} - p_{27}$	0.36	0.78	424	$p_{25} - p_{29}$	0.10	0.81
135	$p_5 - p_{30}$	0.30	0.74	280	$p_{12} - p_{28}$	0.03	0.76	425	$p_{25} - p_{30}$	0.16	0.72
136	$p_6 - p_7$	0.13	0.83	281	$p_{12} - p_{29}$	0.16	0.79	426	$p_{26} - p_{27}$	0.26	0.81
137	$p_6 - p_8$	0.10	0.80	282	$p_{12} - p_{30}$	0.10	0.69	427	$p_{26} - p_{28}$	0.07	0.79
138	$p_6 - p_9$	0.43	0.74	283	$p_{13} - p_{14}$	0.23	0.82	428	$p_{26} - p_{29}$	0.06	0.82
139	$p_6 - p_{10}$	0.07	0.81	284	$p_{13} - p_{15}$	0.23	0.82	429	$p_{26} - p_{30}$	0.20	0.73
140	$p_6 - p_{11}$	0.03	0.82	285	$p_{13} - p_{16}$	0.03	0.83	430	$p_{27} - p_{28}$	0.33	0.79
141	$p_6 - p_{12}$	0.13	0.79	286	$p_{13} - p_{17}$	0.13	0.83	431	$p_{27} - p_{29}$	0.20	0.82
142	$p_6 - p_{13}$	0.20	0.83	287	$p_{13} - p_{18}$	0.33	0.79	432	$p_{27} - p_{30}$	0.46	0.73
143	$p_6 - p_{14}$	0.03	0.82	288	$p_{13} - p_{19}$	0.27	0.81	433	$p_{28} - p_{29}$	0.13	0.80
144	$p_6 - p_{15}$	0.03	0.82	289	$p_{13} - p_{20}$	0.13	0.83	434	$p_{28} - p_{30}$	0.13	0.71
145	$p_6 - p_{16}$	0.17	0.83	290	$p_{13} - p_{21}$	0.17	0.83	435	$p_{29} - p_{30}$	0.26	0.74

*Significant pair.

In an Urban Area of Meerut 93.25% of children in community were found to be completely immunized, 5.25% partially immunized an only 1.5% non-immunized [15]. In a study Jain *et al.* mentioned that 28.9% of children aged 12 - 23 months were fully immunized with BCG, 3 DPT, 3 OPV and Measles vaccines; around 26.5% had not received even a single vaccine and 44.5% were found partially immunized. Around 55.95% of the eligible children were vaccinated for BCG and measles 43.6%. Though nearly 66.8% were covered with first dose of DPT and OPV but about 33.2% children dropped out of the third dose of DPT and OPV for various reasons [16]. In an another study in Gujarat coverage for BCG, OPV3, DPT3 & Measles were 92.04%, 85.23%, 83.71% & 82.20% respectively. Although the vaccination coverage shows higher coverage than previous studies, it is still below the minimum targets set as national goal [17]. Immunization status of children and mothers in the northeastern states (except Assam) was evaluated in comparison with data at the national level using a WHO 30-cluster survey methodology. The proportion of children receiving all the vaccinations like BCG, DPT, OPV, measles in north-eastern states were about 51.9% as against 63.3% achieved at the all India level [18]. In this current study it has been observed that the fully vaccination coverage in the study population is not so high; it is almost same with the previous study reported by Phukan *et al.* [7] with a difference of 1.32% only. The differences between the two survey methods in case of point estimate are not significant and interval estimates has given better estimates in two stage (30 × 30) cluster sampling. Two stage (30 × 30) cluster sampling has given better estimate of variance and design effect of vaccination coverage and design effects are less in two stage cluster sampling vs simple random sampling and cluster sampling vs systematic sampling rather than systematic sampling vs simple random sampling. It has been observed that the clusters are homogeneous (since only 5 pairs of proportions are significant).

6. Conclusion

The finding of the present study revealed that there are no significant differences between the point estimates obtained under two sampling schemes. But there are differences between estimated variance of proportion of children vaccinated in two sampling methods. Also in case of interval estimation two stage (30 × 30) cluster sampling has given better intervals than that of under systematic sampling. Vaccination coverage is high for BCG, OPV and DPT vaccine but it is low for Measles, Hepatitis B, Hib and MMR vaccine and the later doses of OPV and DPT vaccine. Finally the two stage cluster (30 × 30) sampling is more consistent than the systematic sampling as well as simple random sampling for this study population.

Acknowledgements

The research was supported by the grant (number 69/40/2008-ECD-II) from Indian Council of Medical Research (ICMR), New Delhi and UGC-BSR one time grant (No. F.19-145/2015(BSR)) and provided to the first author.

Conflict of Interest

None.

References

[1]   Burton, A., Monasch, R., Lautenbach, B., Gacic-Dobo, M., Neill, M., Karimov, R., Wolfson, L., Jones, G. and Birmingham, M. (2009) WHO and UNICEF Estimates of National Infant Immunization Coverage: Methods and Process. *Bulletin of the World Health Organization*, **87**, 535-541. http://dx.doi.org/10.2471/BLT.08.053819

[2]   Turner, A.G., Magnani, R.J. and Shuaib, M. (1996) A Not Quite as Quick Bit Much Cleaner Alternative to the Expanded Programme on Immunization (EPI) Cluster Survey Design. *International Journal of Epidemiology*, **25**, 198-203. http://dx.doi.org/10.1093/ije/25.1.198

[3]   Luman, E.T., Worku, A., Berhane, Y., Martin, R. and Cairns, L. (2007) Comparison of Two Survey Methodologies to Assess Vaccination Coverage. *International Journal of Epidemiology*, **36**, 633-641. http://dx.doi.org/10.1093/ije/dym025

[4]   Milligan, P., Njie, A. and Benneu, S. (2004) Comparison of Two Cluster Sampling Methods for Health Surveys in Developing Countries. *International Journal of Epidemiology*, **33**, 469-476. http://dx.doi.org/10.1093/ije/dyh096

[5]   Nath, D.C. and Patowari, B. (2014) Estimation and Comparison of Immunization Coverage under Different Sampling Methods for Health Surveys. *International Journal of Population Research*, **2014**, Article ID: 850479. http://dx.doi.org/10.1155/2014/850479

[6]   WHO-SEARO EPI Fact Sheet India, 2011. http://www.searo.who.int/entity/immunization/data/india_epi_factsheet_2011.pdf?ua=1

[7]   Phukan, R.K., Barman, M.P. and Mahanta, J. (2009) Factor Associated with Immunization Coverage of Children in Assam, India: Over the First Year of Life. *Journal of Tropical Pediatrics*, **55**, 249-252. http://dx.doi.org/10.1093/tropej/fmn025

[8]   Lee, E.S. and Forthofer, R.N. (2006) Analyzing Complex Survey Data. 2nd Edition, Sage Publications, Thousand Oaks.

[9]   Levy, P.S. and Lemeshow, S. (2008) Sampling of Populations: Methods and Applications. 4th Edition, John Wiley & Sons, Hoboken. http://dx.doi.org/10.1002/9780470374597

[10] The Marascuillo Procedure. www.itl.nist.gov/div898/handbook/prc/section4/prc474.htm

[11] Katz, J., Yoon, S.S., Brendel, K. and West Jr., K.P. (1997) Sampling Designs for Xerophthalmia Prevalence Surveys. *International Journal of Epidemiology*, **26**, 1041-1048. http://dx.doi.org/10.1093/ije/26.5.1041

[12] Brogan, D., Flagg, E.W., Deming, M. and Waldman, R. (1994) Increasing the Accuracy of the Expanded Programme on Immunization's Cluster Survey Design. *Annals of Epidemiology*, **4**, 302-311. http://dx.doi.org/10.1016/1047-2797(94)90086-8

[13] Rahman, M. and Obaida-Nasrin, S. (2010) Factors Affecting Acceptance of Complete Immunization Coverage of Children under Five Years in Rural Bangladesh. *Salud Pública de México*, **52**, 134-140. http://dx.doi.org/10.1590/S0036-36342010000200005

[14] Chhabra, P., Nair, P., Gupta, A., Sandhir, M. and Kannan, A.T. (2007) Immunization in Urbanized Villages of Delhi. *Indian Journal of Pediatrics*, **74**, 131-134. http://dx.doi.org/10.1007/s12098-007-0004-3

[15] Chopra, H., Singh, A.K., Singh, J.V., Bhatnagar, M., Garg, S.K. and Bajpai, S.K. (2006-2007) Status of Routine Immunization in an Urban Area of Meerut. *Indian Journal of Community Health*, **18**(2)-**19**(1), 19-22.

[16] Jain, S.K., Chawla, U., Gupta, N., Gupta, R.S., Venkatesh, S. and Lal, S. (2006) Child Survival and Safe Motherhood Program in Rajasthan. *Indian Journal of Pediatrics*, **73**, 43-47. http://dx.doi.org/10.1007/BF02758259

[17] Sheth, J.K., Trivedi, K.N., Mehta, J.B. and Oza, U.N. (2012) Assessment of Vaccine Coverage by 30 Cluster Sampling Technique in Rural Gandhinagar. *Gujarat National Journal of Community Medicine*, **3**, 496-501.

[18] Yadav, R.J. and Singh, P. (2004) Immunisation of Children and Mothers in Northeastern States. *Health and Population-Perspectives and Issues*, **27**, 185-193.

Abbreviations

BCG: Bacillis Calmette-Guerin;
OPV: Oral Polio Vaccine;
DPT: Diphtheria-Tetanus-Pertusis;
MMR: Measles Mumps Rubella;
Hib: Haemophilus influenza type b;
WHO: World Health Organization;
EPI: Expanded Programme on Immunization.

8

Community Pharmacists' Strategies in Greece: An Assessment of the Policy Environment and the Mapping of Key Players

Athanassios Vozikis[1]*, Lina Stavropoulou[2], George P. Patrinos[2]

[1]Economics Department, University of Piraeus, Piraeus, Greece
[2]Department of Pharmacy, School of Health Sciences, University of Patras, Patras, Greece
Email: *avozik@unipi.gr

Abstract

The aim of the study was to form and assess the pharmacists' strategies in Greece, by analyzing the policy environment and identifying the role of the key players-stakeholders. For collecting and organizing important information about the pharmacists' policy, the *PolicyMaker's* computerized version of political mapping was used, serving as a database for assessments of the policy's content, the major players, the power and policy positions of key players, the interests of different players, and the networks and coalitions that connect the players. As the research findings show, the initially expected impact of the pharmacists' policy proved to be very optimistic in most of the implemented strategies, as the majority of the strategies have worsened or minimized their success ratio throughout the time in study. Concluding, either the initially set strategies were at the wrong direction or the actions taken to implement them were inappropriate. Moreover, one can suggest that the shifting ability in both the position and the power of the most key players were over-estimated, while they under-estimated the impact of troika-constitutions meddling in the pharmaceutical policymaking and in the health sector cost-containment measures imposing.

Keywords

Community Pharmacy, Stakeholder Mapping, Pharmaceutical Policy, Health Sector, Greece

1. Introduction

In 2012 the recession of the Greek economy was well deeper than initially expected. For the years 2009-2012

---

*Corresponding author.

aggregate, GDP contracted by 20%. At the same time, government consumption continued to fall and investment shrank for the fourth consecutive year. The unemployment rate increased by 15 percentage points to almost 24% [1] [2]. The economic crisis had a dramatic impact in social life, since the reduction and/or lack of income causes losses in welfare and sets large sections of the population in poverty [3].

As the Greek healthcare system is characterized by a large number of regulatory bodies, several ministries shared responsibilities concerning the pharmaceutical policy (the Ministry of Health, the Ministry of Development, the Ministry of Labour and Social Security, the Ministry of Finance, etc.). The above system apart from being very difficult to monitor it was not efficient. Hence, since May 2010 under the MoU all health-related activities were brought under one ministry; the Ministry of Health in order to rationalise licensing, pricing and reimbursement systems for medicines. In this way, the supply side cost containment measures is expected to be reinforced [4].

Public pharmaceutical expenditure followed an upward trend until 2009 reaching the €5 billion or 2% of GDP, in line with developments in overall health expenditure and GDP. However, in 2010-2011 it fell sharply by 22% to reach €3.98 billion in 2011, €2.88 billion or 1.4% of GDP in 2012, €2.44 billion in 2013 and €2 billion or 1% of GDP in 2014 [2] [5]-[7].

The cumulative decrease of €3 billion in (net) public pharmaceutical expenditure in the period 2009/2014 resulted from reforms in the pharmaceutical market (changes in the pricing system, increases in rebates to social security funds, reduction in regulated wholesale and retail margins, reduction in the VAT rates, etc.) [6]-[8].

The Pharmacy Landscape in Greece

The supply of pharmaceutical products in Greece is defined by the pharmaceutical companies that are active in the sector (engaging in the manufacturing or marketing areas) and the distribution chain. More analytically, medicinal products with the exception of those distributed through hospitals, for which no wholesaler intervenes, follow this course: pharmaceutical company—wholesaler—pharmacy. The population density of pharmacies in Greece is the highest among EU Member States, with a ratio of one (1) pharmacy per 1028 inhabitants, compared with the EU-27 average of one (1) pharmacy per 3300 inhabitants (the total number of pharmacies in Greece is over 11.000) [9].

Today in Greece more than 14,000 pharmacists are employed, with the vast majority of those >80% working in independent-community pharmacies. More than 60% of pharmacists are women, while the central tendency in the age distribution is between 55 to 65 years that is very close to the retirement age. Regarding the structure of pharmacies, they are small sized stores which hardly exceed 50 m^2. The legal retail mark-up by pharmacies to the wholesale price is currently set to 35% for medicines that are not reimbursed by Social Security Funds (SSFs), 32.4% for medicines reimbursed by SSFs with a wholesale price of up to €200, 16% for drugs under Law 3816 (having a special wholesale price of up to €200 and a fixed amount of €30 along with a regressive percentage of 8%, 7% and 6% for drugs with a wholesale or special wholesale price of €201 - €500, €501 - €1000 and €1001+, respectively), plus VAT at a rate of 6.5%. Based on the composition of consumption (products with a wholesale price of <€200 have a market share of 91%) and taking into account the pharmacy discounts and rebates, the average profit margin of pharmacies is estimated at about 19% [5]. In summary, along with other countries such as Spain and Italy, pharmacies in Greece follow by the so-called "*Mediterranean*" model in contradiction to the "*North European*" model prevalent in countries of central and northern Europe. Practically this means scattered, many in number, small in size pharmacies in which works only one pharmacist (the owner-the one with the authorization to establish the pharmacy) versus low dispersion, few in number, large in size pharmacies where many pharmacists are working.

Implementation of reforms in pharmaceutical sector has progressed substantially from 2010 and today stands hopefully in the end of a long road. The most remarkable interventions significantly affecting the pharmacy sector refer to the [10] [11]:

1) Implementation of the claw back mechanism (through Ministerial decree) it was set the new-claw back threshold for 2013 (€2.4 bn for outpatient pharmaceutical);

2) New pricing mechanism for medicines (with the new price bulletin the authorities expect a further reduction in prices);

3) Prescription by active substance—Compulsory lowest-priced medicines substitution (since the beginning of 2012, the authorities mandated the substitution of prescribed medicines by the lowest-priced of the same ac-

tive substance in the reference category by pharmacies);

4) Increasing the use of generic medicines (the authorities took further measures to ensure that the target of 60% of the volume of medicines used is made up of generics with a price below that of similar branded products and off-patent medicines, will be accomplished);

5) Reduction of profit margins for medicines (the pharmacies' profit margin was readjusted with the aim of reducing the overall profit margin to no more than 15%, including the most expensive drugs);

6) Prescription budget for each doctor (a prescription budget for each doctor and a target on the average cost of prescription per patient);

7) Regulatory restrictions (deregulation measures as licensing or membership of a professional body, of the professional monopoly, requirements regarding ownership and operating requirements, restrictions on horizontal and vertical integration, etc.);

8) Consolidation in EOPYY (the consolidation of all existing health insurance Funds in a single universal social health insurance organisation—EOPYY); and

9) Electronic prescription (electronic prescription constitutes more than 90% of all prescriptions and can provide real-time information for continuous monitoring and assessment of prescription behavior and pharmaceutical spending by the EOPYY and the Ministry of Health). These measures (and many others) have significantly affected the economic and business sustainability of pharmacies in Greece.

The aim of this study was to form and assess the pharmacists' strategies in Greece, by analyzing the policy environment and identifying the role of the key players-stakeholders. The study also presents the opportunities and obstacles of the community pharmacies and identifies the consequences and impact of the policy formation.

2. Materials and Methods

2.1. Study Design

A list of the main key players-stakeholders (ministries, national & regional pharmacy professional bodies, health professional bodies, universities and research institutes, health insurance funds, the pharmaceutical industry, wholesale drugstores, pharmacy chains, citizens-patients-consumers, the media & press and, finally, political parties) in the pharmacists' policymaking was obtained. The knowledge to identify the key players-stakeholders was created by experts in the field of pharmaceutical policy, by literature review, our previous research expertise in the field and from the opinions of the pharmacists themselves [12]-[16].

For all the above stakeholders, contact details were obtained and a preliminary contact (via email or phone) was performed, in order to identify their willingness and interest to participate in the research. For those accepted to participate, structure interviews were performed or filled questionnaires were obtained [see **Appendix 4**], based on the *PolicyMaker* method for collecting and organizing important information about a policy [17]-[19]. For those who didn't accept to participate or didn't answer to our invitation, their views and roles were identified through their acts and their opinions publicly expressed in media, conferences and professional bodies.

2.2. Data Analysis

PolicyMaker's computerized version of political mapping enhances the flexibility of this method for application to diverse policy environments. *PolicyMaker* serves as a database for assessments of the policy's content, the major players, the power and policy positions of key players, the interests of different players, and the networks and coalitions that connect the players. The *Feasibility Algorithm* is used to calculate the indices of support and opposition shown in the *Feasibility Graph*. The *Feasibility Algorithm* is a mathematical formula involving players' positions and power. The algorithm is applied to each player included in the analysis, producing a value that is added to the appropriate index (support, non-mobilized, or opposition), to create the *Feasibility Graph*. When the *Feasibility Graph—Future* is generated, the program averages the strategy impacts for each player and determines the combined impact. The *Feasibility Algorithm* is then applied to that impact, resulting in a feasibility value for each player. This value is then added to the appropriate index (for support, non-mobilized, or opposition). The three indices are then shown on the *Future Feasibility Graph*. The model embodied in the feasibility algorithm inevitably simplifies reality. However, the multiple uncertainties and informed guesses involved in calculating the *Feasibility Graph* should not be forgotten [17].

In sum, the research method used is intended to help policymakers manage the processes of reform and promote strategic programming as well as strategic thinking [20].

The methodology used, guides the researcher through five analytical steps for assessing the pharmacists' policymaking (**Figure 1**).

All the participants signed the informed consent section and their anonymity and the confidentiality of the questionnaire content was ensured.

3. Results

In the first section of the questionnaire, pharmacists defined the strategic goals of their policymaking. The goals are presented in **Table 1**, along with the proposed achievement mechanism.

The key players-stakeholders in the pharmacy policymaking are presented in **Table 2**.

For every stakeholder its initial (backdated to December 31, 2011):
- territorial Level (*national* or *regional*),
- Sector (*Governmental, Noon-governmental, Political, Media, Commercial, Private, Social*)
- Position (*High Support, Medium Support, Non-Mobilized, Medium Opposition, High Opposition*) and
- Power (*Low, Medium. High*)

is also identified.

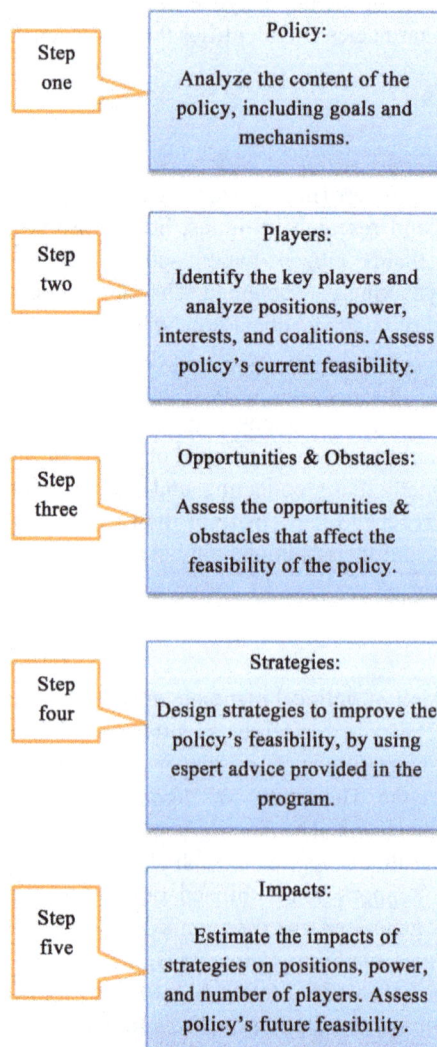

Figure 1. The five steps of analysis.

Taking in consideration the stakeholders' initial position (backdated to December 31, 2011) from **Table 2**, a *Current Position Map* was constructed (**Figure 2**).

As it is shown in the graphical presentation of the stakeholders' initial position, there is a medium to high opposition from the Governmental sector and the media, a neutral position from the other stakeholders of the

Table 1. Policy content.

Goal	Mechanism
Acceptance by the society	Personality Multi-faceted service of patients
Satisfactory working conditions (working hours, etc.)	Through professional body-union Through Pharmaceutical Association
Increase of the role of scientific-professional unions	Pharmacicts' general assemblies
Maintenance—Increase of the profit margins	Through professional body-union, Co-operation (pharmacy chains)
Maintenance of exclusiveness in the provision of pharmaceutical—para-pharmaceutical products	Strikes Professional Unions-Bodies
Maintenance of the existing competition regime	Pharmaceutical Association, professional body-union
Upgrade of the scientific role-position	Lifelong learning, Laboratory Work
Upgrade of the social role-position	Multi-faceted service of patients Advertising, Modernization of pharmacies

Table 2. Player table.

Player name	Level	Sector	Position	Power
Citizens-Patients-Customers	National	Private	Medium Support	Medium
Health Insurance Funds	National	Social	Medium Opposition	High
Hellenic Pharmaceutical Association	National	Non-Governmental	Medium Support	Medium
Media and Press	National	Media	High Opposition	Medium
Medical Association—Doctors	National	Non-Governmental	Non-Mobilized	Medium
Ministry of Development & Competitivess	National	Governmental	Medium Opposition	High
Ministry of Employment and Social Protection	National	Governmental	Medium Opposition	High
Ministry of Finance	National	Governmental	High Opposition	High
Ministry of Health	National	Governmental	Medium Opposition	High
Pharmaceutical Industries	National	Commercial	Non-Mobilized	Medium
Pharmacy Chains	National	Commercial	Non-Mobilized	Medium
Political Parties	National	Political	Non-Mobilized	Medium
Universities	National	Non-Governmental	Non-Mobilized	Low
Wholesale Drugstores	National	Commercial	Medium Support	Medium
Regional Pharmaceutical Association	Regional	Local Non-Governmental	High Support	Medium

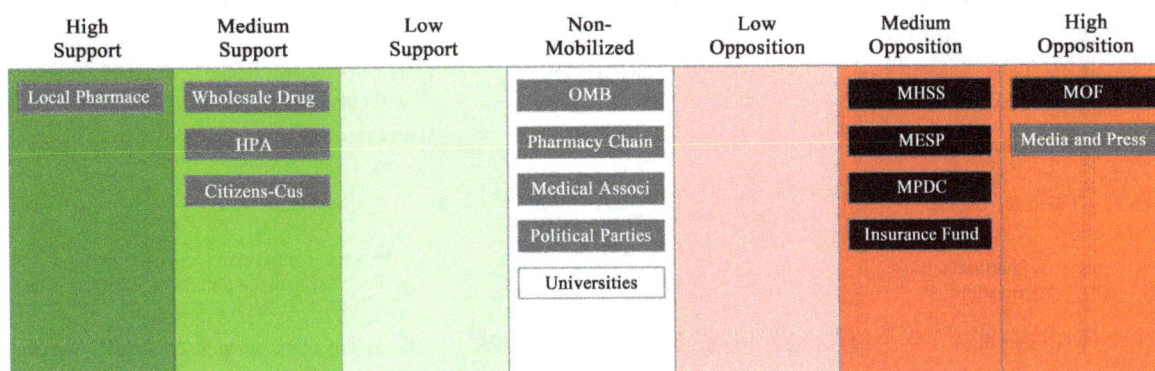

Figure 2. Current position map.

pharmaceutical supply chain and some medium to high support from its professional bodies and—the most promising—the citizens-patients-customers. A more comprehensive graphical presentation of the key players' initial position, but also of the homogeneity of their interests and their grouping is being presented in the Coalition Map in **Figure 3**.

In the Greek community pharmacy environment we discern several opportunities, which should not be unleashed, but also many obstacles that have to cope with (**Table 3**).

The community pharmacies' general strategies were therefore analyzed and connected to certain actions, thoroughly specialized and customized to address each key player position and power [**Appendix 1**].

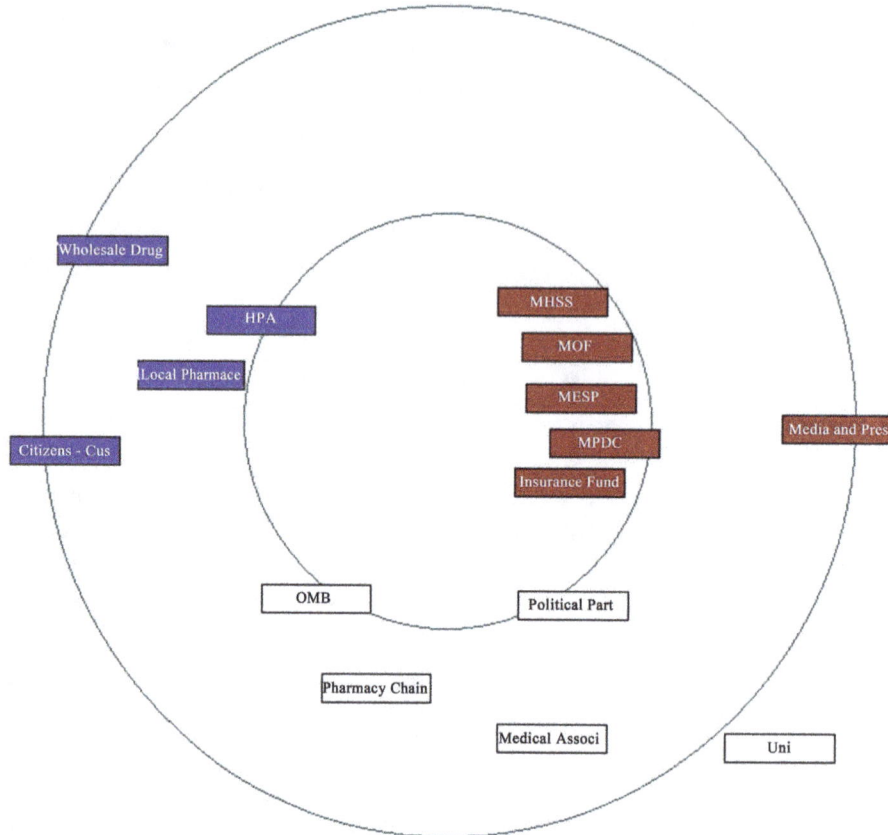

Figure 3. Coalition map.

Table 3. Opportunities and obstacles.

Player name	Opportunity	Obstacle
Citizens-Patients-Customers	Patient-centered approach of the profession	Political and econimic circumstances
Hellenic Pharmaceutical Association	Object enlargement Provision of health services	Expansion of working hours, Entry of non-pharmacists in the profession, Increase of the delinquency
Pharmaceutical Industries	-	Large reduction in profits, Political and economic circumstances
Pharmacy Chains	The economic circumstances encourage the pharmacy chains to flourish	-
Regional Pharmaceutical Association	Provision of health services	Expansion of working schedule, Entry of non-pharmacists in the profession, Increase of the delinquency
Universities	Upgrade of the scientific role of pharmacists	Restriction of the scientific role of pharmacists
Wholesale Drugstores	Increase on sales of para-pharmaceutical products	-

The expected impact of the pharmacists' general strategies, analyzed by each certain strategy and key player is presented in [**Appendix 2**]. The impact is considered as the shift in each player's initial position and power, assuming that pharmacists' certain actions as in [**Appendix 1**], will have a positive impact on key players' future position and a modification in their power of intervention, so as to develop a more friendly policy environment.

Taking in consideration the stakeholders' initial position from **Table 2**, a *Future Position Map* was constructed, expressing the shifts in the key players' position (**Figure 4**).

As it is shown, in this graphical presentation, the pharmacists expected a significant positive shift in the future positions for all key players. More specifically, the Pharmacy sector expected the Government entities to mild their initial high opposite position to medium or low opposition, while non-mobilized positions of other key players to modified to low support and the majority of the pharmaceutical sector players to move to medium or high support. At the same time the pharmacy sector actions were expected to reduce the high power of intervention of the opposition players, while enhancing the power of the supporting players, as presented above in [**Appendix 2**].

We finally assessed in two given distinct time moments (December31, 2012 and June 30, 2013) the success of the pharmacy sector strategy implementation, concerning the degree in which it succeeded in accomplishing the expected impact. The results are presented in [**Appendix 3**], from where it is obvious that the initially expected impact proved to be very optimistic in the most of the implemented strategies. It's worth noting that in the majority of the strategies have worsened or minimized their success ratio throughout the time in study.

4. Discussion

Community pharmacies traditionally have been acting as primary care service points, significantly contributing to the health of citizens not only in Greece, but worldwide [21]-[30].

With the first stormy clouds over the health (and specially over the pharmaceutical) sector, due to initial austerity measures under the Economic Adjustment Programme for Greece [31], community pharmacies turn to their National and Regional professional bodies, in order to preserve their scientific, financial and business interests. Though the reforms to modernize the health care sector were rather general in the MoU, its later in the 2010 reviews, unveiled the severe interventions to the pharmaceutical sector, with significant impact to the community pharmacies as well. Along with the Second Economic Adjustment Programme for Greece [2] and the Medium-Term Fiscal Strategy 2013-2016 [7], the reforms in the Greek health System seem to focus mainly to the pharmaceutical supply chain (from production to community pharmacies) inducing heavy losses to their revenues and profits [6] [8] [32]. Also, the government's drastic measures due to the obligation of the deregulation in the community pharmacies' market, worsen the state of tension in the market [33]-[35]. All these, set in question the feasibility of the community pharmacies in Greece, so the formation of a strategic plan for the community pharmacies was therefore required [36]. The strategic goals set under the pressure of reaction to the initial reforms, could be seen as realistic, comprehensive and in accordance to the vision and mission of other

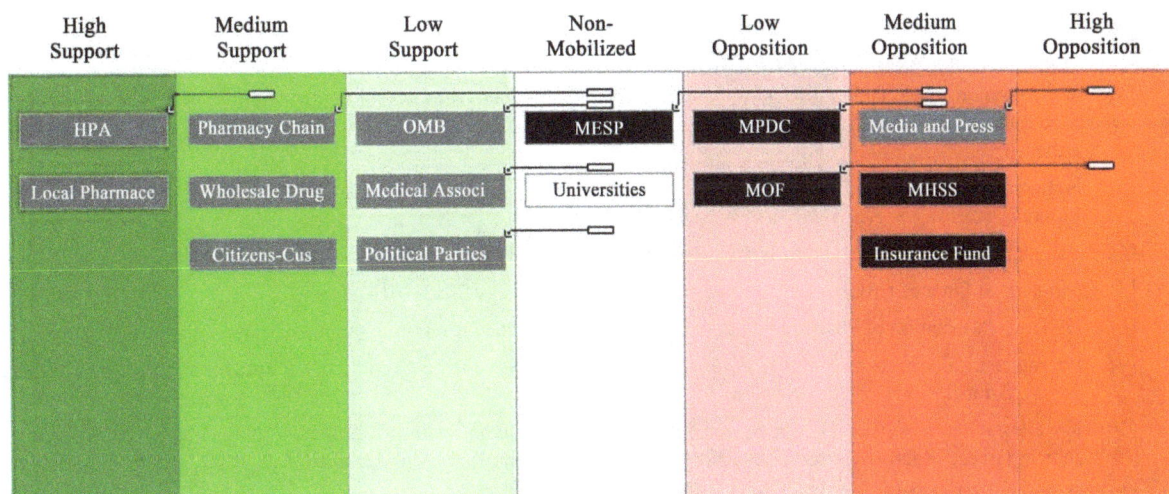

Figure 4. Future position map—all strategies.

European community pharmacists' professional bodies, scientific publications and the PGEU [9] [24] [25] [37]-[50].

But, as the research findings show, either the initially set strategies were at the wrong direction or the actions taken to implement them were inappropriate. Moreover, one can suggest that the shifting ability in either the position or the power of the most key players were over-estimated.

Similar misguided and unsuccessfully developed strategic plans, were also implemented before and in many other countries as well, but never with such a deviance from the initial goals and in such a limited time period [50]-[56].

5. Conclusion

Concluding, on one hand, the community pharmacists proved not to have the ability and the experience to evaluate the current economic and health care environment, while on the other hand, they under-estimated the impact of troika meddling in the pharmaceutical policymaking and in the health sector cost-containment measures imposing.

Competing Interests

The authors declare that they have no competing interests.

Authors' Contributions

AV: Designed the study, the study questionnaire, supervised the analysis and provided comments on the manuscript.

LS: Analyzed literature and participated in the data analysis.

GP: Made major contributions to the background and discussion section and provided comments on the manuscript.

All authors revised the manuscript critically for important intellectual content and approved the final version.

Funding Source

This work was partly funded by the University of Patras research budget.

References

[1]   Eurostat (2013) EU Unemployment Data. Brussels.
      http://appsso.eurostat.ec.europa.eu/nui/show.do?dataset=une_rt_a&lang=en

[2]   European Commission (EC) (2013) The Second Economic Adjustment Programme for Greece: Third Review. European Economy, Occasional Papers 159, European Commission, Directorate-General for Economic and Financial Affairs. Brussels.

[3]   World Health Organization (WHO) (2012) European Health Report. Geneva.
      http://www.euro.who.int/__data/assets/pdf_file/0004/197113/EHR2012-Eng.pdf

[4]   Kanellopoulou, S. (2013) Policies to Contain Public Pharmaceutical Expenditure by Acting Not Only on the Supply-Side but on the Demand Side as Well. Eurobank Economic Research, Greece Macro-Monitor, Focus Notes: Greece, Athens.

[5]   Hellenic Association of Pharmaceutical Companies (SFEE) (2012) The Pharmaceutical Market in Greece_Facts and Figures. Athens.

[6]   Foundation for Economic and Industrial Research (IOBE) (2013) Annual report for the Pharma-Industry 2012. Athens.

[7]   Ministry of Finance (MOF) (2013) Medium-Term Fiscal Strategy 2013-2016. Athens.

[8]   Hellenic Association of Pharmaceutical Companies (SFEE) (2013) A Trip without Compass. Athens. (In Greek)

[9]   Pharmaceutical Group of European Union (PGEU) (2012) Advancing Community Pharmacy Practice in Challenging Times, Annual Report 2012. Brussels.

[10] Kanellopoulou, S. (2012) Health Sector Reforms and the Memorandum of Understanding. Eurobank Economic Research, Greece Macro-Monitor, Focus Notes: Greece, Eurobank Research, Athens.

[11] Roberts, A., Benrimoj, S.I., Dunphy, D. and Palmer, I. (2007) Community Pharmacy: Strategic Change Management. McGraw-Hill Australia Pty Ltd, Sydney.

[12] Gidman, W. (2010) Exploring the Impact of Evolving Health Policy on Independent Pharmacy Ownership in England. Springer Science & Business Media B.V., Netherlands.

[13] McArthur, D. (2007) European Pharmaceutical Distribution: Key Players, Challenges and Future Strategies. Scrip Reports, Informa UK Ltd., London.

[14] Mossialos, E. and Allin, S. (2005) Interest Groups and Health System Reform in Greece. *West European Politics*, **28**, 420-444. http://dx.doi.org/10.1080/01402380500060460

[15] McMillan, S.S., Wheeler, J.A., Sav, A., King, A.M., Whitty, A.J., Kendall, E. and Kelly, F. (2013) Community Pharmacy in Australia: A Health Hub Destination of the Future. *Research in Social and Administrative Pharmacy*, **9**, 863-875. http://dx.doi.org/10.1016/j.sapharm.2012.11.003

[16] Reich, M.R. (1996) Applied Political Analysis for Health Policy Reform. *Current Issues in Public Health*, **2**, 186-191.

[17] Reich, M.R. and Cooper, D.M. (1996) PolicyMaker: Computer-Assisted Political Analysis (Software and Manual). PoliMap, Newton Centre.

[18] Glassman, A., Reich, M.R., Laserson, K. and Rojas, F. (1999) Political Analysis of Health Reform in the Dominican Republic. *Health Policy and Planning*, **14**, 115-126. http://dx.doi.org/10.1093/heapol/14.2.115

[19] Mintzberg, H. (1994) The Rise and Fall of Strategic Planning. Free Press, New York.

[20] Armstrong, M., Lewis, R., Blenkinsopp, A. and Anderson, C. (2005) The Contribution of Community Pharmacy to Improving the Public's Health. Report 3: An Overview of the Evidence-Base from 1990-2002 with Recommendations for Action. Pharmacy Health Link and the Royal Pharmaceutical Society of Great Britain, London.

[21] Kontozamanis, V., Mantzouneas, E. and Stoforos, C. (2003) An Overview of the Greek Pharmaceutical Market. *European Journal of Health Economics*, **4**, 327-333. http://dx.doi.org/10.1007/s10198-003-0206-1

[22] Lluch, M.M. and Kanavos, P. (2010) Impact of Regulation of Community Pharmacies on Efficiency, Access and Equity. Evidence from the UK and Spain. *Health Policy*, **95**, 245-254.

[23] Pharmaceutical Group of European Union (PGEU) (2010) Providing Quality Pharmacy Services to Communities in Times of Change, Annual Report 2010. Brussels.

[24] Pharmaceutical Group of European Union (PGEU) (2012) European Community Pharmacy Blueprint for Optimisation of Health Outcomes to Individual Patients and Value for Health Systems across Europe. Brussels.

[25] Pharmacy Voice (2011) Community Pharmacy: A Blueprint for Better Health. London.

[26] Pharmacy Voice (2012) Community Pharmacy: Our Prospectus for Better Health. Pharmacy Voice Limited, London.

[27] Sainsbury's Pharmacy (2013) The Wells Family Challenge: A Pharmacist First Approach. Collated and Evaluated by 2020 Health, Sainsbury's Co., UK.

[28] Twigg, J.M., Poland, F., Bhattacharya, D., Desborough, A.J. and Wright, J.D. (2013) The Current and Future Roles of Community Pharmacists: Views and Experiences of Patients with Type 2 Diabetes. *Research in Social and Administrative Pharmacy*, **9**, 777-789. http://dx.doi.org/10.1016/j.sapharm.2012.10.004

[29] Moullin, J.C., Sabater-Hernandez, D., Fernandez-Llimos, F. and Benrimoj, S.I. (2013) Defining Professional Pharmacy Services in Community Pharmacy. *Research in Social and Administrative Pharmacy*, **9**, 989-995. http://dx.doi.org/10.1016/j.sapharm.2013.02.005

[30] European Commission, EC (2010) The Economic Adjustment Programme for Greece, European Economy. Occasional Papers 61, European Commission, Directorate-General for Economic and Financial Affairs, Brussels.

[31] OECD (2013) OECD Health Data 2013, OECD Health Statistics (Database). Paris.

[32] Von der Schulenburg, G. and Hodek, J.M. (2008) Costs and Benefits of Pharmacy Regulation in Germany. *Proceedings of the Workshop on Access to High Quality Pharmacy Services*, Brussels, 15 October 2008. http://ec.europa.eu/internal_market/services/docs/pharmacy/20081015_summary_en.pdf

[33] Lluch, M. (2009) Are Regulations of Community Pharmacies in Europe Questioning Our Pro-Competitive Policies? *Eurohealth*, **15**, 26-27.

[34] Vogler, S., Arts, D. and Sandberger, K. (2012) Impact of Pharmacy Deregulation and Regulation in European Countries. Commissioned by Danmarks Apotekerforening (Association of Danish Pharmacies), Gesundheit Österreich GmbH., Vienna.

[35] Business Concept (2012) Pharmacy Feasibility Study. Business Concept Supply Chain, Athens. (In Greek)

[36] Wiedenmayer, K., Summers, S.R., Mackie, A.C., Gous, G.S.A., Everard, M. and Tromp, D. (2006) Developing Pharmacy Practice: A Focus on Patient Care, Handbook—2006 Edition. World Health Organization, Department of Medicines Policy and Standards, Geneva, Switzerland in Collaboration with International Pharmaceutical Federation, The Hague.

[37] Brown, D., Portlock, J., Rutter, P. and Nazar, Z. (2014) From Community Pharmacy to Healthy Living Pharmacy. *Research in Social and Administrative Pharmacy*, **10**, 72-87. http://dx.doi.org/10.1016/j.sapharm.2013.04.014

[38] Deloitte UK, CFHS (2013) Impact of Austerity on European Pharmaceutical Policy and Pricing: Staying Competitive in a Challenging Environment. Deloitte UK Centre for Health Solutions, London.

[39] Department of Health, Social Services and Public Safety (DHSSPSNI) (2013) Making It Better through Pharmacy in the Community. Consultation on Proposals for a Five Year Strategy for Pharmacy in the Community, UK.

[40] Giberson, S., Yoder, S. and Lee, M.P. (2011) Improving Patient and Health System Outcomes through Advanced Pharmacy Practice. A Report to the US Surgeon General, Office of the Chief Pharmacist, US Public Health Service, Rockville.

[41] Pharmaceutical Group of European Union (PGEU) (2012) Sustainable European Community Pharmacies Part of the Solution. Brussels.

[42] ABDA—Federal Union of German Associations of Pharmacists (2012) German Pharmacies Figures Data Facts. Berlin.

[43] Bush, J., Langley, A.C. and Wilson, A.K. 2009) The Corporatization of Community Pharmacy: Implications for Service Provision, the Public Health Function, and Pharmacy's Claims to Professional Status in the United Kingdom. *Research in Social and Administrative Pharmacy*, **5**, 305-318.

[44] Harrison, J., Scahill, S. and Sheridan, J. (2012) New Zealand Pharmacists' Alignment with Their Professional Body's Vision for the Future. *Research in Social and Administrative Pharmacy*, **8**, 17-35. http://dx.doi.org/10.1016/j.sapharm.2010.12.001

[45] Lindberg, K., Nicolini, D., Adolfsson, P., Bergamaschi, M., Delmestri, G., Goodrick, E. and Reay, T. (2008) Exploring the Globalized Face of Pharmacy. In: *Academy of Management "The Questions We Ask"*, Anaheim.

[46] Perepelkin, J. and Manfrin, A. (2012) Pharmacist Service Provision and the Environment of the Community Pharmacy in Canada. *Research in Social and Administrative Pharmacy*, **8**, e53-e54. http://dx.doi.org/10.1016/j.sapharm.2012.08.124

[47] Doucette, R.W., Nevins, C.J., Gaither, C., Kreling, H.D., Mott, A.D., Pedersen, A.C. and Schommer, C.J. (2012) Organizational Factors Influencing Pharmacy Practice Change. *Research in Social and Administrative Pharmacy*, **8**, 274-284. http://dx.doi.org/10.1016/j.sapharm.2011.07.002

[48] NHS Lothian (2013) Pharmacy Strategy 2013-2016. Scotland.

[49] Center for Health Services Management and Evaluation (CHESME) (2001) Expenditure on Pharmaceuticals and the Organizational and Operational Framework of Pharmacies in Greece and the EU. National and Kapodistrian University, Athens.

[50] Co-Operatives Europe (2009) Mapping Exercise: Co-Operatives Working in the Pharmacy Sector in Europe, European Seminar: Cooperative Enterprises in the Pharmacy Sector, Opportunities & Challenges. European House of Co-Operatives, Brussels.

[51] Eyeforpharma (2012) Austerity Agenda Increases Pressure on Pharma Companies to Adopt KAM for Managing Burgeoning Stakeholder Challenges. Eyeforpharma KAM Report 2011/2012, Eyeforpharma, FC Business Intelligence Ltd., London.

[52] Kanavos, P., Vandoros, S., Irwin, R., Nicod, E. and Casson, M. (2011) Differences in Costs of and Access to Pharmaceutical Products in the EU. European Parliament's Committee on Environment, Public Health and Food Safety, D.G. for Internal Policies, Policy Department, Economic and Social Policy, Brussels.

[53] Manhattan Research (2012) Taking the Pulse® Pharmacists 2012: Pharmacist Market Trends. Manhattan Research, New York.

[54] National Pharmacy Association (2012) Community Pharmacy Statistics 2012. http://www.npa.co.uk/About-the-NPA/Media-Centre/Pharmacy-facts/

[55] Sheppard, A. (2010) Generic Medicines: Essential Contributors to the Long-Term Health of Society, Sector Sustainability Challenges in Europe. IMS Health, London.

[56] Schommer, C.J., Yusuf, A.A. and Hadsall, S.R. (2013) Market Dynamics of Community Pharmacies in Minnesota, US from 1992 through 2012. *Research in Social and Administrative Pharmacy*, **10**, 217-231.

Abbreviations

MoU: Memorandum of Understanding; SSFs: Social Security Funds; HPA: Hellenic Pharmaceutical Association; OMB: Pharmaceutical Industries; MHSS: Ministry of Health and Social Solidarity; MESP: Ministry of Employment and Social Protection; MPDC: Ministry of Development & Competitiveness; MOF: Ministry of Finance.

Appendix 1. Strategy Table

Player	Strategy and Actions
Citizens-Patients-Customers, Media and Press	Hire a professional public relations firm to monitor the opposition or to design a negative public relations campaign directed against the opposition.: Feed the press with negative information relating to the government actions and simultaneously positive news for the Pharmacies' issue
Citizens-Patients-Customers, Media and Press, Political Parties	Invoke "Crisis" to Justify Policy: Organize a media campaign to create a sense of public "crisis" regarding access to and costs of pharmaceutical products, in order to justify major policy aims and override opposition.
Citizens-Patients-Customers, Political Parties	Use symbols to Increase public support of the policy: Organizing a media campaign or finding sympathetic victims.
Health Insurance Funds	Get Support from Single Payer Proponents: Persuade single-payer proponents that the policy is the best plan they could hope to achieve.
Hellenic Pharmaceutical Association, Regional Pharmaceutical Association, Citizens-Patients-Customers	Persuade supporters to strengthen their position: Reminding of the promised benefits compared to other policies.
Ministry of Health, Ministry of Finance, Ministry of Employment and Social Protection, Ministry of Development & Competitiveness, Health Insurance Funds	Compromise on Coverage: Compromise on the definition of universal coverage, in order to win support from some critics of the reform effort.
Ministry of Health, Ministry of Finance, Ministry of Employment and Social Protection, Ministry of Development & Competitiveness, Health Insurance Funds	Meet with opponents to seek common goals or mechanisms, and thereby reduce the intensity of their opposition.: Regular meetings with government officials
Ministry of Health, Ministry of Finance, Ministry of Employment and Social Protection, Ministry of Development & Competitiveness, Health Insurance Funds	Reduce the strength of coalitions of opposing groups or individuals, by fostering internal tensions or by winning over a key member.: Appoint their differences in financial and other interests
Ministry of Health, Ministry of Finance, Ministry of Employment and Social Protection, Ministry of Development & Competitiveness, Health Insurance Funds, Media and Press	Undermine the legitimacy of the opposition, by connecting them to negative social values through negative publicity.: Limited access to pharmaceutical products
Universities	Persuade non-mobilized to take a position of support, by adding desired goals and mechanisms to the policy: Provide information and evidence, including technical and political information.
Wholesale Drugstores, Citizens-Patients-Customers, Pharmaceutical Industries, Pharmacy Chains, Medical Association—Doctors	Persuade non-mobilized groups to take a supporting position: Providing incentives, removing objections, or adding desired policy elements.
Wholesale Drugstores, Hellenic Pharmaceutical Association, Regional Pharmaceutical Association, Pharmaceutical Industries, Pharmacy Chains, Medical Association—Doctors, Universities	Strengthen Public Relations: Involve representatives in the working group process to draft the reform policy.
Wholesale Drugstores, Pharmaceutical Industries, Pharmacy Chains, Medical Association—Doctors	Reduce the intensity of their opposition.: Provide compensation for real and perceived harms

Appendix 2. Strategy Impacts

Strategy	Player name	Current Position	Future Position	Current Power	Future Power
Compromise on Coverage	Ministry of Health	Medium Opposition	Non-Mobilized	High	High
Compromise on Coverage	Ministry of Finance	High Opposition	Medium Support	High	High
Compromise on Coverage	Ministry of Employment and Social Protection	Medium Opposition	Low Support	High	Medium
Compromise on Coverage	Ministry of Development & Competitivess	Medium Opposition	Non-Mobilized	High	Medium
Compromise on Coverage	Health Insurance Funds	Medium Opposition	Medium Support	High	High
Get Support from Single Payer Proponents	Health Insurance Funds	Medium Opposition	Medium Opposition	High	High
Hire a professional public relations firm to monitor the opposition or to design a negative public relations campaign directed against the opposition.	Citizens-Patients-Customers	Medium Support	High Support	Medium	Medium
Hire a professional public relations firm to monitor the opposition or to design a negative public relations campaign directed against the opposition.	Media and Press	High Opposition	Low Opposition	Medium	Medium
Invoke "Crisis" to Justify Policy	Citizens-Patients-Customers	Medium Support	Medium Opposition	Medium	Medium
Invoke "Crisis" to Justify Policy	Media and Press	High Opposition	High Opposition	Medium	Medium
Invoke "Crisis" to Justify Policy	Political Parties	Non-Mobilized	Low Opposition	Medium	Medium
Meet with opponents to seek common goals or mechanisms, and thereby reduce the intensity of their opposition.	Ministry of Health	Medium Opposition	Medium Opposition	High	High
Meet with opponents to seek common goals or mechanisms, and thereby reduce the intensity of their opposition.	Ministry of Finance	Medium Opposition	Medium Opposition	High	High
Meet with opponents to seek common goals or mechanisms, and thereby reduce the intensity of their opposition.	Ministry of Employment and Social Protection	Medium Opposition	Low Opposition	High	Medium
Meet with opponents to seek common goals or mechanisms, and thereby reduce the intensity of their opposition.	Ministry of Development & Competitivess	Medium Opposition	Medium Opposition	High	High
Meet with opponents to seek common goals or mechanisms, and thereby reduce the intensity of their opposition.	Health Insurance Funds	Medium Opposition	High Opposition	High	High
Persuade non-mobilized groups to take a supporting position	Wholesale Drugstores	Medium Support	Medium Support	Medium	Medium

Appendix 3. Strategy Impacts

Strategy	Expected Impact	Success (%) 31/12/2011	Success (%) 31/12/2012	Success (%) 30/06/2013
Highlight (emphasize) their differences in financial and other interests	Health Insurance Funds: (No position or change)	25	25	0
Highlight (emphasize) their differences in financial and other interests	Ministry of Development & Competitiveness: (No position or change)	50	25	25
Highlight (emphasize) their differences in financial and other interests	Ministry of Employment and Social Protection: Position weakened to Low Opposition and strengthened to High	50	25	25
Highlight (emphasize) their differences in financial and other interests	Ministry of Finance: Position weakened to Medium Opposition	50	25	25
Highlight (emphasize) their differences in financial and other interests	Ministry of Health: (No position or change)	50	25	25
Compromise on the definition of universal coverage, in order to win support from some critics of the reform effort.	Health Insurance Funds: Position weakened to Medium Support	50	25	25
Compromise on the definition of universal coverage, in order to win support from some critics of the reform effort.	Ministry of Development & Competitiveness: Position weakened to Non-Mobilized and strengthened to Medium	50	25	25
Compromise on the definition of universal coverage, in order to win support from some critics of the reform effort.	Ministry of Employment and Social Protection: Position weakened to Low Support and strengthened to Medium	50	25	25
Compromise on the definition of universal coverage, in order to win support from some critics of the reform effort.	Ministry of Finance: Position weakened to Medium Support	75	50	25
Compromise on the definition of universal coverage, in order to win support from some critics of the reform effort.	Ministry of Health: Position weakened to Non-Mobilized	75	50	50
Feed the press with negative information relating to the government actions and simultaneously positive news for the Pharmacies' issue	Citizens-Patients-Customers: Position weakened to High Support	100	75	50
Feed the press with negative information relating to the government actions and simultaneously positive news for the Pharmacies' issue	Media and Press: Position weakened to Low Opposition	50	50	50
Involve representatives in the working group process to draft the reform policy	Hellenic Pharmaceutical Association: Position weakened to High Support and weakened to Low	50	25	25
Involve representatives in the working group process to draft the reform policy	Medical Association—Doctors: (No position or change)	25	0	0
Involve representatives in the working group process to draft the reform policy	Pharmaceutical Industries: Position weakened to Medium Support and weakened to Low	50	25	25
Involve representatives in the working group process to draft the reform policy	Pharmacy Chains: Position weakened to Medium Support	75	50	50
Involve representatives in the working group process to draft the reform policy	Regional Pharmaceutical Association: weakened to Low	75	75	75
Involve representatives in the working group process to draft the reform policy	Universities: (No position or change)	25	25	25

Continued

Involve representatives in the working group process to draft the reform policy	Wholesale Drugstores: (No position or change)	25	0	0
Limited access to pharmaceutical products	Health Insurance Funds: Position strengthened to High Opposition	50	50	25
Limited access to pharmaceutical products	Media and Press: Position weakened to Medium Opposition	25	25	25
Limited access to pharmaceutical products	Ministry of Development & Competitiveness: Position weakened to Non-Mobilized	50	50	25
Limited access to pharmaceutical products	Ministry of Employment and Social Protection: Position weakened to Non-Mobilized and strengthened to Medium	50	50	25
Limited access to pharmaceutical products	Ministry of Finance: (No position or change)	50	50	25
Limited access to pharmaceutical products	Ministry of Health: Position strengthened to High Opposition	50	50	25
Organize a media campaign to create a sense of public "crisis" regarding access to and costs of pharmaceutical products, in order to justify major policy aims and override opposition.	Citizens-Patients-Customers: Position strengthened to Medium Opposition	100	75	75
Organize a media campaign to create a sense of public "crisis" regarding access to and costs of pharmaceutical products, in order to justify major policy aims and override opposition.	Media and Press: (No position or change)	50	25	25
Organize a media campaign to create a sense of public "crisis" regarding access to and costs of pharmaceutical products, in order to justify major policy aims and override opposition.	Political Parties: Position strengthened to Low Opposition	50	25	25
Organizing a media campaign or finding sympathetic victims	Citizens-Patients-Customers: (No position or change)	75	50	50
Organizing a media campaign or finding sympathetic victims	Political Parties: Position weakened to Medium Support	50	25	25
Persuade single-payer proponents that the policy is the best plan they could hope to achieve	Health Insurance Funds: (No position or change)	50	25	25
Provide compensation for real and perceived harms	Medical Association—Doctors: Position weakened to Low Support	25	0	0
Provide compensation for real and perceived harms	Pharmaceutical Industries: Position weakened to Low Support	50	25	0
Provide compensation for real and perceived harms	Pharmacy Chains: Position weakened to Medium Support and strengthened to High	50	25	25
Provide compensation for real and perceived harms	Wholesale Drugstores: (No position or change)	50	25	0
Provide information and evidence, including technical and political information.	Universities: (No position or change)	75	50	50
Providing incentives, removing objections, or adding desired policy elements.	Citizens-Patients-Customers: (No position or change)	50	50	50

Continued

Providing incentives, removing objections, or adding desired policy elements.	Medical Association—Doctors: Position weakened to Low Support	25	25	0
Providing incentives, removing objections, or adding desired policy elements.	Pharmaceutical Industries: Position weakened to Low Support	50	25	25
Providing incentives, removing objections, or adding desired policy elements.	Pharmacy Chains: Position weakened to Low Support and strengthened to High	75	50	50
Providing incentives, removing objections, or adding desired policy elements.	Wholesale Drugstores: (No position or change)	50	25	25
Regular meetings with government officials	Health Insurance Funds: Position strengthened to High Opposition	50	25	25
Regular meetings with government officials	Ministry of Development & Competitiveness: (No position or change)	75	50	25
Regular meetings with government officials	Ministry of Employment and Social Protection: Position weakened to Low Opposition and strengthened to Medium	50	25	25
Regular meetings with government officials	Ministry of Finance: Position weakened to Medium Opposition	75	50	25
Regular meetings with government officials	Ministry of Health: (No position or change)	75	50	25
Reminding of the promised benefits compared to other policies	Citizens-Patients-Customers: Position weakened to High Support	75	75	75
Reminding of the promised benefits compared to other policies	Hellenic Pharmaceutical Association: Position weakened to High Support and weakened to Low	100	100	100
Reminding of the promised benefits compared to other policies	Regional Pharmaceutical Association: weakened to Low	100	75	75

Appendix 4. Research Questionnaire

1) **To your opinion, what are the main goals associated with the community pharmacists' implementation policy and define the priority for each of them (check the appropriate cell).**

Goals	Priority		
	Low	*Medium*	*High*

2) What are the mechanisms that the community pharmacists' implementation policy (must) use to achieve the above mentioned goals? (Note, each mechanism must refer to a certain goal).

	Mechanism	Goal
1)		
2)		
3)		
4)		
5)		
6)		
7)		
8)		
9)		
10)		

3) Please, identify all the players that might be affected by or might affect the community pharmacists' implementation policy, and assess their position on the policy (check the appropriate cell).

Stakeholders	Qualitative assessment of the strength of a player's support or opposition				
	high *supporter*	*Medium supporter*	*Non-mobilizied*	*medium opponent*	high *opponent*

4) **Please, estimate how much power each particular player has over the outcome of the community pharmacists' implementation policy debate (check the appropriate cell).**

Stakeholders	Qualitative assessment of a player's power over the outcome		
	Low	Medium	High

5) **Please, fill in the Interests Table below by estimating each player's level of interest in certain types of interest fields, concerning the community pharmacists' implementation policy debate (use L (Low), M (Medium) or H (High)).**

Stakeholders	Qualitative assessment of a player's interest on various Fields							
	Financial	Political	Personal	Scientific	professional	Moral		

6) Please, identify the <u>Strengths</u> of the community pharmacists' Sector (up to 5 Strengths).

1)	
2)	
3)	
4)	
5)	

7) Please, identify the <u>Weaknesses</u> of the community pharmacists' Sector (up to 5 Weaknesses).

1)	
2)	
3)	
4)	
5)	

8) Please, identify and assess transitions that may present opportunities (Opportunities) to enhance the political feasibility of the community pharmacists' implementation policy (up to 5 Opportunities).

1)	
2)	
3)	
4)	
5)	

9) Please, identify and assess transitions that may create significant obstacles (Threats) to enhance the political feasibility of the community pharmacists' implementation policy (up to 5 Threats).

1)	
2)	
3)	
4)	
5)	

9

Empathy Levels of Dental Students of Central America and the Caribbean

Víctor Patricio Díaz-Narváez[1,2*], Ana María Erazo Coronado[3], Jorge Luis Bilbao[4], Farith González[5], Mariela Padilla[6], Madeline Howard[7], Guadalupe Silva[8], Joel Arboleda[8], Mirian Bullen[9], Robert Utsman[6], Elizabeth Fajardo[10], Luz Marina Alonso[11], Marcos Cervantes[12]

[1]Facultad de Odontología, Universidad San Sebastián, Santiago, Chile
[2]Universidad Autónoma de Chile, Santiago, Chile
[3]Universidad Metropolitana, Barranquilla, Colombia
[4]Facultad de Medicina, Universidad Libre Seccional Barranquilla y Fundación Universitaria San Martín Sede Puerto Colombia, Barranquilla, Colombia
[5]Facultad de Odontología, Universidad de Cartagena, Cartagena, Colombia
[6]Universidad Latinoamericana de Ciencia y Tecnología, San José, Costa Rica
[7]Facultad de Odontología, Universidad de Costa Rica, San José, Costa Rica
[8]Universidad Central del Este, San Pedro de Macorís, República Dominicana
[9]Facultad de Odontología, Universidad de Panamá, Ciudad de Panamá, República de Panamá
[10]Faculty of Health Sciences, Universidad del Tolima, Ibagué, Colombia
[11]División de Salud, Universidad del Norte, Barranquilla, Colombia
[12]Facultad de Ciencias Sociales, Universidad del Norte, Barranquilla, Colombia

Email: *victor.diaz@uss.cl, amec1708@gmail.com, jbilbao55@hotmail.com, fgonzalezm1@unicartagena.edu.co, mpadilla@ulacit.ac.cr, mhowarducr@gmail.com, guadalupesilva1@gmail.com, Jarboleda@uce.edu.do, ladymi516@yahoo.com, rutsmana282@ulacit.ed.cr, efajardo@ut.edu.co, lmalonso@uninorte.edu.co, marcos.cervantes@gmail.com

Abstract

Objective: The aim of this study is to check whether there are differences in the distribution of empathy levels in dental students from nine faculties of dentistry Colombia, Panama, Costa Rica and Dominican Republic. Methods: The levels of empathy and matrices of empathy construct matrices are estimated dental students by using the Jefferson Scale of Physician Empathy, the Spanish version for students (S version) culturally validated in Colombia, Panama, Costa Rica and Dominican Republic measured by arbitrator criteria. Cronbach α is estimated. Data of empathic orientation of the studied factors between faculties are analyzed and compared by ANOVA and Duncan

---

*Corresponding author.

test and matrices of empathy construct using discriminant analysis. **Results:** We find that there are differences in levels of empathy between universities, courses, gender and interaction between the Dental Faculty (University) and Course. The comparison between matrices shows unexplained variances and differences observed between the levels of empathy in student populations. **Conclusions:** Variability in empathy is observed in the studied factors and among student populations. The variability is an empirical finding, but is not possible in this work, to explain why.

Keywords

Empathy, Jefferson Scale of Physician Empathy (JSPE), Levels of Empathy

1. Introduction

Empathy is an attribute that contributes positively [1]-[5] in the process of patient care by the health professional. Empathy should also be given attention in the process of formation of these health professionals [6]. Empathy is defined based on three dimensions: a) to put into perspective, b) care with compassion and c) the ability to "step into the shoes of the patient" [7] [8]; as a result, they are involved in complex cognitive and emotional processes.

The empirical evidence observed in several studies of faculties of various health careers appears to be contradictory in relation to the examination of, at least, two factors: year (academic year) and gender [1]-[5] [7]-[10]. The possible explanation for this diversity of results may be due to the varying components of empathy maybe, in turn, influenced by other variables that affect the structure of the components of empathy [5]. According to Silva *et al.* [11], these differences open new areas of investigation concerning the possible socio-cultural implications that can influence the empathy. However, there are no studies comparing the empathy between different higher education institutions within a country and between countries. The existence of such differences may constitute empirical evidence of socio-cultural factors that affect the structuring of empathy in ontogenetic processes in the subjects. The aim of this study is to test whether there are differences in levels of empathy among student populations of nine dental schools from four countries of Central America and the Caribbean.

2. Materials and Methods

This study, an exploratory, cross-sectional and ex post facto cause-effect [12], (was approved by the Ethics Committee of Research, University of Development and German Clinic with approval of code CAS-UDD approval: 2011-64 in Santiago de Chile). It addresses students composed by levels from first through fifth years of Dental School, from the Faculty of Dentistry of Metropolitan University (Erazo *et al.*) [13] and San Martin de Barranquilla (Bilbao *et al.*) [3], University of Magdalena (sent to publish) and University of Cartagena (sent to publish) of the Republic of Colombia; Universidad Latina (sent to publish) and University of Panama (sent by publish) of the Republic of Panama; Latin University of Science and Technology (Sanchez *et al.*) [14] and the University of Costa Rica (Howard *et al.*) [15] of the Republic of Costa Rica, and the Universidad Central del Este (Silva *et al.*) [11] of the Dominican Republic. Data collection was conducted from June to August 2012, simultaneously at designated schools. The sample was comprised of those subjects who could be evaluated on the day the instrument was applied. All students, upon the application of the scale, were attending the last part of the first semester of each course. Participants from each of the samples were applied the Jefferson Scale of Physician Empathy (JSPE), the Spanish version for students (S version), and culturally appropriate in each of the countries studied by Committee Criteria [7] [16] [17]. There were no exclusion criteria, since the object was to evaluate the variable of interest of the majority of students. Consistent with referred to above, a single anonymous and confidential measurement (after signing informed consent), performed by a neutral operator, was first applied to students of fourth year classes. In the case of fifth year students, the instrument was administered on a visit to the clinical setting, with the same indications previously mentioned.

3. Statistical Methods

The data were subjected to a Cronbach α (reliability by internal consistency) [18]-[20] and Cronbach α based on established elements. Subsequently, it estimated with Cronbach α that removing an item (question applied instrument) for each estimate, in order to verify the explanatory role of each question.

The summation score of raw data of empathy levels obtained were initially subjected to an Shapiro-Wilk normality test [21] and Levene test of homoscedasticity [22] on the three factors studied: University (Faculty), Course (Academic Year) and Gender. The descriptive statistics were estimated; arithmetic mean and standard deviation. The comparison of means among the factors within the levels of the main factors and the interactions between the main factors were performed using a general linear model and Duncan test for unbalanced data [12]. Observed power (1-β) and the effect size (η2) [12] [23] were evaluated. Subsequently, a discriminant analysis was performed. The λ statistic of Wilks [24] was used in order to measure the proportion of the total variance of the discriminant scores not explained by differences in the factors examined. To test whether the variance and covariance matrices of each University (School of Dentistry) come from or not the same population, Box's M test [24] [25] was used. Data were analyzed using the SPSS 20.0 statistical program. The level of significance was set at $\alpha \leq 0.05$ and $\beta \leq 0.20$ in all cases.

4. Results

The general value of Cronbach α was 0.775 and evidence of internal consistency can be characterized as good and the value of this statistic, based on established elements, resulted similar to the non-typified (0.782), all of which show that the variances are similar between elements [25] [26]. When the Cronbach α values were eliminated they fluctuated between 0.752 - 0.784, all of which indicates that all elements are providing some degree of explanation of the construct studied. The statistic F = 6363.07; of a Hotelling T2 test, was highly significant ($p < 0.0005$), and shows that the means of the elements are distributed differently and indicates that the questions, possibly associated with some dimensions, are contributing in different ways to the explanation of the construct. All this, in general, shows that the scale is reliable in the data analyzed in this study.

The application of a three-factor model allowed to observe that the factors "University", "Course", Gender and, finally, "University" in interaction with the factor "Course" (University * Course), were highly significant ($p < 0.0005$), which indicates that there are differences between the universities studied, between courses, between gender and between courses of different universities. However, the η2 statistic, which indicates the magnitude of the effect size, is small (0.104, 0.009, 0.007 and 0.061 respectively). The observed values of the power of the test was 1.00; 0.903; 0.937 and 1.00 respectively; all of which show that there is low risk of committing a Type II error. The R2 value was 0.217 uncorrected and corrected 0,177; which show that the model does not explain all the variation, but also shows the existence of other factors (other than those studied) that are influencing the determination of the values of the observed levels of empathy.

In **Table 1**, the mean values of the variable levels of empathy in every University studied are presented. In **Table 2**, the results of applying the Duncan test are presented. It is noted that four groups are formed. The first consists of the means of the University of Magdalena (Colombia), that was significantly different ($p < 0.05$) from the means of the Universities of Metropolitan and San Martin (Colombia) and Central del Este (Dominican Republic), which form a second group and, among them, there are no significant differences (p > 0.05). Later a third group was composed of the means of the Universities America (Panama), ULACIT of Costa Rica, Cartagena (Colombia) and the University of Panama, among which there are no significant differences ($p > 0.05$). Finally, a fourth group was formed, only consisting of the means of the University of Costa Rica, which differed significantly ($p < 0.05$) of all previously formed groups.

Table 3 shows the mean results of the factor "Course". It is noted that two groups are formed, which differ significantly among them ($p < 0.05$).The first consists of the average of the "first year"; while the second group consists of the rest of the means of which between them there are no significant differences ($p > 0.05$). Regarding the "gender" factor, an average of 104.265 for the female gender (typical error = 0.446; confidence interval with a Lower Limit = 103.351 and Upper Limit = 105.179) and, for males, the average was 101.446 (typical error = 0.79; confidence interval Lower Limit = 99.517 and Upper Limit = 102.615), with significant differences ($p < 0.05$) between them. In **Table 4**, the results of the estimation of means between the University and Course factors (University * Course) are presented.

The comparison between the complete data arrays of the instruments applied permit the estimation of the Box M statistic (3947.847), which was highly significant ($p < 0.005$); indicating that the covariance matrices between

Table 1. Results of the estimation of mean, standard error and confidence interval of empathic orientation in each of the Dental University studied.

Dental University	Median	Standard Error	Confidence Interval 95%	
			Lower Limit	Upper Limit
Universidad Latina de Panamá	102.637	2.312	98.102	107.172
Universidad de Cartagena (Colombia)	105.525	0.794	103.968	107.081
Universidad de Magdalena (Colombia)	92.490	1.098	90.336	94.644
Universidad Metropolitana (Colombia)	100.061	1.224	97.659	102.462
Universidad Central del Este (Dominicana)	101.724	1.120	99.528	103.921
ULACIT de Costa Rica	103.468	1.179	101.156	105.780
Universidad de Costa Rica	111.888	.940	110.045	113.732
Universidad de Panamá	105.198	1.818	101.633	108.762
Universidad San Martín (Colombia)	100.999	1.228	98.590	103.408

Table 2. Results of the comparison between the means of empathic orientation between different universities studied.

Dental University	N	Subset			
		1	2	3	4
Universidad de Magdalena	173	92.48			
Universidad Metropolitana	154		99.41		
Universidad San Martín	168		100.92		
Universidad Central del Este	239		101.26		
Universidad Latina de Panamá	92			104.55	
ULACIT de Costa Rica[*]	225			105.49	
Universidad de Cartagena	360			105.99	
Universidad de Panamá	133			107.67	
Universidad de Costa Rica	290				111.88
Sig.		1.000	0.255	0.062	1.000

[*]In the case of ULACIT Costa Rica, being a 4-year program, students will be distributed in 5 groups, according to school cycles.

Table 3. Results of the comparison of means between courses by Duncan's test.

Course	N	Subset	
		1	2
First	377	99.62	
Second	439		104.08
Fourth	323		105.10
Fifth	330		105.30
Third	365		106.28
Sig.		1.000	0.057

universities compared differ. X^2 tests, associated with the contrasts of the discriminant functions were highly significant ($p < 0.0005$) and fluctuated between 884.263 and 31.92; all of which show that the unexplained va the presence of different populations. Something similar occurs when comparing the data of the populations riance between the matrices is higher than the explained variance within these matrices, and in most cases are in

Table 4. Results for the estimation of means of empathic orientation. Standard error and Confidence Intervals for each level of combination of the factors University and Course.

Dental University	Course	Median	Standard Error	Confidence Interval of 95%	
				Lower Limit	Upper Limit
Universidad Latina de Panamá	First	100,833	5450	90,144	111,522
	Second	101,806	5578	90,865	112,746
	Third	102,056	7331	87,677	116,434
	Fourth	98,769	3345	92,208	105,330
	Fifth	109,722	2814	104,202	115,242
Universidad de Cartagena	First	100,618	1593	97,494	103,743
	Second	106,634	1561	103,572	109,696
	Third	107,509	2044	103,499	111,518
	Fourth	105,146	1828	101,561	108,732
	Fifth	107,715	1804	104,178	111,253
Universidad de Magdalena	First	92,977	2323	88,421	97,533
	Second	98,272	2611	93,151	103,394
	Third	98,100	2421	93,352	102,849
	Fourth	88,881	2543	83,894	93,868
	Fifth	84,220	2368	79,576	88,864
Universidad Metropolitana	First	97,615	2799	92,126	103,105
	Second	98,023	2314	93,485	102,561
	Third	100,089	2298	95,582	104,596
	Fourth	95,185	2833	89,629	100,740
	Fifth	109,392	3316	102,889	115,895
Universidad Central del Este	First	93,043	2247	88,636	97,449
	Second	97,783	1829	94,195	101,370
	Third	105,474	1894	101,759	109,189
	Fourth	105,050	2985	99,195	110,905
	Fifth	107,272	3234	100,930	113,614
ULACIT de Costa Rica	First	98,291	2515	93,358	103,224
	Second	103,847	2130	99,669	108,025
	Third	102,063	3474	95,249	108,877
	Fourth	105,188	2436	100,410	109,966
	Fifth	107,951	2423	103,199	112,703

Continued

	First	107,463	2209	103,130	111,796
	Second	109,383	1772	105,908	112,859
Universidad de Costa Rica	Third	109,290	1846	105,669	112,911
	Fourth	116,570	2382	111,899	121,242
	Fifth	116,733	2233	112,354	121,113
	First	106,899	2885	101,241	112,557
	Second	106,795	3368	100,191	113,400
Universidad de Panamá	Third	110,926	3965	103,149	118,704
	Fourth	100,317	4080	92,315	108,319
	Fifth	101,050	5527	90,209	111,891
	First	97,038	2424	92,285	101,792
	Second	99,625	2764	94,205	105,045
Universidad San Martín	Third	99,222	3761	91,846	106,598
	Fourth	112,655	2310	108,125	117,185
	Fifth	96,455	2177	92,185	100,724

formed by the interaction between the factors "Universities * Courses". The value of the Box M statistic (15553.48) was highly significant ($p < 0.005$); also indicating that the covariance matrices between populations, resulting from the combinations between the University and Course factors, differ.

5. Discussion

The results observed in the statisticians estimate for the variables of empathic orientation, comparing averages of this variable and the resulting matrix values and comparing these estimates between dental schools studied in Colombia, Panama, Costa Rica and Dominican Republic, allow the following generalizations: a) there are differences between dental schools of the universities studied; b) There are differences between courses, c) females have higher levels empathic orientation then males; d) interactions between factors (University and Course) were observed and, therefore, differences between populations derived from a combination at both levels; e) the existence of a coefficient of determination (R^2) relatively low and observation of a unexplained variance could be the expression of unknown factors or those not considered in this study and that they are influencing the variable factors of the level of empathy.

The variability of results observed in other studies, in which empathy levels were studied within each University or Faculty [11] [13]-[16] [27]-[38], allowed different findings. These differences are expressed in the factors studied, considering the course and gender. In some populations women were more empathic than men and in others the opposite occurred or simply there were no differences between genders. In the course factor, in some of the student populations, increasing with the elapsed academic years, in others it decreased and others remained stable. Besides the differences within these populations, we have found that they also occur among populations of students of the same career; possibley meaning, differences exist between schools within a country and between schools from different countries. One possible explanation for this variability is that the structure of each component of empathy depends on the influence of factors other than those of the other component. At the same time, empathy itself depends on the interaction between these components. Therefore, it is hypothetically possible to induce what is actually measured, with the applied scale, is the result of a complex process consisting in structuring and interaction of the components of empathy, a process that occurs in the context of another dimension: ontogenetic. As a consequence, the explanation of the variability between populations of students in relation to empathy is a complex problem [5]. The theory of mind and mirror neurons [39]-[46] can try to explain the processes occurring within the mind and there is empirical evidence to support it, but does not explain the entire process of formation of empathy. In this regard, the development process of the anatomical, psychological and neural basis of a subject, the way these are constructed and interact, are subjected to the action of external factors that act on the dialectical process [5]. As a result of the complex action of these factors, the way to integrate cognitive and affective components of empathy should be different among individuals, but also among populations, as these populations may have different economic standards and conditions, cultural, moral, educational, among others [1] [5]; which, can also differentially influence the building process of empathy. Therefore, the differences cannot be explained in this work; at best, be apprehended and a limitation of this study, which opens the doors to the need for further research to answer the question: What are all the factors responsible for these differences and how exactly do these modulate the process of the formation of empathy?

Current knowledge about empathy allows us to a firm that the formation of this construct in dentists (and in all professions in the area of health) is part of the responsibility of the universities [5] and, in this sense, some authors suggest that empathy can be learned [47] [48]. Therefore, the university has the task of studying the action of concrete practices that are possible to perform in order to raise levels of empathy in students, considering two aspects: a) that students who come to universities already have some empathic structure obtained by a previous experience of life and b) that the teaching of empathy in higher education (and in all educational systems) cannot be assumed with mechanistic conceptions. However, this work has restrictions which can be summarized as: a) the design used is cross-sectional and longitudinal study is needed to confirm whether these observed facts are maintained over time or vary with him and b) is necessary to study factors that could explain the behavior of the observed levels of empathy.

6. Conclusion

In accordance with the objective of this work, it was established that there was variability among student populations composed of dental schools in the same country and between schools from different countries. These differences could be empirical evidence of social and cultural factors that shaped empathy levels of a population and constituted a working hypothese for the future to clarify why this phenomenon occurred.

Competing Interests

The authors declare that they have no competing interests.

Financing

Research funded by the authors.

References

[1]   Hojat, M., Gonella, J.S., Nasca, T.J., Mangione, S., Vergare, M. and Magee, M. (2002) Physician Empathy: Definition, Components, Measurement and Relationship to Gender and Specialty. *American Journal of Psychiatry*, **159**, 1563-1569. http://dx.doi.org/10.1176/appi.ajp.159.9.1563

[2]   Morales, S. (2012) Study of Empathy Level and Achievement Motivation in Students of Dentistry in University of Concepcion. *Revista Educación en Ciencias de la Salud*, **9**, 121-125.

[3]   Bilbao, J., Alcócer, A., Salazar, G., Rivera, I., Zamorano, A. and Díaz-Narváez, V.P. (2013) Measurement of Empathetic Orientation in Dentistry Students of Fundación Universitaria San Martín. Puerto Colombia (Atlántico, Colombia). (Atlántico, Colombia). *Salud Uninorte (Barranquilla)*, **29**, 34-41.

[4]   Kane, G.C., Gotto, J.L., Mangione, S., West, S. and Hojat, M. (2007) Jefferson Scale of Patient's Perceptions Empathy: Preliminary Psychometric Data 2007. *Croatian Medical Journal*, **48**, 81-86.

[5]   Díaz-Narváez, V.P., Alonso, L.M., Caro, S.E., Silva, M.G., Arboleda, J., Bilbao, J.L. and Iglesias, J. (2014) Empathic Orientation among Medical Students from Three Universities in Barranquilla, Colombia and One University in the Dominican Republic. *Archivos Argentinos de Pediatría*, **112**, 41-49.

[6]   Stephenson, A., Higgs, R. and Sugarman, J. (2001) Teaching Professional Development in Medical Schools. *The Lancet*, **357**, 867-870. http://dx.doi.org/10.1016/S0140-6736(00)04201-X

[7]   Alcorta-Garza, A., González-Guerrero, J.F., Tavitas-Herrera, S.E., Rodríguez-Lara, F.J. and Hojat, M. (2005) Validation of the Scale of Empathy Medical Jefferson Medical Students in Mexico. *Salud Mental*, **28**, 57-63.

[8]   Hojat, M., Mangione, S., Kane, G.C. and Gonnella, J.S. (2005) Relationship between Scores of the Jefferson Scale of

Physician Emphaty (JSPE) and the Interpersonal Reactivity Index (IRI). *Medical Teacher*, **27**, 625-628.
http://dx.doi.org/10.1080/01421590500069744

[9]   Roh, M., Hahm, B., Lee, D. and Suh, D. (2010) Evaluation of Empathy among Korean Medical Students: A
      Cross-Seccional Study Using the Korean Version of the Jefferson Scale of Physician Empathy. *Teaching and Learning
      in Medicine*, **22**, 167-171. http://dx.doi.org/10.1080/10401334.2010.488191

[10] Kataoka, H., Koide, N., Ochi, K., Hojat, M. and Gonnella, J. (2009) Measurement of Empathy among Japanese Medi-
      cal Student. Psychometrics and Score Differences by Gender and Level of Medical Education. *Academic Medicine*, **84**,
      1192-1197. http://dx.doi.org/10.1097/ACM.0b013e3181b180d4

[11] Silva, M.G., Arboleda, J. and Díaz-Narváez, V.P. (2013) Empathic Orientation Dental Students from the Universidad
      Central Del Este. *Odontoestomatología*, **15**, 24-33.

[12] Díaz-Narváez, V.P. (2009) Scientific Research Methodology and Biostatistics for Professionals and Students of Health
      Sciences. 2ed, RiL Editores, Santiago.

[13] Erazo, A.M., Alonso, L.M., Rivera, I., Zamorano, A. and Díaz-Narváez, V.P. (2012) Measuring Empathic Orientation
      Dental Students Barranquilla Metropolitan University (Colombia). *Revista Salud Uninorte*, **28**, 354-363.

[14] Sánchez, L., Padilla, M., Rivera, I., Zamorano, A. and Díaz-Narváez, V.P. (2013) Evaluation of Empathetic Orienta-
      tion in Odontology Students. *Educación   Médica Superior*, **27**, 216-225.

[15] Howard, M., Navarro, S., Rivera, I., Zamorano, A. and Díaz-Narváez, V.P. (2013) Measuring the Level of Empathic
      Orientation in the Student of the Faculty of Dentistry, University of Costa Rica. *Revista Odovtos*, **15**, 21-26.

[16] Rivera, I., Arratia, R., Zamorano, A. and Díaz-Narváez, V.P. (2011) Evaluación del nivel de orientación empática en
      estu-diantes de Odontología. *Salud Uninorte (Barranquilla, Colombia)*, **27**, 63-72.

[17] Leyva, Y.E. (2011) A Review of the Construct Validity of Criterion-Referenced Tests. *Perfiles Educativos*, **33**, 131-
      154.

[18] Cervantes, V. (2005) Interpretations of Cronbach's Alpha Coefficient. *Avances en Medición*, **3**, 9-28.

[19] Oviedo, H.C. and Campo-Arias, A. (2005) An Approach to the Use of Cronbach's Alfa. *Revista Colombiana de Psi-
      quiatría*, **34**, 572-580.

[20] Streiner, D.L. (2003) Starting at the Beginning: An Introduction to Coefficient Alpha and Internal Consistency. *Jour-
      nal of Personality Assessment*, **80**, 99-103. http://dx.doi.org/10.1207/S15327752JPA8001_18

[21] Shapiro, S.S. and Wilk, M.B. (1965) An Analysis of Variance Test for Normality (Complete Samples). *Biometrika*, **52**,
      591-611. http://dx.doi.org/10.1093/biomet/52.3-4.591

[22] Hair, J.F., Anderson, R.E., Tatham, R.L. and Black, W.C. (2001) Multivariate Analysis. Prentice-Hall, Madrid.

[23] Frías, M.D., Llobell, J.P. and García, J. (2000) Size of Treatment Effect and Statistical Significance. *Psicothema*, **2**,
      236-240.

[24] Levy, J.P. and Varela, J. (2003) Multivariate Analysis for the Social Sciences. Pearson Prentice-Hall, Madrid, 249-257.

[25] Visauta, B. (1998) Statistical Analysis with SPSS: Vol. II. McGraw-Hill, Madrid, 135-137.

[26] Palacios, S. (2007) Development and Validation of the Scale of Values Domains Television (DETV). *Revista Investi-
      gación en Educación*, **25**, 403-420.

[27] Silva, H., Rivera, I., Zamorano, A. and Díaz-Narváez, V.P. (2013) Evaluation of Empathetic Orientation in Dentistry
      Students of Finis Terrae University in Santiago, Chile. *Revista Clínica de Periodoncia, Implantología y Rehabilitación
      Oral*, **6**, 130-133.

[28] Carrasco, D., Bustos, A. and Díaz, V. (2012) Empathetic Orientation of Chilean Dental Students. *Revista Estoma-
      tológica Herediana*, **22**, 145-151.

[29] Oviedo, M. (2011) Empathy Training of Students in the Faculty of Dentistry at the University of Carabobo. Univer-
      sidad Autónoma de Madrid, 158.
      http://biblioteca.universia.net/html_bura/ficha/params/title/empatia-estudiantes-formacion-facultad-odontologia-univer
      sidad-carabobo/id/55311551.html

[30] Alonso, L.M., Caro, S.E., Erazo, A.M. and Díaz-Narváez, V.P. (2013) Evaluación de la orientación empática en estu-
      diantes de medicina de la Universidad del Norte. Barranquilla (Colombia). *Revista Salud Uninorte*, **29**, 22-33.

[31] Rojas-Serey, A.M., Castañeda-Barthelemiez, S. and Parraguez-Infiesta, R.A. (2009) Empathetic Orientation of the
      Physical Therapist's Students from Two Schools of Chile. *Educación Médica*, **12**, 103-109.

[32] Chen, D., Lew, R., Hershman, W. and Orlander, J. (2007) A Cross-Sectional Measurement of Medical Student Empa-
      thy. *Journal of General Internal Medicine*, **22**, 1434-1438. http://dx.doi.org/10.1007/s11606-007-0298-x

[33] Bellini, L. and Shea, J. (2005) Mood Change and Empathy Decline Persist during Three Years of Internal Medicine
      Training. *Academic Medicine*, **80**, 164-167. http://dx.doi.org/10.1097/00001888-200502000-00013

[34]   Chen, J., LaLopa, J. and Dang, D. (2008) Impact of Patient Empathy Modeling on Pharmacy Students Caring for the Underserved. *American Journal of Pharmaceutical Education*, **72**, Article 40. http://dx.doi.org/10.5688/aj720240

[35]   Nunes, P., Willians, S., Sa, B. and Stevenson, K. (2011) A Study of Emphaty Decline in Students from Five Health Disciplines during Their First Year of Training. *International Journal of Medical Education*, **2**, 12-17. http://dx.doi.org/10.5116/ijme.4d47.ddb0

[36]   Hojat, M., Vergare, M.J., Maxwell, K., Brainard, G., Herrine, S.K., Isenberg, G.A., Veloski, J. and Gonnella, J.S. (2009) The Devil Is in the Third Year: A Longitudinal Study of Erosion of Empathy in Medical School. *Academic Medicine*, **84**, 1182-1191. http://dx.doi.org/10.1097/ACM.0b013e3181b17e55

[37]   Sherman, J. and Cramer, A. (2005) Measurement of Changes in Empathy during Dental School. *Journal of Dental Education*, **69**, 338-345.

[38]   Beattie, A., Durham, J., Harvey, J., Steele, J. and McHanwell, S. (2012) Does Empathy Change in First-Year Dental Student? *European Journal of Dental Education*, **16**, e111-e116. http://onlinelibrary.wiley.com/doi/10.1111/j.1600-0579.2011.00683.x/full

[39]   Gutiérrez-Ventura, F., Quezada-Huerta, B., López-Pinedo, M., Méndez-Vergaray, J., Díaz-Narváez, V., Zamorano, A. and Rivera, I. (2012) Measuring the Level of Empathic Perception of Students of the Faculty of Dentistry Robert Beltrán. Cayetano Heredia Peruvian University. *Revista Estomatológica Herediana*, **22**, 91-99.

[40]   Varela, T., Villalba, R.H., Gargantini, P., Quinteros, S., Villaba, S.B. and Díaz-Narváez, V.P. (2012) Levels of Empathic Orientation Dental Students at the Catholic University of Cordoba, Argentina (UCC). *Claves de Odontología*, **70**, 15-22.

[41]   Rivera, I., Arratia, R., Zamorano, A. and Díaz-Narváez, V.P. (2011) Measurement of Empathetic Orientation in Dentistry Students. *Revista Salud Uninorte*, **27**, 63-72.

[42]   Garaigordobil, M. and García de Galdeano, P. (2006) Empathy in Children Aged 10 to 12 Years. *Psicothema*, **18**, 180-186.

[43]   Rizzolatti, G., Fogassi, L. and Gallese, V. (2001) Neurophisiological Mechanisms Underlying the Understanding and Imitation of Action. *Nature Reviews Neuroscience*, **2**, 661-670. http://dx.doi.org/10.1038/35090060

[44]   García-García, E., González, J. and Maestú-Unturbe, F. (2011) Mirror Neurons and Theory of Mind in Explaining Empathy. *Ansiedad y Estrés*, **17**, 265-279.

[45]   Arán, V., López, M.B. and Richaud, M.C. (2012) Neuropsychological Approach to the Empathy Construct: Cognitive and Neuroanatomical Aspects. *Cuadernos de Neuropsicología*, **6**, 63-83.

[46]   Smith, A. (2006) Cognitive Empathy and Emotional Empathy in Human Behavior and Evolution. *The Psychological Record*, **56**, 3-21.

[47]   Almonte, C. and Montt, M.A. (2012) Child and Adolescent Psychopathology. 2ª Ed, Mediterráneo, Santiago, 45-58.

[48]   Schwartz, B. and Bohay, R. (2012) Can Patients Help Teach Professionalism and Empathy to Dental Students? Adding Patient Videos to a Lecture Course. *Journal of Dental Education*, **76**, 174-184.

10

Understanding the Experiences of Heavy Smokers after Exercise

Mary Hassandra[1], Athanasios Kolovelonis[2], Stiliani Ani Chroni[3], Alkistis Olympiou[4], Marios Goudas[2], Yiannis Theodorakis[2]

[1]Department of Sports, University of Jyväskylä, Jyväskylä, Finland
[2]Department of Physical Education & Sport Science, University of Thessaly, Trikala, Greece
[3]Department of Sports & Physical Education, Hedmark University College, Elverum, Norway
[4]School of Sport and Exercise Science, College of Social Science, University of Lincoln, Lincoln, UK
Email: mgoudas@pe.uth.gr

Abstract

There is now strong evidence that exercise has an acute effect on the urge to smoke and the accompanying withdrawal symptoms. However, the perceptions by heavy smokers of exercise and its relationship to the urge to smoke have not been well documented. The aim of the present study is to understand the experiences of heavy smokers with regard to exercise and its effect on their urge to smoke. Five physically inactive, heavy smokers are asked to abstain from smoking the night before exercising on a cycle ergometer under two conditions (one at medium and one at vigorous intensity done a week apart). Semi-structured, in-depth interviews are conducted after the second exercise session. Thematic analysis reveals six themes describing the participants' experience of exercise, urge to smoke, exercise preferences, exercise and smoking relationship, exercise as an aid to quit smoking, and the effects of the experimental procedure. Overall, the participants' experiences support the existing literature, which has posited affective, biological, and cognitive mechanisms contributing to a delay in the urge to smoke after exercise. The main findings pertain to: (1) the "feel-good" effect after exercise as a relief from the "feel-bad" effect during exercise; (2) the decreased urge to smoke after exercise, stated by all participants regardless of reported positive and negative feelings; and (3) exercise as a "clearing the mind" mechanism rather than an attention-distracting mechanism.

Keywords

Physical Activity, Smoking, Perceptions, Intensity, Urge to Smoke

1. Introduction

Physical activity and smoking are among those modifiable behaviors that have a positive impact on health. Today, there is abundant evidence for the positive effect of physical activity on health [1] [2]. However, only 15% of Greeks take some forms of physical activity 5 times a week and only 3% play sport at least once a week [3]. With regard to smoking, research has shown that it exacerbates the prevalence of various functional problems, leading to serious diseases and an increased mortality rate [4] [5]. Indeed, according to the HEART-funded Hellas Tobacco Survey in a nationwide household survey conducted in 2010, the prevalence of smoking in Greece was calculated at 41% (45% among men and 38% in women, $p = 0.04$). It is considered as one of the highest per capita consumption rates of tobacco products among European Union member states [6].

Although research examining physical activity and smoking behaviors started during the 1980s [7] [8], for some years the relationship between these behaviors was not clarified. Over the last decade, studies have supported an existing inverse relationship between the two variables [9] [10]. Despite the fact that studies of exercise-based treatments for substance use disorders have, in general, provided limited and inconsistent evidence, there are several theoretical and practical arguments in favor of such interventions [11]. Today, there are two groups of studies that have examined exercise interventions in relation to smoking: those examining the acute effects e.g. [12] and those examining the long-term effects e.g. [13]. Their respective results can enhance our understanding of how exercise can be used as treatment for smoking. However, there is little information from the acute-effect exercise studies about smokers' perception of exercise. Such information may improve the effectiveness of exercise-aided, smoking-cessation interventions.

In the last few years, three reviews on the acute effects of exercise on smoking-related measures were published: Haasova *et al.* [12], Roberts, Maddison, Simpson, Bullen, and Prapavessis [14], and Taylor, Ussher, and Faulkner [15]. Taylor *et al.* [15] reviewed 14 studies, 12 of which compared exercise bout with a passive condition; they reported a positive effect of exercise on cigarette craving, withdrawal symptoms, and smoking behavior. The other two studies compared exercise bout with two different intensities, revealing no differences in smoking-related outcomes. In all the studies reviewed, cigarette craving, withdrawal symptoms, and negative affect decreased during exercise and remained low for up to 50 minutes after it. Specifically, cravings and withdrawal symptoms were reduced after an exercise bout with intensity ranging from 60% - 85% of the heart rate reserve (HRR) (lasting 30 - 40 min) to 24% of the HRR (lasting 15 min), and similarly with isometric exercise (for 5 min). Taylor *et al.* [15] concluded that even relatively small doses of exercise should be recommended as an aid for managing cigarette craving and withdrawal symptoms. For future research, they suggested that the mechanisms involved, such as stress reduction and neurobiological mechanisms should be explored further because these could lead to the development of more effective and practical methods for managing withdrawal phenomena.

The review of Haasova *et al.* [12] used individual participants' data from 17 studies and compared participants engaging in physical activity with control group participants, using post-intervention measurements of strength of desire to smoke with baseline adjustments. Despite a high degree of between-study heterogeneity, their results showed physical activity groups achieving a greater reduction in cravings compared with the controls. The latest review by Roberts *et al.* [14] revealed similar findings: cigarette craving was reduced after exercise for a wide range of intensities, ranging from isometric exercise and yoga to vigorous activity of 80% - 85% of the HRR. However, they reported that tobacco withdrawal symptoms and negative affect increased during vigorous exercise. They highlighted that, although we have evidence for the acute effect of exercise on reducing cigarette craving, it remains unclear which is the most effective exercise intensity to reduce the craving and what the underlying mechanisms associated with these effects are.

In an effort to identify potential mechanisms that could explain why exercise alleviates tobacco craving, Roberts *et al.* [14] clustered the most recent research findings into three hypothetical explanatory mechanisms: the affective, the biological, and the cognitive. According to the affective hypothetical mechanism, research evidence supports the claim that an increase in positive affect could result in a decreased desire to smoke. However, results from different studies disagree on the optimal level of intensity required to create an increase in positive effect, e.g., according to Bock, Marcus, King, Borrelli, and Roberts [16] and Harper [17] a bout of vigorous exercise reduced the negative affect and psychological withdrawal symptoms, respectively, in smokers undertaking an exercise-aided program for quitting smoking. Yet, in Everson, Daley, and Ussher's study [18], both moderate and vigorous intensity exercise conditions yielded similar effects on cravings and a notably adverse effect on mood. Everson *et al.* [18] suggested that perhaps moderate intensity exercise rather than vigorous exercise should be prescribed. They attributed the contradictory findings mainly to the participants' varying levels of motivation, and hypothesized that less tolerance to the vigorous exercise can be explained by the fact that these participants were abstaining from smoking for research purposes and so were not truly motivated to quit.

The biological hypothetical mechanism, which concerns the link between physiological exercise and smoking-related variables, remains uncharted territory. It is hypothesized that psychobiological changes (such as β-endorphins, opioids, and cortisol) can mediate the changes in withdrawal symptoms associated with exercise. Studies have supported changes in heart rate variability, caused by short or long abstinence and acute bouts of exercise, possibly having an immediate effect [19]-[21]. For example, a single session of exercise (e.g. a self-paced 15-min walk) can attenuate or reduce both post-exercise systolic and diastolic blood pressure responses to stress [22] [23].

The cognitive perspective, which claims that exercise may influence cognitive demands in such a way that it acts as a distraction from smoking-related thoughts, has not gained support recently due to no studies reporting an effect on distraction from cigarette craving [17] [24]-[26]. Roberts *et al.* [14] postulated that expectancy and credibility are two factors that need further examination as possible regulating factors in future research on the cognitive hypothesis. At the same time, the study [27] revealed varying cognitive activation of smokers towards smoking images after exercise when compared with control treatment. This finding suggests a neurocognitive process possibly being initiated after exercise, which mediates an effect on cigarette craving.

In conclusion, according to the research evidence it can be postulated that an acute bout of exercise reduces cigarette craving and other smoking-related variables, whereas part of the variation in the magnitude of the effects depends on the exercise intensity. But the question remains: How is this information linked to the knowledge that we need for promoting the adoption and maintenance of exercise among smokers who try to quit? To enrich our knowledge, we employed a qualitative methodological approach to explore answers to the following research question: How are acute bouts of exercise (of two different intensities) experienced by physically inactive, heavy smokers? We deemed that new information could possibly help researchers consider the potential pitfalls of acute exercise studies conducted in laboratory settings, because often laboratory effects do not translate well to the real world, when smokers try to quit using exercise as an aid. This approach can also provide a platform for rich participant-based information, from which new variables could emerge that act as potential moderators and mediators in the link between exercise and smoking behaviors.

2. Methods

The present study was part of a larger project aiming to examine the effects of exercise on physiological and psychological parameters related to smoking. The project consisted of a series of laboratory and field experiments which employed various exercise regimes.

2.1. Participants

The participants were five healthy Greek adults (four males and one female; mean age 36.00 ± 3.39 years), recruited through advertisements in the press offering a small monetary incentive to participate in the study. They obtained a doctor's permission to participate in the study. They were heavy smokers (mean number of cigarettes per day 24 ± 5.48; mean score on the Fagerstrom Nicotine Dependence Scale 6.80 ± 1.64) and physically inactive (as assessed by the International Physical Activity Questionnaire—short form—IPAQ, www.ipaq.ki.se), and were asked to abstain from smoking the night before the exercise. Their CO levels showed (PICO Smokerlyser, Bedfont, Rochester, UK) that they had indeed followed instructions and abstained from smoking (<15 p.p.m. [parts per million], mean = 11.7 ± 6.14 p.p.m. for vigorous and 12.6 ± 5.37 p.p.m. for moderate exercise).

2.2. Setting—Procedure—Data Collection

Ethical approval for the current study was granted by the University of Thessaly Ethics Review Committee. Participants signed consent forms which informed them of their participation and withdrawal rights. They exercised on a cycle ergometer (Monark874E, Sweden) for 30 min under two different intensity conditions, with a 1-week interval between the two sessions. In one condition they were required to exercise at a medium intensity, maintaining their heart rate (HR) at an estimated 50% - 60% of their HRR. In the other they were required to exercise at vigorous intensity, maintaining their HR at an estimated 65% - 75% of their HRR. The order of medium and vigorous exercise intensities was counterbalanced across the participants. **Table 1** displays the physiological measures recorded during the two exercise conditions for each participant. In the vigorous-intensity condition the average HR and workload were higher and the average CO and carboxyhemoglobin levels were lower, although these values were the reverse of those seen in the medium-intensity condition.

Interviews were conducted immediately after completion of the second exercise session in a quiet setting. The duration of the interviews ranged from 45 min to 60 min. The main interview questions were:

"How did you perceive the exercise experience you just completed?"

"What were your feelings/thoughts before and during the exercise session in comparison to what they are now–after the exercise?"

"Can you make a comparison between the two exercise sessions, last week and this week?"

"Being a smoker, do you think it affected your exercise experience? If yes, how?"

"Did the exercise sessions impact your urge to smoke immediately after the exercise? If yes, how?"

"If you chose to exercise in everyday life, what would you choose to do?"

"Would you in the future choose exercise as a supportive aid to quit if you decided to quit smoking?"

As the main perspective in qualitative research interviewing is personal meaning [28], the interviews conducted aimed to capture how the participants interpreted and understood the exercise experience through their own personal meaning. Follow-up probes were also used to promote dialogue and to obtain more detailed descriptions of the smokers' experiences during and after the exercise sessions, considering their perceptions, feelings, thoughts, interpretations, etc. Examples of probes include: "Can you tell me more about…?", "Can you give me an example of…?" The interviews were conducted by the second author, they were audio recorded and then transcribed verbatim. The transcriptions yielded 72 pages of single-spaced text.

2.3. Data Analysis

Thematic analysis [29] was used to analyze the transcribed interviews. Analysis took place "at the end" [30]—the coders—researchers analyzed the data after completion of data collection. Two of the authors read the transcriptions and identified higher-order themes, based on the research questions that had been developed initially. At the next step, lower-order themes within each higher-order theme were identified inductively. The data-driven lower-order themes were identified within the raw information and were grouped under each higher-order theme. The purpose was to search for patterns based on the information being studied [29]. During the categorization of the lower-order themes, the two authors discussed all themes exhaustively to reach a consensus. To enhance the reliability of themes and coding, a third author commented and the appropriate corrections were made until the three researchers had reached agreement.

Peer debriefing sessions were also conducted (with a researcher external to the study who was competent in qualitative methodology) to examine the methodological procedures and interpretations of the data coding [31]. To achieve trustworthiness [32], the following methods were used: (a) checking of members was carried out during and after the interviews; (b) the second researcher—interviewer kept notes of personal thoughts and nonverbal forms of communication during the exercise sessions and interviews, which comprised a reflexive

Table 1. Physiological measures for each participant and exercise intensity.

	Medium intensity						Vigorous intensity					
	HR (beats/min)		WL (W)		CO (p.p.m.)	COHb (%)	HR (beats/min)		WL (W)		CO (p.p.m.)	COHb (%)
Participants	Mean	SD	Mean	SD			Mean	SD	Mean	SD		
Participant 1	133.33	6.86	88.10	11.36	7	1.6	148.17	15.05	96.53	12.36	5.5	1.5
Participant 2	128.83	6.85	107.05	9.12	15	3	142.67	5.43	101.33	11.38	20	3.4
Participant 3	127.50	7.69	83.73	18.92	7	1.8	151.83	6.97	109.00	22.26	6	1.6
Participant 4	127.83	6.55	75.53	8.24	19	3.7	138.83	14.91	106.95	17.40	15	3
Participant 5	133.00	6.00	84.63	12.85	15	3	142.33	16.51	102.50	16.76	12	2.6

Note: CO: carbon monoxide; COHb: carboxyhemoglobin; HR: heart rate; p.p.m.: parts per million; SD: standard deviation; WL: workload.

journal; (c) triangulation of the data [3] analysis was achieved by examining the participants' data on the physiological and psychological measures and the notes of the interviewer.

3. Results and Discussion

Analysis of the data produced the thematic structure shown in **Table 2**. Six higher-order themes were labeled: (1) experience of the exercise; (2) the urge to smoke; (3) exercise preferences; (4) the exercise and smoking rela-

Table 2. Thematic structure of data analysis.

Experience of exercise			
During exercise	Affective	Negative	Hard, tired, unpleasant, pressure, wish to finish soon, negative thoughts
		Positive	Happy
	Biological	Negative	Heavy legs
After exercise	Affective	Negative	Tired, exhausted, stressed, difficult, tension, weak (immediately after)
		Positive	Relaxed, satisfied, optimistic, better mood, positive, calm, more energy, more alive mentally and physically, more vivid, think better, active (after 15 mins)
	Biological	Negative	Heavy and tired legs, hard even to walk, high heart rate, sweaty, painful
	Cognitive		Is it because we forget or a relief from a false alert?
Urge to smoke			
During exercise	Affective	Higher urge	Stress, anxiety, need to relax from the tension (high intensity), pressure (high intensity)
	Cognitive	Low urge	Not thinking of smoking at all
		Higher urge	As an escape from exercise pressure
After exercise	Affective	Low urge	Need to relax and calm down first, tired, exhausted, feelings of wellness, relaxed
	Biological	Low urge	Sweaty, out of breath, "open" lungs, breathing difficulties, need to rest first
	Cognitive	Low urge	No thoughts of smoking, clears your mind, not to waste the effort and satisfaction from accomplishment to finish the exercise
Exercise preference			
Preferred intensity	Vigor	Affective	Better when I feel tense, difficult at first but then much better, more self-satisfaction, more enjoyable, gives more energy
	Moderate	Affective	More pleasant, easier, less tired
		Cognitive	As beneficial as vigor
Preferred type of exercise and intensity in everyday life	Unsupervised	Outdoors	Walking, jogging, gardening
	Supervised	Indoors	Gym
	Gradual increase		Gradual increase in both intensity and duration
Exercise and smoking relationship			
Effects of exercise on smoking behavior	Does not affect		Unrelated behaviors, compatible behaviors (if light physical activity or light smoker), no effect on managing desire to smoke
	Does affect		Positive effect on general sense of self-control, increase in self-efficacy over behavioral control
Effects of smoking on exercise behavior			Breathing problems, discomfort, low endurance, negative thoughts, difficult

Continued

Exercise as an aid to quitting smoking	
Would use under conditions	Moderate in intensity
	Gradually increased intensity and duration
	In combination with medicine
	In combination with a strong will to quit
Reasons to use exercise as an aid to quitting smoking	Escape from sedentary routine
	Feel healthier
	Realize the harm of smoking
	Social support/comparison
	Empowerment to quit
	Distraction from smoking
	Feel-good effect
Effects of experimental procedure	
On stress	During their first exercise experience, feelings of tension, stress
On urge to smoke	Increased urge to smoke due to unfamiliar environment
Momentum	Exercising as an experience to realize the negative effects of smoking on physical condition

tionship; (5) exercise as an aid to quitting smoking; and (6) the effects of the experimental procedure. A presentation of the themes follows, describing the meaning that participants attributed to the experience of not smoking from the previous night until after the morning of moderate- or vigorous-intensity exercise. Discussion of the findings has been incorporated into the results section to help the reader place the findings and their interpretations within the existing related literature.

3.1. The Experience of Exercise

Participants described their exercise experience using both positive and negative words. Comments related to their somatic condition were mostly negative about how they felt during the exercise or immediately after. Their responses reflected the increased fatigue or perceived exertion:

"*During cycling I felt exhausted, but after I finished it feels OK, back to normal*".

"*In the beginning, I was feeling happy but as time was passing by I was very tired and wished to finish as soon as possible*".

Similar experiences have been reported extensively by physically inactive smokers in previous research [24] [33] and are considered to be the main reason for limited compliance with the exercise programs [34]. Affective comments were also both positive and negative, with the negative ones referring to feelings during exercise as well us on completion, whereas positive ones referred to the period during which the participants' HR dropped. Similarly, in the relevant literature findings, exercise-related affective responses were positive [16] [35] or negative [18].

A comment made by a participant, who tried to explain why he thought he had negative feelings during exercise and positive ones after, could be a topic for further investigation:

"*Is it because we forget? Maybe we think that it is OK when the pain (in the legs) is gone and then you say to yourself it is OK, it was nothing*".

Thus, he explained that this happened possibly because he forgot the negative feelings he had during exercise with the relief of the positive feelings after the exercise, which compensated for the intense negative feelings during exercise.

3.2. Urge to Smoke

Consistent with results from previous studies that suggest that exercise might reduce the urge to smoke and the accompanying withdrawal symptoms [25], most of our participants reported a decrease in the urge to smoke for a period ranging from 15 min to half a day. Participants' attributions for this delay in the urge to smoke related not only to affective and biological reasons but also to cognitive ones:

"... *because you made a conscious effort to exercise and you felt satisfied with yourself that you did it*".

It is interesting that both positive (e.g. wellness) and negative (e.g. exhaustion, tiredness) feelings were used as explanations for the decreased urge to smoke. When affect is changed during or after exercise (positively and/or negatively), it appears to decrease one's urge to smoke at that moment. Nevertheless, negative affect experienced after a vigorous exercise session can also have a detrimental influence on future exercise adoption and maintenance [35] [36]. According to a recent systematic review [37], a positive change in the basic affective response during moderate exercise was linked to future physical activity, but the post-exercise affect had a null relationship. They also found that affective responses during and after exercise correlated reliably with affective judgments about future physical activity. Other participants in our study provided answers that are more aligned with the biological approach, such as breathing difficulties and a sense of deep breathing, or "open" lungs as they described it. McClernon, Westman, and Rose [38] also detected this effect of (controlled) deep breathing on decreased withdrawal symptoms in dependent smokers.

A cognitive approach-related explanation was provided by some participants who elaborated on the absence of thoughts about smoking. The previous literature suggests that exercise acts as a mechanism that distracts attention; however, it was questioned whether this explanatory mechanism had been tested in an experiment [25]. In a research report, Daniel *et al.* [25] concluded that the effect of exercise in reducing both the desire to smoke and cigarette withdrawal symptoms is not caused by distraction. Based on contradictory findings, and due to the absence of adequate empirical evidence, further investigations should explore exercise as a "clearing the mind" procedure immediately after the exercise.

Some of our participants shared thoughts of smoking being present, but they tried to manage and control them. According to Ekkekakis and Acevedo [39], exercise acts as a thought suppressant, shifting one's attention from cognitive to somatic thoughts. The thought-suppression mechanism in smokers has generated quite controversial results in the literature. There are findings in support of the notion that thought suppression leads to a decreased desire to smoke [40], whereas other findings postulate that suppression of smoking thoughts results in increased subsequent smoking behavior [41]. Participants in the present study stated that they were trying to manage their smoking thoughts by rationalizing why they should not smoke after participating in an exercise session:

"... *because you made a conscious effort to exercise and you felt satisfied with yourself that you did it*".

It would be interesting, in future studies, to examine the effectiveness of suppression of smoking thoughts after an exercise session.

Although four participants reported a delay in the smoking urge, one of them indicated that he experienced an increase in his urge to smoke, especially during the vigorous exercise session:

"... *the urge to smoke was higher before exercise as well as during exercise but lower after exercise*".

Then he explained the increased urge as a reaction to the pressure that he felt during the exercise sessions. He specifically said:

"*I would like to have a cigarette to relax from the tension of exercise*".

Feelings of distress during vigorous exercise have been reported by smokers [18], and smoking is commonly explained by them as a stress management reaction [42].

3.3. Exercise Preference

With regard to the preferred intensity of the condition, most participants favored the medium intensity and explained their preference with both affective and cognitive statements, e.g.:

"*I prefer the medium intensity, because as I said I am not used to exercise and it was an easier task for me than the intense*".

The affective statements pertained to the differential feelings experienced during the two conditions, with greater emphasis on the more negative ones during vigorous exercise. Consistent with results from previous studies [18], moderate intensity was preferable because it was accompanied by more positive feelings and perceived benefits. The cognitive statement supporting the perceived positive benefits (or outcome expectancies) suggested that medium intensity was preferable. Outcome expectancies have been studied in the previous literature in relation to cravings or other tobacco withdrawal symptoms [17] [26], but not to the preferred exercise condition.

Preference for high-intensity exercise under specific conditions was reported by one participant who explained his choice through the affective perspective:

"... *high intensity is preferable, difficult at first but then much better; the first 5 minutes makes you feel exhausted–tired causing breathing difficulties but after that point it was enjoyable. High-intensity exercise gives me more energy*".

This participant was physically inactive, similar to the other participants, but during the interview he shared that he had been an athlete in the past. It is possible that the exercise-induced increase in his positive affect was triggered by his positive memory traces related to his past experiences as a competitive athlete. According to existing studies [37] [43], it is possible for an exerciser's memory to consciously or subconsciously influence the affect.

Statements about participants' preferences for physical activities in everyday life varied, depending on the type and duration of exercise; however, with regard to exercise intensity, most of the participants favored a gradual increase:

"*I do not like to feel pushed (during exercise). I want to gradually increase the intensity*".

Gradual increase in exercise intensity has been found to be beneficial for smokers who attended a program to quit smoking using exercise as an aid [16] [17]. When the participants attempted to explain their preferences over the type, duration, and intensity of exercise, their words reflected feelings of autonomy ("*I would rather choose a mix of intensities according to my mood*"), relatedness ("*socializing while exercising is preferable*"), and competence ("*my physical condition is not good, so I easily get tired*"). These quotes reflect a basic tenet of self-determination theory [44], which posits that one's intrinsic motivation for participation in a given activity is contingent on the satisfaction of one's basic needs of competence, autonomy, and relatedness.

3.4. Exercise and Smoking Relationship

Negative effects of smoking on exercise behavior were reported by the participants, e.g.:

"*Cigarettes had an effect on my negative thoughts ... more negative thoughts than a non-smoker; it would be easier had I been a non-smoker*".

These negative effects are consistent with what is found in the literature, for example [45]. However, two participants shared their physical activity and smoking behaviors being unrelated to each other, although the two behaviors coexist:

"*I do not believe that exercise can make me stronger at managing my desire to smoke; it is just the good mood feeling at this moment*".

When probed, they elaborated further that these behaviors can coexist when engaged in a lighter type of physical activity:

"*I can smoke at the same time when gardening or biking, but it is not as enjoyable*".

According to Boutelle, Murray, Jeffery, Hennrikus, and Lando [46], there may be a threshold level of exercise that must be reached for either physiological changes to occur in smokers' behavior or a negative effect on other behaviors to occur.

On the contrary, another participant stated that being physically active could be beneficial for his sense of self-efficacy and self-control, in general:

"*... exercise had a positive effect on my perceived sense of control ... increased my sense of being effective over controlling my health behavior even if this is not the smoking behavior itself but maybe in general*".

It should be noted here, and it is discussed again later, that this participant was the one who reported the momentum effect of the exercise experimental procedure on him outside the lab exercise behavior. It has been stated that changes in a harmful behavior (such as inactivity) may serve as a "gateway" for changing other behaviors (such as smoking), whereas increased self-efficacy, motivation, or self-confidence acts as a mediating mechanism [47]-[49].

3.5. Exercise as an Aid to Quitting Smoking

When asked if they would choose exercise as an aid to quitting smoking, most participants answered that they would use it under certain conditions:

"*I would choose a moderate exercise due to my low fitness levels*" or "*Exercise might help me quit smoking but only if I had a strong will to quit*".

The participants reported the following mechanisms with regard to how exercise might help them: the "feel-good" effect of exercise, distraction of attention, empowerment of changing one behavior for another (the "gateway" effect), routine changes to everyday life, recognition of benefits for a healthy lifestyle, realization of the harmful effect of smoking, and social support that they could get in group-based exercise programs. For example, one participant, when explaining how exercise might aid his effort to quit smoking, said:

"*... because it would make me escape from the sedentary everyday routine and later, when I feel healthier and more active, then it might make me think that the smoking habit holds me back and I have to stop [smoking]*".

Participants' statements about the link between their experiences of the acute effects of exercise and possible future attempts to quit smoking using exercise as a supportive method were related to the intensity of the proposed exercise program, their motivation to quit, and the additional support that could be received during the program (e.g. drug support). Existing empirical results suggest that the most effective programs for quitting smoking used a combined methods approach [50] [51], which appeared to be what our participants favored.

3.6. Effects of the Experimental Procedure

An unanticipated higher-order theme, relating to the experimental procedure itself, which appeared to have an effect on two participants, was identified in their answers without any probing or questioning. The theme was about the unfamiliar laboratory environment and experimental protocol, especially during their first visit, which pressured the participants:

"*... during the first time, the lab, the experimental environment and procedure had an effect on the urge to smoke because I was unfamiliar and I felt a lot of pressure*".

This might have had an effect on the exercise experience, which they shared with us. However, for another participant the experimental procedure had a different effect:

"*I already started walking, four days now. I was never doing this before. The reason was: the first session was very tough on me when after 15 minutes on the bike I started feeling tired. And this made me think. And this thinking is working now a little and the only problem is smoking*".

The first exercise session provided the momentum for him to continue, and soon after he realized that his fitness level was very low. This increased awareness motivated him to make an effort to increase his physical activity during the week between the two exercise sessions.

In general, the findings of the present study are in accordance with previous studies investigating the acute effects of exercise on abstinent smokers using a quantitative approach. Nevertheless, our findings also offer insights into and raise concerns about particular issues that should be taken into account when studying the mechanisms of acute exercise-induced effects on smokers' behaviors.

4. Limitations

Our study had several limitations: first, it is limited by its retrospective design for one of the two exercise sessions because the interviews were conducted after the second session. Participants were asked to recall their thoughts and feelings for the first of the two sessions in addition to the one they had just completed, which may have produced errors in inherent cognitive recall (especially errors of attribution) and time recall, and selective perception biases might have had an effect on their descriptions of what and when they felt or thought. However, by counterbalancing the order of medium and vigorous exercise intensities across participants and using probes for crucial answers, e.g. "How long after the end of the exercise session you ..." we partially controlled for these limitations and their effects on the data. A second limitation relates to the sample size, which was small, so the results could be limited in scope or applicability when addressing a wider population of smokers; therefore, it would be particularly useful in future studies to interview larger numbers of participants selected using a stratified sampling procedure, which will group participants according to key characteristics (e.g. stage of behavior change, motivation to quit, and exercise history), allowing comparisons at various levels.

5. Conclusions

In summary, our findings highlight the participants' interpretations of their experience of the acute effects of exercise on their bodies, thoughts, and feelings. These interpretations and the meaning assigned to them are based on individuals' previous knowledge, experiences, emotions, beliefs, and attitudes about those two behaviors. Most of the interpretations have direct or indirect links to the existing literature in this research area. Participants' preferences for exercise intensity, type, and duration, in relation to the perceived effects of exercise on smoking urges, seem also to be related to individuals' past exercise experiences, general attitude, and beliefs. According to Stelter [52], personal meaning integrates the past, present, and future. It emerges, on the basis of earlier experiences, that the participant integrates into the current situation and, through this, integrates a possible or expected future into the current action. Overall, the variability of the participants' perspectives on the themes of exercise preference, exercise-smoking relationship, and exercise as an aid to quitting smoking seems to either directly or indirectly relate to their motivation to quit, and their stage of change for smoking and physical activity behavior. Moreover, there are some shared ideas that may be useful in generating possible future research ideas: a. the "feel-good" effect after exercise as a relief from the "feel-bad" effect during exercise; b. the decreased urge to smoke as an effect after exercise, stated by all participants regardless of reported positive or negative feelings; and c. exercise as more of a "clearing the mind" mechanism than one that distracts attention.

The main strength of the present study is the qualitative approach to a fairly well-researched topic, which until now involved quantitative approaches. By giving voice to participants, we are able to arrive at the personal meaning, which can lead to new research on the acute effects of exercise and the underlying mechanisms behind these effects.

Acknowledgements

Funding for this study was provided through the European Union (European Social Fund—ESF) and Greek national funds through the Operational Program "Education and Lifelong Learning" of the National Strategic Reference Framework (NSRF)—Research Funding Program: THALES. Investing in knowledge society through the European Social Fund.

We would like to thank Theodora Tzatzaki, Anastasia Tsiami, Eirini Manthou, and Kalliopi Georgakouli for running the exercise protocols and collecting the physiological data.

References

[1]   Dishman, R.K., Washburn, R.A. and Heath, G.W. (2004) Physical Activity Epidemiology. Human Kinetics, Champaign.

[2]   Khan, K.M., Thompson, A.M., Blair, S.N., Sallis, J.F., Powell, K.E., Bull, F.C. and Bauman, A.E. (2012) Sport and Exercise as Contributors to the Health of Nations. *The Lancet*, **380**, 59-64. http://dx.doi.org/10.1016/S0140-6736(12)60865-4

[3]   European Commission (2010) Special Eurobarometer: Sport and Physical Activity. Brussels.

[4]   Doll, R., Peto, R., Boreham, J. and Sutherland, I. (2004) Mortality in Relation to Smoking: 50 Years' Observations on Male British Doctors. *British Medical Journal*, **328**, 1519-1528. http://dx.doi.org/10.1136/bmj.38142.554479.AE

[5]   Ezzati, M., Henley, S.J., Thun, M.J. and Lopez, A.D. (2005) Role of Smoking in Global and Regional Cardiovascular Mortality. *Circulation*, **112**, 489-497. http://dx.doi.org/10.1161/CIRCULATIONAHA.104.521708

[6]   Center for Global Tobacco Control (2011) The Greek Tobacco Epidemic. http://www.who.int/fctc/reporting/party_reports/greece_annex1_the_greek_tobacco_epidemic_2011.pdf

[7]   Blair, S.N., Jacobs, D.R. and Powell, K.E. (1985) Relationships between Exercise or Physical Activity and Other Health Behaviors. *Public Health Report*, **100**, 172-180.

[8]   Conway, T.L. and Cronan, T.A. (1992) Smoking, Exercise, and Physical Fitness. *Preventive Medicine*, **21**, 723-734. http://dx.doi.org/10.1016/0091-7435(92)90079-W

[9]   Paavola, M., Vartiainen, E. and Haukkala, A. (2004) Smoking, Alcohol Use, and Physical Activity: A 13-Year Longitudinal Study Ranging from Adolescence into Adulthood. *Journal of Adolescent Health*, **35**, 238-244. http://dx.doi.org/10.1016/S1054-139X(04)00059-X

[10]   Kaczynski, A.T., Manske, S.R., Mannell, R.C. and Grewal, K. (2008) Smoking and Physical Activity: A Systematic Review. *American Journal of Health Behavior*, **32**, 93-110. http://dx.doi.org/10.5993/AJHB.32.1.9

[11]   Linke, S.E. and Ussher, M. (2014). Exercise-Based Treatments for Substance Use Disorders: Evidence, Theory, and Practicality. *The American Journal of Drug and Alcohol Abuse*, **41**, 7-15. http://dx.doi.org/10.3109/00952990.2014.976708

[12] Haasova, M., Warren, F.C., Ussher, M., Janse Van Rensburg, K., Faulkner, G., Cropley, M., *et al.* (2013) The Acute Effects of Physical Activity on Cigarette Cravings: Systematic Review and Meta-Analysis with Individual Participant Data. *Addiction*, **108**, 26-37. http://dx.doi.org/10.1111/j.1360-0443.2012.04034.x

[13] Ussher, M.H., Taylor, A. and Faulkner, G. (2012) Exercise Interventions for Smoking Cessation. *Cochrane Database of Systematic Reviews*, **1**, Article ID: CD002295. http://dx.doi.org/10.1002/14651858.CD002295.pub4

[14] Roberts, V., Maddison, R., Simpson, C., Bullen, C. and Prapavessis, H. (2012) The Acute Effects of Exercise on Cigarette Cravings, Withdrawal Symptoms, Affect, and Smoking Behavior: Systematic Review and Meta-Analysis. *Psychopharmacology*, **222**, 1-15. http://dx.doi.org/10.1007/s00213-012-2731-z

[15] Taylor, A.H., Ussher, M.H. and Faulkner, G. (2007) The Acute Effects of Exercise on Cigarette Cravings, Withdrawal Symptoms, Affect and Smoking Behavior: A Systematic Review. *Addiction*, **102**, 534-543. http://dx.doi.org/10.1111/j.1360-0443.2006.01739.x

[16] Bock, B.C., Marcus, B.H., King, T.C., Borrelli, B. and Roberts, M.R. (1999) Exercise Effects on Withdrawal and Mood among Women Attempting Smoking Cessation. *Addictive Behaviors*, **24**, 399-410. http://dx.doi.org/10.1016/S0306-4603(98)00088-4

[17] Harper, T.M. (2011) Mechanisms behind the Success of Exercise as an Adjunct Quit Smoking Aid. Doctoral Dissertation, Retrieved from Electronic Thesis and Dissertation Repository. http://ir.lib.uwo.ca/etd/198

[18] Everson, E.S., Daley, A.J. and Ussher, M. (2008) The Effects of Moderate and Vigorous Exercise on Desire to Smoke, Withdrawal Symptoms and Mood in Abstaining Young Adult Smokers. *Mental Health and Physical Activity*, **1**, 26-31. http://dx.doi.org/10.1016/j.mhpa.2008.06.001

[19] Niedermaier, O.N., Smith, M.L., Beightol, L.A., Zukowskagrojec, Z., Goldstein, D.S. and Eckberg, D.L. (1993) Influence of Cigarette-Smoking on Human Autonomic Function. *Circulation*, **88**, 562-571. http://dx.doi.org/10.1161/01.CIR.88.2.562

[20] Lucini, D., Bertocchi, F., Malliani, A. and Pagani, M. (1996) A Controlled Study of the Autonomic Changes Produced by Habitual Cigarette Smoking in Healthy Subjects. *Cardiovascular Research*, **31**, 633-639. http://dx.doi.org/10.1016/0008-6363(96)00013-2

[21] Stein, P.K., Rottman, J.N. and Kleiger, R.S. (1996) Effect of 21 mg Transdermal Nicotine Patches and Smoking Cessation on Heart Rate Variability. *American Journal of Cardiology*, **77**, 701-705. http://dx.doi.org/10.1016/S0002-9149(97)89203-X

[22] Hamer, M., Taylor, A.H. and Steptoe, A. (2006) The Effect of Acute Aerobic Exercise on Blood Pressure Reactivity to Psychological Stress: A Systematic Review and Meta-Analysis. *Biological Psychology*, **71**, 183-190. http://dx.doi.org/10.1016/j.biopsycho.2005.04.004

[23] Taylor, A. and Katomeri, A. (2006) Effects of a Brisk Walk on Blood Pressure Responses to the Stroop, a Speech Task and a Smoking Cue among Temporarily Abstinent Smokers. *Psychopharmacology*, **184**, 247-253. http://dx.doi.org/10.1007/s00213-005-0275-1

[24] Ussher, M., Nunziata, P., Cropley, M. and West, R. (2001) Effect of a Short Bout of Exercise on Tobacco Withdrawal Symptoms and Desire to Smoke. *Psychopharmacology*, **158**, 66-72. http://dx.doi.org/10.1007/s002130100846

[25] Daniel, J.Z., Cropley, M. and Fife-Schaw, C. (2006) The Effect of Exercise in Reducing Desire to Smoke and Cigarette Withdrawal Symptoms Is Not Caused by Distraction. *Addiction*, **101**, 1187-1192. http://dx.doi.org/10.1111/j.1360-0443.2006.01457.x

[26] Daniel, J.Z., Cropley, M. and Fife-Schaw, C. (2007) Acute Exercise Effects on Smoking Withdrawal Symptoms and Desire to Smoke Are Not Related to Expectation. *Psychopharmacology*, **195**, 125-129. http://dx.doi.org/10.1007/s00213-007-0889-6

[27] Janse Van Rensburg, K., Taylor, A., Benattayallah, A. and Hodgson, T. (2012) The Effects of Exercise on Cigarette Cravings and Brain Activation in Response to Smoking-Related Images. *Psychopharmacology*, **221**, 659-666. http://dx.doi.org/10.1007/s00213-011-2610-z

[28] Kvale, S. (1996) Interviews: An Introduction to Qualitative Research Interviewing. Sage, Thousand Oaks.

[29] Boyatzis, R.E. (1998) Transforming Qualitative Information: Thematic Analysis and Code Development. Sage, London.

[30] Rossman, B.G. and Rallis, S.F. (1998) Learning in the Field: An Introduction to Qualitative Research. Sage, London.

[31] Patton, M.Q. (1990) Qualitative Evaluation and Research Methods. 2nd Edition, Sage, Newbury Park.

[32] Lincoln, Y.S. and Guba, E. (1985) Naturalistic Enquiry. Sage, Beverly Hills.

[33] Daniel, J.Z., Cropley, M., Ussher, M. and West, R. (2004) Acute Effects of a Short Bout of Moderate versus Light Intensity Exercise versus Inactivity on Tobacco Withdrawal Symptoms in Sedentary Smokers. *Psychopharmacology*, **174**, 320-326. http://dx.doi.org/10.1007/s00213-003-1762-x

[34] Hughes, J.R., Crow, R.S., Jacobs, D.R., Mittelmark, M.B. and Leon, A.S. (1984) Physical Activity, Smoking, and Exercise-Induced Fatigue. *Journal of Behavioral Medicine*, **7**, 217-230. http://dx.doi.org/10.1007/BF00845388

[35] Ekkekakis, P. and Petruzzello, S.J. (1999) Acute Aerobic Exercise and Affect: Current Status, Problems, and Prospects Regarding Dose-Response. *Sports Medicine*, **28**, 337-374. http://dx.doi.org/10.2165/00007256-199928050-00005

[36] Dishman, R.K. (1990) Determinants of Participation in Physical Activity. In: Bouchard, C., Shephard, R.J., Stephens, T., Sutton, J.R. and McPherson, B.D., Eds., *Exercise, Fitness, and Health: A Consensus of Current Knowledge*, Human Kinetics, Champaign, 75-101.

[37] Rhodes, R.E. and Kates, A. (2015) Can the Affective Response to Exercise Predict Future Motives and Physical Activity Behavior? A Systematic Review of Published Evidence. *Annals of Behavioral Medicine*, **49**, 715-731. http://dx.doi.org/10.1007/s12160-015-9704-5

[38] McClernon, F.J., Westman, E.C. and Rose, J.E. (2004) The Effects of Controlled Deep Breathing on Smoking Withdrawal Symptoms in Dependent Smokers. *Addictive Behaviors*, **29**, 765-772. http://dx.doi.org/10.1016/j.addbeh.2004.02.005

[39] Ekkekakis, P. and Acevedo, E.O. (2006) Affective Responses to Acute Exercise: Toward a Psychobiological Dose-Response Model. In: Acevedo, E.O. and Ekkekakis, P., Eds., *Psychobiology of Physical Activity*, Human Kinetics, Champaign, 91-109.

[40] Erskine, J.A.K., Ussher, M., Cropley, M., Elgindi, A., Zaman, M. and Corlett, B. (2012) Effect of Thought Suppression on Desire to Smoke and Tobacco Withdrawal Symptoms. *Psychopharmacology*, **219**, 205-211. http://dx.doi.org/10.1007/s00213-011-2391-4

[41] Erskine, J.A.K., Georgiou, G. and Kvavilashvili, L. (2010) I Suppress Therefore I Smoke: The Effects of Thought Suppression on Smoking Behavior. *Psychological Science*, **21**, 1225-1230. http://dx.doi.org/10.1177/0956797610378687

[42] Kassel, J.D., Stroud, L.R. and Paronis, C.A. (2003) Smoking, Stress, and Negative Affect: Correlation, Causation, and Context across Stages of Smoking. *Psychological Bulletin*, **129**, 270-304. http://dx.doi.org/10.1037/0033-2909.129.2.270

[43] Ekkekakis, P., Parfitt, G. and Petruzzello, S.J. (2011) The Pleasure and Displeasure People Feel when they Exercise at Different Intensities. Decennial Update and Progress towards a Tripartite Rationale for Exercise Intensity Prescription. *Sports Medicine*, **41**, 641-671. http://dx.doi.org/10.2165/11590680-000000000-00000

[44] Ryan, R.M. and Deci, E.L. (2000) Self-Determination Theory and the Facilitation of Intrinsic Motivation, Social Development, and Well-Being. *American Psychologist*, **55**, 68-78. http://dx.doi.org/10.1037/0003-066X.55.1.68

[45] Sandvik, L., Erikssen, G. and Thaulow, E. (1995) Long Term Effects of Smoking on Physical Fitness and Lung Function: A Longitudinal Study of 1393 Middle Aged Norwegian Men for Seven Years. *British Medical Journal*, **311**, 715-718. http://dx.doi.org/10.1136/bmj.311.7007.715

[46] Boutelle, K.N., Murray, D.M., Jeffery, R.W., Hennrikus, D.J. and Lando, H.A. (2000) Associations between Exercise and Health Behaviors in a Community Sample of Working Adults. *Preventive Medicine*, **30**, 217-224. http://dx.doi.org/10.1006/pmed.1999.0618

[47] Emmons, K.M., Marcus, B.H., Linnan, L., Rossi, J.S. and Abrams, D.B. (1994) Mechanisms in Multiple Risk Factor Interventions: Smoking, Physical Activity, and Dietary Fat Intake among Manufacturing Workers. *Preventive Medicine*, **23**, 481-489. http://dx.doi.org/10.1006/pmed.1994.1066

[48] King, T.K., Marcus, B.H., Pinto, B.M., Emmons, K.M. and Abrams, D.B. (1996) Cognitive-Behavioral Mediators of Changing Multiple Behaviors: Smoking and a Sedentary Lifestyle. *Preventive Medicine*, **25**, 684-691. http://dx.doi.org/10.1006/pmed.1996.0107

[49] Sherwood, N.E., Hennrikus, D.J., Jeffery, R.W., Lando, H.A. and Murray, D.M. (2000) Smokers with Multiple Behavioral Risk Factors: How Are They Different? *Preventive Medicine*, **31**, 299-307. http://dx.doi.org/10.1006/pmed.2000.0710

[50] Ferguson, J., Bauld, L., Chesterman, J. and Judge, K. (2005) The English Smoking Treatment Services: One-Year Outcomes. *Addiction*, **100**, 59-69. http://dx.doi.org/10.1111/j.1360-0443.2005.01028.x

[51] Fiore, M.C., Jaen, C.R., Baker, T.B., Bailey, W.C., Benowitz, N.L., Curry, S.J., *et al.* (2008) Treating Tobacco Use and Dependence: 2008 Update, Clinical Practice Guideline, US Department of Health and Human Services, Public Health Service, Rockville.

[52] Stelter, R. (2008) Exploring Body-Anchored and Experience-Based Learning in a Community of Practice. In: Schilhab, T., Juelskjær, M. and Moser, T., Eds., *Learning Bodies*, Danmarks Pædagogiske Universitetsforlag, Copenhagen, 111-129.

11

Empathy Gender in Dental Students in Latin America: An Exploratory and Cross-Sectional Study

Víctor Patricio Díaz-Narváez[1,2*], Ana María Erazo Coronado[3], Jorge Luis Bilbao[4], Farith González[5], Mariela Padilla[6], Madeline Howard[7], María Guadalupe Silva[8], Mirian Bullen[9], Fredy Gutierrez[10], Teresa Varela de Villalba[11], Mercedes Salcedo Rioja[12], Joyce Huberman[13], Doris Carrasco[14], Robert Utsman[15]

[1]School of Dentistry, Universidad San Sebastián, Santiago, Chile
[2]Associate Investigator, Universidad Autónoma de Chile, Santiago, Chile
[3]Universidad Metropolitana, Barranquilla, Colombia
[4]School of Medicine, Universidad Libre Seccional Barranquilla y Fundación Universitaria San Martín Sede Puerto Colombia, Barranquilla, Colombia
[5]School of Dentistry, Universidad de Cartagena, Campus de la Salud Barrio Zaragocilla, Cartagena, Colombia
[6]School of Health Sciences, Universidad Latinoamericana de Ciencia y Tecnología, San José, Costa Rica
[7]School of Dentistry, Universidad de Costa Rica, San Pedro de Montes de Oca, San José, Costa Rica
[8]Institute for Scientific Research, Universidad Central del Este, San Pedro de Macorís, Dominican Republic
[9]School of Dentistry, Universidad de Panamá, Panama City, Panama
[10]Facultad de Estomatología Roberto Beltrán, Universidad Peruana Cayetano Heredia, Lima, Peru
[11]School of Medicine, Universidad Católica de Córdoba, Córdoba, Argentina
[12]Department of Pediatric Dentistry, School of Dentistry, Universidad Nacional Mayor de San Marcos, Lima, Peru
[13]School of Dentistry, Faculty of Clinical Medicine, Universidad del Desarrollo, Santiago, Chile
[14]School of Dentistry, Universidad de Concepción, Concepción, Chile
[15]Investigation of the School of Health Sciences, Universidad Latinoamericana de Ciencia y Tecnología, San José, Costa Rica

Email: *victor.diaz@uss.cl, amec1708@gmail.com, jbilbao55@hotmail.com, fgonzalezm1@unicartagena.edu.co, mpadilla@racsa.co.cr, mhowarducr@gmail.com, guadalupesilva1@gmail.com, ladymi516@yahoo.com, fredy.gutierrez@upch.pe, tebeva@hotmail.com, ritasalcedor@hotmail.com, jhuberman@udd.cl, doriscarrasco@udec.cl

Abstract

Background: It is well-founded that empathy is an attribute that increases the likelihood of good

---

*Corresponding author.

communication between health professionals and patients, and it is usual that there is the conviction that empathy levels are higher in women than in men. **Aims:** A study comparing levels of empathy gender of students in 18 schools of dentistry from six Latin American countries was conducted. **Method:** An exploratory cross-sectional study of which empathy levels were measured by the Jefferson Scale of Empathy for dental students (S version) and these levels were compared between genders by t-student test, after verification of normal distribution and homoscedasticity. **Results:** Variability was found in the results of the comparisons. In some cases, empathy levels were higher in women, others in men and in most of them there were no differences between genders. **Conclusions:** The observed results do not support the belief that women are more empathetic than men. However, more studies must be performed in more powers and countries to verify that the results described constitute a scientific fact and not just a feature of dental students specifically in the countries studied.

Keywords

Empathy, Gender, Dental Students

1. Background

The professional relationship between health practitioner and patient must be considered a two person interaction of which both have different personal interests [1], constitutes a human encounter. This relationship contains, itself, an eminent subjectivity and inter-subjectivity that goes beyond the purely clinic dimension of a treatment [2].

The empathy during health care can be understood as a cognitive and behavioral attribute, which implies the capacity to understand how the experiences and feelings of a patient can influence and can be influenced by illness and its symptoms, and the capacity to communicate that understanding to the patient [3]. This constitutes one of the elements needed to develop basic communication skills for the human relationship that is performed, voluntarily in form [4].

Investigations in the professional area of health show that the empathy has been related, theoretically and empirically, to diverse attributes, such as the pro-social behavior, the ability to obtain clinical history, has increased the level of patient and doctor satisfaction, as well as good clinical results [2] [5] [6].

Various authors have proposed that women show higher levels of empathy compared to men [7]-[9] and those empathy measurements, of those investigations, have been performed with different instruments developed for the general population and the medical field. On the other hand, some authors have proposed, with theoretical basis and less empirical evidence, that empathy could be a "variable" that is subjected to the influence of several factors, in addition to the gender [10]-[12], as well as age, intent about the specialty to follow in the future, the current course the student is taking, structure and family environment, personality, empathetic experiences, socio-cultural environment, scale of ethical and moral values, among others; which could act as independent "variables" or confounding variables, and at the same time, could contribute to explain the variability observed in empathetic orientation levels found in some research [13]-[16].

There are many researches in which empirical results have been found that contradict the fact that women are more empathetic than men [17]-[19]. However, more empirical evidence is required to demonstrate the real existence of this contradiction. The purpose of this investigation is to determine if indeed the levels of empathy are higher in women, in relation to the male students of 18 dental faculties of six countries in Latin America.

2. Materials and Methods

This is an exploratory, non-experimental, descriptive, transversal and ex post facto cause-effect investigation, bio-ethically governed by the rules of Helsinki(was approved by the Ethics Committee of Research, Development University and German Clinic with code CAS-UDD approval: 2011-64 in Santiago de Chile).The studied population was composed of students of first through fifth year from 18 dental faculties of six countries in Latin America (Dominican Republic, Costa Rica, Panama, Colombia, Argentina and Chile) (n_{total} = 4407) (**Table 1**).

Table 1. Estimation results of the descriptive statistics of the levels of gender empathy in each of the universities studied.

School of Dentistry	Gender	Median	Standard Error	Confidence Level of 95%			
				Inferior Limit	Superior Limit	Standard Deviation	n
Universidad de Antofagasta (Chile)	Female	110,518	1.312	107,945	113,090	14,262	114
	Male	110,144	1.477	107,249	113,040	13,393	90
Universidad Latina de Panamá (Panamá)	Female	104,971	1.675	101,688	108,255	14,051	70
	Male	101,826	2.922	96,098	107,554	15,831	23
Universidad de Cartagena (Colombia)	Female	107,869	0.940	106,026	109,713	12,518	222
	Male	103,190	1.197	100,843	105,537	12,396	137
Universidad de Magdalena (Colombia)	Female	96,080	1.494	93,151	99,008	18,544	88
	Male	88,753	1.520	85,774	91,732	16,758	85
Universidad Metropolitana (Barranquilla, Colombia)	Female	98,826	1.461	95,962	101,690	16,175	92
	Male	100,274	1.779	96,786	103,763	13,541	62
Universidad Central de Este (República Dominicana)	Female	102,000	1.091	99,862	104,138	13,424	165
	Male	99,622	1.629	96,428	102,815	18,358	74
Universidad de Concepción (Chile)	Female	117,364	0.976	115,450	119,278	11,880	206
	Male	113,756	1.206	111,391	116,120	13,036	135
Universidad del Desarrollo (Chile)	Female	116,296	0.983	114,368	118,224	12,444	203
	Male	110,983	1.307	108,421	113,544	11,573	115
Universidad Finis Terrae (Chile)	Female	113,464	0.974	111,555	115,373	13,307	207
	Male	110,098	1.387	107,378	112,818	13,905	102
Universidad ULACIT (Costa Rica)	Female	106,735	1.075	104,629	108,842	14,350	170
	Male	101,636	1.889	97,932	105,340	10,913	55
Universidad Andrés Bello (Sede Viña del Mar) (Chile)	Female	112,958	1.016	110,965	114,951	14,160	190
	Male	112,231	1.295	109,691	114,770	12,432	117
Universidad Católica de Córdova (Argentina)	Female	108,134	1.210	105,761	110,507	15,195	134
	Male	98,527	1.889	94,823	102,231	15,206	55
Universidad Peruana Cayetano Heredia (Perú)	Female	110,511	1.016	108,518	112,503	13,712	190
	Male	107,176	1.699	103,845	110,508	13,427	68
Universidad de Costa Rica (Costa Rica)	Female	112,762	0.986	110,830	114,695	14,516	202
	Male	109,841	1.494	106,913	112,769	14,417	88
Universidad De Panamá (Panamá)	Female	108,318	1.336	105,699	110,937	15,901	110
	Male	104,565	2.922	98,838	110,293	15,249	23
Universidad San Martín (Barranquilla, Colombia)	Female	100,431	1.387	97,712	103,151	13,996	102
	Male	101,667	1.725	98,285	105,048	19,233	66
Universidad de San Marcos (Perú)	Female	108,471	1.387	105,751	111,190	12,934	102
	Male	109,939	1.415	107,164	112,714	15,208	98
Universidad Andrés Bello (Sede Santiago) (Chile)	Female	112,692	0.864	110,998	114,386	12,977	263
	Male	109,810	1.033	107,785	111,835	14,653	184

Stratified samples by gender were obtained from this population. The collection of data was performed between July and August 2012. Since the students were able to visit different clinic areas, attend classes in different places, in addition to be absent from classes, among other circumstances, it was not possible to apply the scale to all the students. The scale was not applied to the ones who were absent, (due to the reasons before mentioned) nor on the second time in order to avoid possible skewed answers. The Jefferson Scale of Empathy (JSE) in the Spanish version for students of Medicine (version S) was used in each of the participating countries, based on criteria Alcorta-Garza *et al.* [10] and Rivera *et al.* [20], was applied to those participating students in classrooms or clinic rooms, using just one anonymous and confidential measurement by a neutral operator. Before the Jefferson Scale of Empathy (JSE) was applied, it was submitted to board (a committee composed of five relevant academic members of the Psychology and Dentistry field or related to), in order to verify the cultural and content validity [2]. A pilot study was created for the purpose of checking the students comprehension of the scale culturally adapted. There was not judgment of exclusion, since the objective was to evaluate the variable of interest of as many students as possible.

Statistical Analysis

The primary and original data from the empathy levels of each university examined were submitted to the Cronbach's alpha test (reliability by internal consistency). The sum of the primary data score, obtained using the scale previously mentioned, was initially submitted to the Kolmogorov-Smirnov normality test (K-S) in both types and to the Homoscedasticity Levene test. Descriptive statistics were estimated, arithmetic mean, absolute deviation and standard deviation of these sum. Comparisons between both genders mean were performed by Student's t-test, considering the presence of equal variances. The effect size was measured by the Hedges g. Data was processed by the statistical program SPSS 20.0 TM. The significance level used was ≤ 0.05 in each case.

3. Results

The K-S test was not significant ($p > 0.05$), in any of the data groups, which means that the data observed were distributed normally. The Cronbach's alpha test estimated for each gender and university fluctuated between 0.768 and 0.834, which shows that the data have values of acceptable internal consistency. **Table 1** shows the results of the descriptive statistics estimation of empathy levels, estimated for each gender and each of the studied universities, and **Table 2** shows the results of the total mean estimation in both examined gender. This last table shows that women have superior empathy levels compared to the men, and that the student's t-test was highly significant ($p < 0.0001$); however, the value statistically adjusted was 0.199, which shows that the effect size is low, therefore, the magnitude of the differences between means is small.

The results of estimation of equal variances between the studied gender in each university, the comparison of the means between the gender in each university and the effect size corresponding to each of the comparisons are presented in **Table 3**. The F-Test was not significant ($p > 0.05$) in all cases, with the exception of the comparison between the gender variances in the San Martin University (Barranquilla, Colombia) ($p < 0.01$).

The student's t-test was not significant ($p > 0.05$) in the following universities: Antofagasta (Chile), Andrés Bello (Viña del Mar branch, Chile), Universidad Latina and from Panama (Panama), Universidad Metropolitana and San Martin (Barranquilla, Colombia), Universidad Nacional Cayetano Heredia and Nacional Mayor de San Marcos (Lima, Peru), Universidad de Costa Rica (San José, Costa Rica) and Universidad Central del Este (Dominican Republic).

Significant differences ($p < 0.05$) were found in the rest of compared universities. Of all the universities where no significant differences were found, five of these absolute values of the means were higher in women; in three of them the absolute values were higher in men and in two of them, the means were practically the same (**Table 1**).

The effect size sample was low (lower then 0.2) in six of them and in the rest the effect was medium-sized (between 0.2 and 0.5) (**Table 3**). In the case of the universities where statistical differences were found, in all cases the values of the empathy levels were higher in women than in men (**Table 1**). However, from these statistical differences, the only one that had a high effect size was the University Católica de Córdoba ($g = 0.632$); meanwhile in the rest of the universities the value of the effect size sample fluctuated between 0.209 and 0.438 which is considered medium-sized (**Table 3**).

4. Discussion

The studies of gender empathy level distribution initiated with works of Block [21] and followed by Hoffman [22]. The first one did not find differences between men and women; however, the second one found that women had more points than men regarding Affective Empathy (AE), but the opposite happened regarding Cognitive Empathy (CE). Later on, Eisenberg and Lennon [23] had the same results as Hoffman [22]. Those differences were attributed to the gender role stereotypes.

Table 2. Estimation results of the total median for each gender.

Gender	Median	Standard Error	Confidence Level of 95%	
			Inferior Limit	Superior Limit
Female	108,244	0.283	107,690	108,798
Male	105,224	0.408	104,425	106,024

T Test = 6.4; p < 0.0001; g = 0.199.

Table 3. Results of the comparison of means of both genders in each of the universities studied and estimation of the effect size (g).

Universities	F test	Signification	T Value-student	Signification	g
Universidad de Antofagasta (Antofagasta, Chile)	0.138	p = 0.711 ns	0.191	p = 0.849 ns	0.0272
Universidad Latina (Ciudad de Panamá, Panamá)	0.001	p = 0.975 ns	0.503	p = 0.616 ns	0.217
Universidad de Cartagena (Cartagena, Colombia)	0.024	p = 0.877 ns	3.606	p = 0.0001**	0.375
Universidad de Magdalena (Santa Marta, Colombia)	3.585	p = 0.060 ns	2.723	p = 0.007**	0.414
Universidad Metropolitana (Barranquilla, Colombia)	1.467	p = 0.228 ns	−0.578	p = 0.562 ns	−0.095
Universidad Central del Este (San Pedro de Macorí, República Dominicana)	4.228	p = 0.041 ns	1.001	p = 0.319 ns	0.158
Universidad de Concepción (Concepción, Chile)	0.397	p = 0.529 ns	2.639	p = 0.009**	0.292
Universidad del Desarrollo (Santiago, Chile)	0.172	p = 0.678 ns	3.751	p = 0.0001**	0.438
Universidad Finis Terrae (Santiago, Chile)	1.011	p = 0.315 ns	2.060	p = 0.040*	0.302
Universidad Latinoamericana de la Ciencia y Tecnología (San José, Costa Rica)	3.040	p = 0.083 ns	2.417	p = 0.016*	0.375
Universidad Andrés Bello, Sede Viña del Mar (Viña del Mar, Chile)	3.256	p = 0.702 ns	0.457	p = 0.648 ns	0.054
Universidad Católica de Córdoba (Córdoba, Argentina)	0.115	p = 0.735 ns	3.947	p = 0.001**	0.632
Universidad Peruana Cayetano Heredia (Lima, Perú)	0.119	p = 0.731 ns	1.73	p = 0.085 ns	0.244
Universidad de Costa Rica (San José, Costa Rica)	0.526	p = 0.469 ns	1.579	p = 0.115 ns	0.202
Universidad de Panamá (Ciudad de Panamá, Panamá)	0.162	p = 0.688 ns	1.036	p = 0.302 ns	0.261
Universidad San Martín (Barranquiilla, Colombia)	9.491	p = 0.002**	−0.481	p = 0.631 ns	−0.076
Universidad Nacional Mayor de San Marcos (Lima, Perú)	1.21	p = 0.273 ns	−0.736	p = 0.462 ns	−0.104
Universidad Andrés Bello, Sede Santiago (Santiago, Chile)	1.031	p = 0.31 ns	2.19	p = 0.029*	0.209

ns: not significant (p > 0.05); *p < 0.05; **p < 0.01.

Other studies have supported those conclusions [24]-[26], but using different measurement tools. Fernández-Pinto et al. [27], suggested two possible generalizations of these results: 1) that the empathy seems to be connected to individual differences, such as personality and gender differences, and 2) the results of the research made seem insufficient to come to a conclusion about the interrelationships named, since the results come from the measurement of empathy using different tools and, therefore, underlie different concepts of conceptualizations of the empathy behind each one of the measurement types. This situation makes these results incomparable, stimulates the ambiguity and even its apparent contradiction.

Additional studies developed with students from different health and geographic areas [28]-[30], agree with the fact that women score higher empathy measures than men, with the exception of a study realized with dental students in Malaysia, in which differences between both genders were not found and men scored absolute values higher than women [31]. In Latin America (LA) some studies were developed about the empathy levels in different schools of dentistry and the results around the gender differences are contradictory. Studies have been performed by Gutierrez et al. [32], Salcedo et al. (results sent to publish) in Perú; Carrasco et al. [33], Huberman et al. [34], López et al. (results not published), González et al. (results not published), and Silva et al. [35] en Chile; Silva et al. [36] in Dominican Republic; Bilbao et al. (results sent to publish), Erazo et al. [37], González et al. (data sent to publish), Pérez et al. (data sent to publish) in Colombia; Howard et al. [38], Sánchez et al. [39]

in Costa Rica, Bullen *et al.* (results sent to publish); Gordon *et al.* (results not published) in Panamá, Varela *et al.* [40] in Argentina. All these results show that there is variability in the answer of empathy levels in both students outside and inside from all the different universities considered in this study [41]. The totality of authors previously mentioned developed their research in LA with the Jefferson Scale of Empathy (JSE), adapted to the health area researched, therefore, the difference of tools seems not to be the variability source and they can be compared not only by the scale used, but by the same methodological conceptions and statistics with which these studies were developed.

Vera [41], analyzing some of these studies about empathy in dental students from LA, sets three generalizations: 1) the empathy represents a variable behavior; 2) there is a tendency to show higher levels of empathy in female and in higher courses and 3)these variables do not explain more than 20% of the variation found. The authors from this study completely agree with the generalization 1) and 3), but the data observed in this current study shows variability in the gender and, therefore, it is not possible to coincide with the generalization 2), in relation to the "gender" factor. The studies previously mentioned, show that the variability is necessary to be explained, mostly, if required to make interventions that try to increase empathy levels in students of health science, by active processes of empathy teaching-learning.

The differences found could have some sources of explanation. Mercadillo *et al.* [42] propose that compassion is a moral emotion that determines a help behavior and the observation of the brain activity, after the students were submitted to watch images triggered to compassion; it showed that the compassion experience triggers by the experience of physical pain or illness, and it is associated to the experience of dislike, anxiety and dominance, characteristics of negative emotions. On other hand, the brain maps of this experience [42] show that women expressed a higher and more diverse activity in the basal and limbic zones of the brain, such as parahippocampal and temporal cortex (anger and sadness) and frontal areas involved in processing learned information and carrying out (intentions and making decisions). Men showed predominant activity in the orbitofrontal cortex (learning of moral concepts and social rules), but the behavioral results of their emotional experience did not show differences, which creates contradiction between what the students said what they felt and what their brains reflected.

Two proposals exist to explain this difference. Men as well as women feel compassion in similar ways, but feelings are processed by different ways in the brain: compassion felt by women goes with an empathy that can benefit the spread, and in men the feeling of compassion and their decision to help is directed by the moral judgment of the situation: "when someone suffers one has to help". The described differences can be explained by two proposals: 1) the evolutionist in which a woman owns a more sensible empathic system that assists the nurturing system; the high levels of oxytocin in women produce reactions like inhibiting pain faced with intruders, increases the anger to protect her children and builds an emotional bond towards them [43] and 2) the cultural proposal indicates that both the family and social education teach women and men to express their emotions in different ways. Both proposals do not have to be observed mostly as contradictions. Mercadillo *et al.* [42] comes to the conclusion that "even though the brain and body are different between genders, those differences do not determine the way we behave, they just lead the members of a gender to respond in an easier way to specific types of situations."

These situations are valued as concepts, rules and ways of expression that get into our brains and we learn during our daily lives, culturally and can create ways of response and perception throughout human development [42]. However, to obtain a major approach of which is the empathic behavior between gender, longitudinal studies are required, but not only related to location, since the result of this type would explain the local situation and what can be valid for a population not necessarily is valid for others, because of the possible influxes of some factors regarding the conformation of empathy. The social stereotypes (sexual role) influence the answers, since these stereotypes assign women the tendency of caring and supporting weak people, a bigger capacity to detect feelings and nonverbal signs and a major concern about the social aspects of interaction and other's feelings [43] [44].

On the other hand, other authors proposed that empathy has an impact in the emotional health and in the social field throughout culture [4] [43]-[46], besides it is correlated with the pro-social behavior and altruism and also inhibits the unsocial and aggressive behavior [47] [48]. There are circumstances that negatively influence empathy: levels of anxiety, claustrophobia, obesity, depression and stress [47]-[49]. In summary, the variability of observed empathy levels in this study, related to gender, cannot be explained. This variability constitutes empirical evidence that the empathy construct is difficult to elucidate and that some of the possible explanations that have been used so far, do not have a general character (for example, gender role).

5. Conclusions

It is still early to make generalizations regarding the distribution of the empathy levels in gender, because of the possible following reasons: 1) the observed variability between the genders in different universities of LA can be just a limited fact of the studied countries and, therefore, other studies are required in order to confirm that this variability is a general characteristic in LA, or is only endorsed to the six countries studied in this document, and even, it could be just a characteristic of the students of dentistry; 2) at least, in the studied region in this current document, intervention with teaching-learning processes associated with empathy should not occur without a prior study of what are the factors of influence, how they influence and by how much.

Acknowledgements

I wish to thank Dr. Aracelis Calzadilla Nuñez (Department of Child and Adolescent Psychiatry, Hospital Félix Bulnes, Santiago, Chile) for critically reading the final manuscript and considerations made for her.

Authors' Contributions

All authors designed the study. They participated in the statistical analysis, drafting of the components of this work and final review and final approval of the article.

Conflicts of Interest

The authors declare that they have no competing interests.

References

[1]   Dörr, A. (2004) Acerca de la comunicación médico-paciente desde una perspectiva histórica y antropológica. *Revista médica de Chile*, **132**, 1431-1436. http://dx.doi.org/10.4067/S0034-98872004001100014

[2]   Kane, G.C., Gotto, J.L., Mangione, S., West, S. and Hojat, M. (2007) Jefferson Scale of Patient's Perceptions of Physician Empathy: Preliminary Psychometric Data. *Croatian Medical Journal*, **48**, 81-86.

[3]   Hojat, M., Gonnella, J.S., Mangione, S., Nasca, T.J. and Magee, M. (2003) Physician Empathy in Medical Education and Practice: Experience with the Jefferson Scale of Physician Empathy. *Seminars in Integrative Medicine*, **1**, 25-41. http://dx.doi.org/10.1016/S1543-1150(03)00002-4

[4]   Moya-Albiol, L., Herrero, N. and Bernal, M.C. (2010) The Neural Bases of Empathy. *Revue Neurologique*, **50**, 89-100.

[5]   Squier, R.W. (1990) A Model of Empathic Understanding and Adherence to Treatment Regimens in Practitioner-Patient Relationships. *Social Science & Medicine*, **30**, 325-339. http://dx.doi.org/10.1016/0277-9536(90)90188-X

[6]   Hojat, M., Mangione, S., Nasca, T.J., Cohen, M.J.M., Gonnella, J.S., Erdmann, J.B., *et al.* (2001) The Jefferson Scale of Empathy: Development and Preliminary Psychometric Data. *Educational and Psychological Measurement*, **61**, 346-365. http://dx.doi.org/10.1177/00131640121971158

[7]   Halpern, J. (2001) From Detached Concern to Empathy: Humanizing Medical Practice. Oxford University Press, New York.

[8]   Neuwirth, Z.E. (1997) Physician Emphathy—Should We Care? *Lancet*, **350**, 606. http://dx.doi.org/10.1016/S0140-6736(05)63323-5

[9]   Arnold, I. (2002) Assessing Professional Behavior: Yesterday, Today and Tomorrow. *Academic Medicine*, **77**, 502-515. http://dx.doi.org/10.1097/00001888-200206000-00006

[10]   Alcorta-Garza, A., González-Guerrero, J.F., Tavitas-Herrera, S.E., Rodríguez-Lara, F.J. and Hojat, M. (2005) Validación de la escala de empatía médica de Jefferson en estudiantes de Medicina mexicanos. *Salud Mental*, **28**, 57-63.

[11]   Smith, M. and Dundes, L. (2008) The Implications of Gender Stereotypes for the Dentist-Patient Relationship. *Journal of Dental Education*, **72**, 5562-5570.

[12]   Retuerto, A. (2004) Diferencias en empatía en función de la variables género y edad. *Apuntes de Psicología*, **22**, 323-339.

[13]   Rahimi-Madiseh, M., Tavakol, M., Dennick, R. and Nasiri, J. (2010) Empathy in Iranian Medical Students: A Preliminary Psychometric Analysis and Differences by Gender and Year of Medical School. *Medical Teacher*, **13**, e471-e478. http://dx.doi.org/10.3109/0142159x.2010.509419

[14] Schwartz, B. and Bohay, R. (2012) Can Patients Help Teach Professionalism and Empathy to Dental Students. Adding Patient Videos to a Lecture Course. *Journal of Dental Education*, **76**, 174-184.

[15] Garaigordobil, M. and García de Galdeano, P. (2006) Empatía en niños de 10 a 12 años. *Psicothema*, **18**, 180-186.

[16] Sánchez-Queija, I., Oliva, A. and Parra, A. (2006) Empatía y conducta prosocial durante la adolescencia. *Revista de Psicología Social*, **21**, 259-271. http://dx.doi.org/10.1174/021347406778538230

[17] Glaser, K., Markham, F.W., Adler, H.M., McManus, R.P. and Hojat, M. (2007) Relationships between Scores on the Jefferson Scale of Physician Empathy, Patient Perceptions of Physician Empathy, and Humanistic Approaches to Patient Care: A Validity Study. *Medical Science Monitor*, **13**, 291-294.

[18] Mercer, S.W. and Reynolds, W.J. (2002) Empathy and Quality of Care. *The British Journal of General Practice*, **52**, S9-S12.

[19] Halpern, J. (2003) What Is Clinical Empathy? *Journal of General Internal Medicine*, **18**, 670-674. http://dx.doi.org/10.1046/j.1525-1497.2003.21017.x

[20] Rivera, I., Arratia, R., Zamorano, A. and Díaz-Narváez, V.P. (2011) Measurement of Empathetic Orientation in Dentistry Students. *Revista Salud Uninorte*, **27**, 63-72.

[21] Block, J.H. (1976) Assessing Sex Differences: Issues, Problems and Pitfalls. *Merril-Palmer Quarterly*, **22**, 283-308.

[22] Hoffman, M.I. (1977) Sex Differences in Empathy and Related Behaviours. *Psychological Bulletin*, **84**, 712-722. http://dx.doi.org/10.1037/0033-2909.84.4.712

[23] Eisenberg, N. and Lennon, R. (1983) Sex Differences in Empathy and Related Capacities. *Psychological Bulletin*, **94**, 100-131. http://dx.doi.org/10.1037/0033-2909.94.1.100

[24] Mestre, M.V., Samper, P., Frías, M.D. and Tur, A.M. (2009) Are Woman More Empathetic than Men? A Longitudinal Study in Adolescence. *The Spanish Journal of Psychology*, **12**, 76-83. http://dx.doi.org/10.1017/S1138741600001499

[25] Hojat, M., Mangione, S., Nasca, T.J., Cohen, M.J.M., Gonnella, J.S., Erdmann, J.B., *et al.* (2001) The Jefferson Scale of Empathy: Development and Preliminary Psychometric Data. *Educational and Psychological Measurement*, **61**, 346-365. http://dx.doi.org/10.1177/00131640121971158

[26] Rojas, A.M., Castañeda Barthelemiez, S. and Parraguez-Infiesta, R.A. (2009) Orientación empática de los estudiantes de dos escuelas de kinesiología de Chile. *Educación Médica*, **12**, 103-109.

[27] Fernández-Pinto, I., López-Pérez, B. and Márquez, M. (2008) Empatía: Medidas, teorías y aplicaciones en revisión. *Anales de Psicología*, **24**, 284-298.

[28] Hojat, M., Mangione, S., Nasca, T.J., Rattner, S., Erdmann, J.B., Gonnella, J.S., *et al.* (2004) An Empirical Study of Decline in Empathy in Medical School. *Medical Education*, **38**, 934-941. http://dx.doi.org/10.1111/j.1365-2929.2004.01911.x

[29] Sherman, J. and Cramer, A. (2005) Measurement of Changes in Empathy during Dental School. *Journal of Dental Education*, **69**, 338-345.

[30] Chen, D., Lew, R. and Hershman, W. (2007) A Cross-Sectional Measurement of Medical Student Empathy. *Journal of General Internal Medicine*, **22**, 1434-1438. http://dx.doi.org/10.1007/s11606-007-0298-x

[31] Babar, M.G., Omar, H., Lim, L.P., Khan, S.A., Mitha, S., Ahmad, S.F.B., *et al.* (2013) An Assessment of Dental Students' Empathy Levels in Malaysia. *International Journal of Medical Education*, **4**, 223-229.

[32] Gutierrez, F., Quezada, B., López, M., Méndez, J., Díaz Narváez, V.P., Zamorano, A. and Rivera, I. (2012) Medición del nivel de percepción empática de los estudiantes de la Facultad de Estomatología Roberto Beltrán. Universidad Peruana Cayetano Heredia. *Revista Estomatológica Herediana*, **22**, 91-99

[33] Carrasco, D.E., Bustos, A. and Díaz, V. (2012) Orientación empática en estudiantes de odontología chilenos. *Revista Estomatológica Herediana*, **22**, 145-151.

[34] Huberman, J., Rodríguez, M.P., González, S. and Díaz Narváez, V.P. (2014) Empathetic Orientation Levels in Odontology Students of the Universidad del Desarrollo, sede Santiago (Chile). *Revista Clínica de Periodoncia, Implantología y Rehabilitación Oral*, **7**, 169-174. http://dx.doi.org/10.1016/j.piro.2014.11.001

[35] Silva, H., Rivera, I., Zamorano, A. and Díaz Narváez, V.P. (2013) Evaluation of Empathetic Orientation in Dentistry Students of Finis Terrae University in Santiago, Chile. *Revista Clínica de Periodoncia, Implantología y Rehabilitación Oral*, **6**, 130-133.

[36] Silva, M.G., Arboleda, J. and Díaz Narváez, V.P. (2013) Empathic Orientation Dental Students from the Universidad Central del Este. *Odontoestomatología*, **15**, 24-33.

[37] Erazo, A.M., Alonso, L.M., Rivera, I., Zamorano, A. and Díaz Narváez, V.P. (2012) Measurement of Empathetic Orientation in Dentistry Students of Metropolitana University of Barranquilla (Colombia). *Revista Salud Uninorte*, **28**, 354-363.

[38] Howard, M., Navarro, S., Rivera, I., Zamorano, A. and Díaz-Narváez, V.P. (2013) Medición del nivel de orientación empática en el estudiantado de la Facultad de odontología, Universidad de Costa Rica. *Odovtos*, **15**, 21-29.

[39] Sánchez, L., Padilla, M., Rivera, I., Zamorano, A. and Díaz Narváez, V.P. (2013) Niveles de orientación empática en los estudiantes de odontología. *Educación Médica Superior*, **27**, 216-225.

[40] Varela, T.B., Villaba, R.H., Gargantini, P., Quinteros, S. and Díaz Narváez, V.P. (2012) Niveles de orientación empática en estudiantes de Odontología de la Universidad Católica de Córdoba, Argentina (UCC). *Claves de Odontología*, **19**, 15-22

[41] Vera, C. (2014) Empathetic Orientation in Dentistry Students from Latin America. Literature Review. *Journal of Oral Research*, **3**, 123-127. http://dx.doi.org/10.17126/joralres.2014.029

[42] Mercadillo, R.E., Díaz, J.L. and Barrios, F.A. (2007) Neurobiología de las emociones morales. *Salud Mental*, **30**, 1-11.

[43] Bartels, A. and Zeki, S. (2004) The Neural Correlates of Maternal and Romantic Love. *Neuroimage*, **21**, 1155-1166. http://dx.doi.org/10.1016/j.neuroimage.2003.11.003

[44] Michalska, K.J., Kinzler, K.D. and Decety, J. (2013) Age-Related Sex Differences in Explicit Measures of Empathy Do Not Predict Brain Responses across Childhood and Adolescence. *Development Cognitive Neuroscience*, **3**, 22-32. http://dx.doi.org/10.1016/j.dcn.2012.08.001

[45] Mercadillo, R. (2006) Evolución del comportamiento. De monos, simios y humanos. Editorial Trillas, México DF.

[46] Nanda, S. (2013-2014) Are There Gender Differences in Empathy? *Undergraduate Journal of Psychology at Berkeley*, **7**, 22-42.

[47] Cassels, T.G., Chan, S., Chung, W. and Birch, S.A. (2010) The Role of Culture in Affective Empathy. Cultural and Bicultural Differences. *Journal of Cognition and Culture*, **10**, 309-326. http://dx.doi.org/10.1163/156853710X531203

[48] Carlo, G., Hausmann, A., Christiansen, S. and Randall, B.A. (2003) Sociocognitive and Behavioral Correlates of a Measure of Prosocial Tendencies for Adolescents. *The Journal of Early Adolescence*, **23**, 107-134. http://dx.doi.org/10.1177/0272431602239132

[49] Fonseca, J., Divaris, K., Villaba, S., Pizarro, S., Fernández, M., Codjambassis, A., *et al.* (2012) Perceived Sources of Stress amongst Chilean and Argentinean Dental Students. *European Journal of Dental Education*, **17**, 30-38. http://dx.doi.org/10.1111/eje.12004

12

Culture Circle as a Teaching Approach in the Education of Teenager Health Multipliers on Leprosy Awareness

Estela Maria Leite Meirelles Monteiro[1,2*], Amanda Araújo das Mercês[3],
Amanda Carla Borba de Souza Cavalcanti[3], Ana Márcia Tenório de Souza Cavalcanti[1],
Ana Catarina Torres de Lacerda[3], Rosália Daniela Medeiros da Silva[2],
Andrea Rosane Sousa Silva[1], Waldemar Brandão Neto[2]

[1]Graduate Program in Nursing, Federal University of Pernambuco (UFPE), Recife, Brazil
[2]Graduate Program in Child and Adolescent Health, Centre of Health Sciences, Federal University of Pernambuco, Recife, Brazil
[3]Nursing Department at the Federal University of Pernambuco, Recife, Brazil
Email: *estelapf2003@yahoo.com.br

Abstract

Objective: The study aims to evaluate the use of a teaching method proposed by Paulo Freire, Culture Circles, in the education of teenagers multipliers on leprosy awareness. **Methods:** It is an action-research study with a qualitative approach developed in a public school in Pernambuco, Brazil. Five Culture Circles were conducted involving the participation of 26 teenagers. The followings were used as data collection tools: observation, field notes, photography and filming. **Results:** The educational intervention on health addressed the following topics: 1) Definition and transmission of leprosy; 2) Characteristics and diagnosis of leprosy; 3) Treatment of leprosy; 4) Aesthetics, prejudice and mental health related to leprosy; and 5) Planning of educational activities for teenagers as health multipliers on leprosy awareness. The educational action on health provided this age group to perceive themselves, act as political subjects in the development of Culture Circles, and act as protagonists in the dissemination of knowledge on leprosy. **Conclusions:** This study highlights that the application of active methodologies, such as Culture Circles, is able to encourage the engagement of young people in community empowerment and bring together health professionals and the school community in an intersectoral work in order to develop action strategies involving the promotion of health in the context of neglected diseases such as leprosy.

---

*Corresponding author.

Keywords

Adolescents, School Health, Leprosy Awareness, Culture Circles, Health Promotion

1. Introduction

Leprosy is an infectious disease transmitted by the contact with untreated people or people with its transmissible forms. Today, it still represents a serious public health problem in Brazil and in developing countries. It is a condition that affects the lives of people more in a psycho-emotional sense than in health impairment due to the constant threat of prejudice, suffering, abandonment, deformity and psychosocial problems [1].

Inequalities, determinants and socially decisive aspects portray the epidemiological data on leprosy, which leads us to think about how health policies still need to be contextualized considering the culture, customs, socio-economic aspects and the disease's own behavior in each territory [1] [2].

In Brazil, the occurrence of new leprosy cases is increasing, mostly between the 10 to 15 age group. These cases are directly related to active transmission focuses and socioeconomic conditions. It is known that the most vulnerable populations are in less favored areas and since they are closely related to endemicity of the region, they have a great relevance for the epidemiology of the disease [3].

Considering cases of leprosy in Pernambuco, it occupies the tenth position in the coefficient of detection of this disease in Brazil. 36 cases in each group of 100,000 Pernambuco inhabitants are diagnosed with the disease and may suffer some sort of disability in the future, with often irreversible physical and psychological consequences. When analyzing it within the state according to its regions, the metropolitan area of Recife concentrates 55% of cases of the disease. Of cases classified as new, 27% already have disease consequences with regard to developmental disabilities. Within the Northeast region, Pernambuco occupies the third position with a higher leprosy detection rate, second only to Maranhão and Piauí. It is estimated that there are 14 cases per 100,000 aged under 15 in the state of Pernambuco [4].

There is not a specific form of prevention of leprosy, but there are measures that may prevent new cases, such as early diagnosis and treatment, monitoring of contacts and effective actions of health education. Leprosy diagnosis and the correct treatment without interruptions have a great importance in the prevention of physical disabilities. Prevention is primarily made through guidelines for self-care, psychologic and social support, measures that reduce prejudiced behavior towards people with leprosy and encourage family and friends not to repel patients by minimizing or preventing possible sequelae [5].

Understanding the epidemiology and the clinical characteristics of leprosy patients is paramount to design actions addressing the needs of these patients. They are developed together with the population and managers through social control and drafting of effective public policies on the activities of disease prevention and health promotion of the population affected [1].

In this context, there is a need to understand the dynamics of the disease by the teenager, since this stage of life is characterized by a period marked by a set of socio-psychological transformations. It leaves the young person exposed to a model of life until then unknown, full of uncertainties and insecurities that make it more vulnerable to situations of personal and interpersonal conflicts and establishing at the same time behavioral patterns that will become traces of its personality [6].

For a teenager who is in a phase of changes and adaptations, the beginning of a disease such as leprosy has negative repercussions such as truancy, depreciation of self-image with consequent change in the self-esteem and self-exclusion from the social environment. The person may become sad and without encouragement to perform daily activities, which is emphasized by the stigmatizing nature of the disease [7].

In this sense, social devices play a fundamental role in helping teenagers to face different situations. Most important is the role of the school. Upon recognizing the importance of this environment, the school has constituted a fruitful scenario for intersectoral actions between education and health with a focus on educational strategies to promote the health of this age group. The potential of teenagers to act as disseminators of knowledge in their family and social context should also be considered.

In order to establish strategies that promote the health of the teenage population with a focus on prevention and control of leprosy, there is the need to develop health education actions based on active methodologies, which provide a collective knowledge committed to social transformation. In this context, Culture Circles permeate a participatory educational experience with an emphasis on dialogue, autonomy and interaction between the popular and the scientific knowledge. It is a fruitful field for action-reflection-action in the preparation of a systematic proposal for an emancipatory health education [8].

Culture Circles are a teaching tool that breaks the curricular rigidity of academic formalism and provides necessary conditions for the actors involved—students and teachers—to feel familiarized to discuss significant issues for both groups, disregarding issues pre-fixed by a static curriculum regulation. The Culture Circle leads to critical thinking and different understandings on the part of its participants. It also enables a cognitive effervescence, involving problem-situations inherent to a same cultural universe. Thus, it constitutes a favorable arena for a group, with an in-depth process of communion around mutual learning, to produce knowledge from the elements of its culture [9].

Within the presented context and the experience of the authors in health education actions with Culture Circles, this study aims to evaluate the implementation of Culture Circles as a teaching approach in the education of teenagers multipliers on leprosy awareness.

2. Methods

It is an action-research study with a qualitative approach [10], based on the Paulo Freire Method: Culture Circles. For the development of the action-research, it was necessary to reconcile the role of the researcher and the animator of the Culture Circles, establishing an interaction with school teenagers, social actors of the study, determining a research collaboration with broader processes of educational activities and collective construction of knowledge. The choice of the Culture Circle as a theoretical and methodological framework in the development of educational intervention in health was established in order to provide teenagers to perceive themselves and act as agents of change regarding situations of vulnerability experienced in the community [11], inviting them at the same time to take the lead of disseminating knowledge on leprosy awareness.

The study was developed from August to November 2013 in a public school in the municipality of Camaragibe-PE, Brazil, which offers elementary school I and II. For the selection of the 26 teenagers in the study, the intentional sampling technique was used. The following inclusion criteria were adopted: 12 - 18 years age group of both sexes regularly enrolled in the mentioned school and teenagers showing a personal interest to actively participate in the health educational proposal.

The educational intervention occurred with the implementation of Culture Circles, in which the data produced in the group were recorded. For this collection of data, besides the researcher and animator of the Circle, there was the participation of other components with specific tasks such as filming, photographic record and taking of field notes.

There were five Culture Circles, each lasting two hours, which took place in the auditorium and in the school yard. The educational intervention addressed the following topics: 1) Definition and transmission of leprosy; 2) Characteristics and diagnosis of leprosy; 3) Treatment of leprosy; 4) Aesthetics, prejudice and mental health related to leprosy; and 5) Planning of educational activities for teenagers as health multipliers on leprosy awareness. To conduct the educational intervention in health, eight cyclical, inter-related phases were adopted as proposed by Monteiro and Vieira [8], adapted from the Paulo Freire method, as shown in **Figure 1**.

The previous knowledge phase was intensely experienced by the authors and was essential to the planning of the Culture Circles. It required an initial insertion of animators/researchers into the school scenario to raise and record cognitive, socio-cultural and psycho-emotional issues that involved the reality of adolescents participating in the Circles and the previous knowledge about leprosy.

For the analysis of the data, the data triangulation method [12] was used in order to achieve a greater validity and reliability of qualitative data. The organization of empirical material occurred with the detailed description of all the events of the Culture Circle through the transcription of the information collected with speeches record in full, narration of information contained in field notes, transcription of the filmed material ordered by narration and discussion, following the sequence of the Culture Circles. The analysis and interpretation synthesis occurred in a dialogue with the related literature and the experience of educational action, from which the cultural meanings on the approach to leprosy emerged.

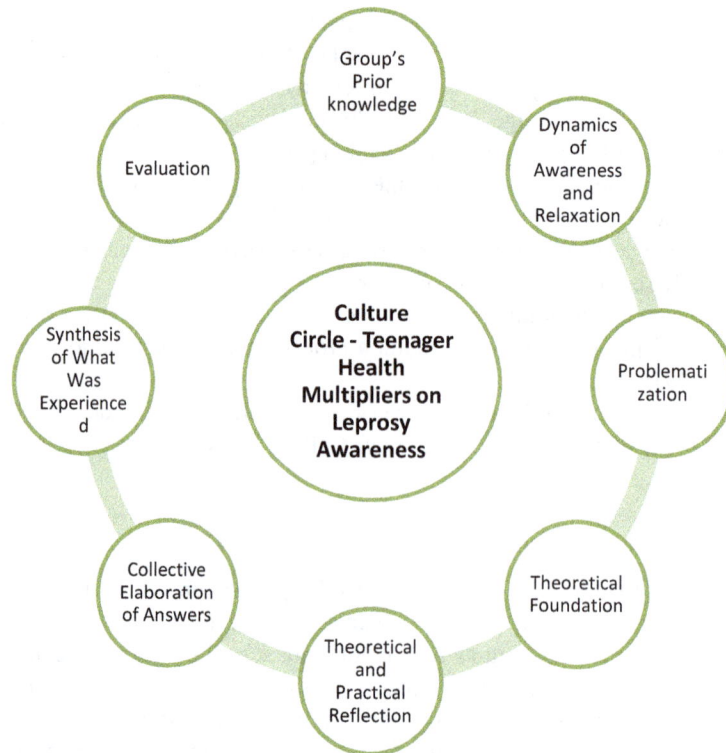

Figure 1. Phases of the Paulo Freire Method as proposed by Monteiro and Vieira (2010) and used in this study.

The study followed the advocated by the resolution no. 466/12 of the National Health Council [13], with the approval of the Ethics Committee of the Health Sciences Center of the Federal University of Pernambuco by the CAAE record (Presentation Certificate for Ethics Considerations) No. 16095013.5.0000.5208.

3. Results

The planning of educational activities took into account the desire and expectation of adolescents, and approached researchers and school management in a collaborative work of health promotion. The presentation of the results obeyed the order of the development of phases of each Circles, which outlined the educational process in the education of teenagers multipliers of health on leprosy.

All adolescents live in the community surrounding the school, considered of low economic status. As for the socio-demographic profile of the participants, it is described in **Table 1**.

1) The first Culture Circle dealt with the theme Definition and transmission of leprosy.

The awareness dynamics provided an integration among teenagers, where everyone was arranged in a circle. A person who was inside the circle should leave and walk around to choose a participant. This should tell its name and a characteristic with the first letter of its name, leaving to the person chosen the ability to follow up the activity.

The Problematization brought the following generative question: What do you understand about leprosy? Each teen was asked to answer the question with a drawing and then explain its meaning. Then, a poster was designed with the collective production of drawings. Most teenagers drew faces with expressions of sadness and doubt represented by question marks. Of the 26 teenagers, only three had some knowledge about the disease because they had experienced cases in the family or had access to posters on leprosy at health centers. They expressed this knowledge by producing drawings representing people crying with spots on the body.

Regarding the theoretical foundation, a contextualized scientific content was presented using a flipchart with colorful and simple illustrative photos and a clear language so that they could deepen the understanding of the disease and its means of transmission.

Table 1. Characterization of the demographic data of the study sample.

Variables	Adolescents (N = 26) %
Gender	
Female	80.8
Male	19.2
Age	
12 years	19.2
13 years	50.0
14 years	30.8
Religion	
Catthcolic	57.7
Evangelical	34.6
Referred not have	7.7
Who do you live with	
Parents	80.8
Mother and Stepfather	11.5
Mother	3.8
Father	3.8
Those who work	
Parents	23.1
Father	50.0
Mother	19.2
Parents and brothers	7.7
How many people live in the residence	
3 to 4 people	50.0
5 to 6 people	42.3
7 or morepeople	7.7

The theoretical and practical Reflection was the resume of the guiding question seeking to identify the knowledge and opinions of teenagers on the theme, thus creating a relation between the experienced reality and the contextualized content. At this phase, teenagers expressed that the discussions produced in the Circle led to changes and advances in the knowledge acquired. They reported that they previously believed that the spread of leprosy occurred by hug, kiss, handshake, touching skin injuries and/or that it was a sexually transmitted disease.

For the collective preparation of answers, it was requested that each teenager said a word to define leprosy. Two categories were identified: 1) Teenagers expressed words of encouragement such as perseverance, determination, strength, focus, faith. 2) Teenagers also portrayed an awareness regarding the prejudice and the exclusion experienced by people who have leprosy represented by the words sadness, exclusion, prejudice.

In the synthesis phase, a poster/mural was prepared with drawings, encouragement sentences, words that retake the theme addressed in the Circle.

At the time of the evaluation, an informative booklet containing crossword puzzles related to the theme of the circle was delivered to the teenagers. It was answered by the participants complementing the knowledge addressed in the Circle.

2) The second Culture Circle dealt with the theme Characteristics and Diagnosis of Leprosy.

In the awareness-raising dynamic, teenagers chose magazine pictures that portrayed similarities or differences in relation to the theme considering the popular knowledge.

In the questioning phase, the following question was addressed: What are the characteristics of leprosy? How can it be diagnosed? It stimulated the identification of knowledge, doubts and concerns of the participants.

For the theoretical and practical basis, an album-series exploring the clinical and diagnostic features of the disease was used. At the theoretical and practical reflection phase, a playful activity regarding the questions about leprosy was conducted. They were addressed in this Circle. The playful activity was the application of a board game, for which the group was organized into three subgroups with a choice of one representative for each of them. The rules were: each participant rolls the dice and move the respective number of spaces. In some spaces, there are questions. If the player correctly answers the question, it remains in that space. If the player wrongly answers the question, it moves back two spaces. Upon reaching the end of the board, the player drew a question and answered it.

During the collective preparation of answers phase, teenagers resumed the initial questioning, allowing the re-elaboration of a more scientific-based answer. Then, educational materials were delivered containing a list of the addressed knowledge, as well as the Internet address of the website and the Facebook group, a virtual environment to streamline communication and clarification of doubts.

In the synthesis phase, the expectations of multipliers in relation to the issue addressed during the round were taken into account, clarifying their questions about the function of the multiplier and the relevant topic. The group demonstrated an acceptance of the methodology applied to the association of leaflets and the interaction with social networks.

The evaluation of the Circle was conducted through a dynamic in which teenagers reported what they felt about the development of the Circle phases, opting to "like it" or not. The evaluations were positive, since all have chosen to mark "like it". An open dialog was conducted for teenagers to express the appreciation of the dynamics presented.

3) The third Culture Circle addressed the topic Leprosy treatment.

The Circle began with an awareness dynamic, in which each student received a sheet of paper and a pencil, and then was asked: What do you want your friend that is at your right to do? They answered the question and signed their names. Then, after everyone had delivered the sheets of paper, the facilitator asked each person to do what the friend asked for and finished by explaining the objective of the dynamic: What I do not want for myself, I do not do to others.

At the problematization phase, the students were divided into five groups and received a cardboard and colored pencils. Each group was asked to discuss how to treat leprosy and register on cardboard what the group thought. Afterwards, each group presented their poster. The following statements were recorded:

The treatment is expensive, but in some cases, the health center provides it. (E1)
If the person has no money to buy the medicine, it can seek it at the health center (E2).
In some cases, people seek the medicine at the health center, but sometimes it does not have the medicine. Then, the person has to buy it, but one has no money and one leaves the disease there [...] (E3).
[...] there is indeed treatment and the medicine is free (E4).
Our group thinks the treatment is done by drugs in pills and it is prepared in the health center and it is free (E5).

At the theoretical basis phase, a flip chart was used to explain the treatment of the disease. The medication blister pack was presented, differentiating the paucibacillary and multibacillary method for child and adult treatment. Supervised doses were highlighted. They are at the top of the blister pack and should be taken in the presence of nurses. The continuous medication can be used at home. During the explanations, several questions emerged, such as:

Do other drugs that are not taken in front of the nurse have to be taken every day? (E5)Can people with anemia take the medicine? (E8)
Is there an illness that interferes with it, and you cannot take the medicine? (E11)
If the person is thinking that it has the disease and the health center is closed, can I go to a hospital? (E19)
If one takes the red medicine and the pee color changes, must one continue using the medicine? (E24)

All doubts were clarified, and the importance of not interrupting the treatment was stressed. The side effects of medications and other necessary precautions during treatment were also explained. It was stressed that leprosy is curable.

To support the theoretical and practical reflection, a game in which students were divided into five groups was elaborated. A blister pack with an increased size, made of rubber produced by the facilitators, was put on the ground. The dynamic was to roll a dice and walk on the pills. The person that fell on top of a pill with a question should answer it correctly to advance. The questions addressed the treatment of leprosy.

For the collective elaboration of answers, the facilitator of the Circle asked several questions about the treatment of the disease, obtaining a consistency in the responses given by the group.

At the synthesis phase, the facilitator used a parody of the treatment of leprosy and distributed the lyrics to students so everyone could sing.

In the evaluation phase, the teenagers expressed that they liked the different learning methods using music and educational games, highlighting the importance of using a playful method to facilitate learning, as was evident in some opinions:

[...] so we learn playing [...] (E17)
[...] it was one of the best, because there were many different activities such as music and games on the same day [...] (E26).

4) The fourth Culture Circle addressed Mental health and Prejudice towards leprosy.

The dynamics of awareness and casualness aimed to educate teenager participants in relation to situations of stigma and prejudice experienced by people with leprosy. In the awareness dynamics, it was presented to every teenager, following its placement in a circle, a hat that had a mirror on the inside reflecting the teenager's own face, and another hat with a picture of an individual with a leonine face characteristic of leprosy in an advanced stage without treatment. Then, teenagers were asked to talk a little about each image.

A dialogue followed, in which participants expressed their feelings and opinions regarding the experienced activity. The following was reported: conflicting feelings of insecurity and fear at the prospect of interacting with people with leprosy. This led the group to think about how society can be prejudiced and insensitive, having an excluding attitude and potentiating negative feelings towards a person with leprosy.

The problematization led to a discussion and a broad concept of health and disease, in which health was defined as the balance between physical, psychological and social well-being. This concept was discussed considering that leprosy affects the individual in its entirety. In preparing the understanding of prejudice, the predominance of the society's posture was evidenced based on ignorance and lack of knowledge about the disease.

In the theoretical basis, the video series—Heirs of Prejudice-Part 2 was presented. It is available at the following address: https://youtu.be/sOPwb_EG6E8. It portrays in the speech of former patients the isolation and social prejudice evidenced by the compulsory relocation of patients to the Colônia de Mirueira, located in the State of Pernambuco, Brazil.

In the theoretical practical reflection, teenagers demonstrated a visible sensitivity to deepen the discussions on the stigma experienced by patients with leprosy considering the construction of knowledge grounded on the prior knowledge plus the reports presented by protagonist patients of their exclusion stories for having leprosy.

Teenagers highlighted that people with leprosy needed support to continue the treatment and that in addition to physical problems resulting from the pathology, patients with the disease are emotionally shaken. This contributes to a feeling of low self-esteem and contribute to a greater difficulty in adherence to drug therapy.

At the time of the collective elaboration of answers, the teenagers were encouraged to reflect on the problem-situation raised earlier in the Circle regarding exclusion and prejudice situations experienced by leprosy patients. Discussions in the group fostered the development of broader thoughts, triggered by an articulated composition of responses by the teenagers.

In the synthesis of what was experienced, the materials were made available for teenagers to collectively produce a poster with the knowledge acquired during the Culture Circle. They explained with ease and with a critical reflection that prejudice is wrong, that the incentive to treatment is important and that a carrier of the disease can lead a normal life provided it is treating the disease regularly.

In the evaluation stage of the Circle, the knowledge about leprosy and prejudice was evaluated. Teenagers demonstrated a fluency on the subject. They answered all questions with ease and security, as well as designing posters that encouraged an unprejudiced conduct towards people with the disease. The learning triggered by the construction of collective knowledge and social responsibility to seek knowledge about leprosy aiming to overcome a prejudice posture that is fruit of ignorance and lack of solidarity was notorious.

5) The fifth Culture Circle addressed the Planning of an educational action by teenagers as multipliers in leprosy awareness.

In the dynamics of awareness/casualness, five sheets of craft paper were scattered on the floor. In each, a name of a playful activity was written: theater, dance, music, drawing and puppet theater. They were asked to group themselves according to their skills. The largest group went to theater, followed by drawing. Only one person chose dance, two chose music and none chose puppet theater.

The problematization phase presented a discussion of the presentation method to be used by teenagers as multipliers on leprosy awareness. When considering the proposal of a group action, the teenagers listed theater as a form of popular expression regarding health.

The theoretical basis was a brief explanation of the elaboration of the scenic text, construction of the characters, setting the stage, spoken and unspoken communication and interaction with the public.

At the time of theoretical and practical reflection, the initial question was resumed with the definition of the play's central idea by the multipliers. The facilitators assisted in the composition of the text, with the lines of the characters that each teenager was responsible for playing.

The play told the story of a teenager who had stains throughout the skin and so friends did not want to approach her. Then, the teacher notes that she has a sad countenance and advises her to talk to her mother in order to take her to the Family Health Unit. When she is taken to the health service, the teenager sees a nurse who carries out an inspection and an evaluation of the sensitivity of the stain. With the reception, necessary guidance about leprosy and necessary referrals, she is happy to know that it is a curable disease and has a treatment offered for free.

For the collective preparation of answers, teenagers resumed the preliminary question, defining the knowledge about their characters and lines, as well as setting the stage, asking the facilitators of Culture Circles for another meeting to correctly play their character.

In synthesis phase, the importance of acting as multipliers and everything that was experienced was emphasized. Finally, in evaluating the Circle, facilitators questioned what they thought about the Circle and obtained the following statements:

[...] I'm happy with what I learned [...] (E15)
[...] I'm feeling very special to be part of the project and to be able to say what I've learned to other teens [...] (E18)

The teenagers acted as multipliers in leprosy awareness in their school (municipality of Camaragibe) and in other public schools in the Distrito Sanitário V (Municipality of Recife, Pernambuco, Brazil), which had no coverage of the Health in School Program during the National Pre-Campaign on Leprosy and Geohelminth Infections held in August 2013.

4. Discussion

Schools are a favorable scenario for health education interventions with teenagers, providing an intersectoral action to promote health for this age group. As a place of unique opportunities in the development of educational activities, schools should invest more in activities that promote health in partnership with institutions linked to health services due to their strategic role in the development of actions and in the implementation of educational programs that could improve health conditions such as the Health in School Program ("Programa Saúde na Escola", PSE). Therefore, such actions must value partnerships for a participatory, interdisciplinary cross development, and provide playful and interactive processes [14].

As an active methodology, the Culture Circle favored the learning process upon ensuring the autonomy and the main role of adolescents as multipliers in health on leprosy awareness, changing the prejudice attitudes towards individuals with the disease. The organization of teenagers in a circle maintains a possibility of dialog in the process of building a collective, shared and contextualized knowledge, which led students to an inner journey towards personal, formal, informal experiences. The development of Culture Circles requires the work of animators/facilitators in the collective construction of knowledge, providing a link between the popular and the scientific knowledge.

Creativity is of fundamental importance to the Culture Circle coordinator. It must seek to grasp the totality of human expressions that are embedded in the cultural universe of the group, considering everything that the body produces and signals such as gestures, language expressions, attitudes and silence [9].

The steps that guide the Culture Circles as proposed by Freire are composed of Thematic Research, The matization and Problematization. In this study, we used the phases as proposed by Monteiro and Vieira [8], which systematically address the phases proposed by Freire in youth and adult literacy, explaining in detail how the health educator might base its planning during an educational activity.

The Thematic Research requires that the facilitator/animator consider the prior knowledge of teenagers, the Thematization of the interests and their demands regarding the contents to be addressed. The Problematization causes participants to express their experience and/or opinion before a contextual questioning of a topic, allowing the construction of a dialogical understanding of the cultural universe of teenagers. Freire [15] defined culture as the way people understand and express their world and how people can understand themselves in their relations with their world.

The study requires to "take a serious and curious attitude towards a problem" ([16], p. 58). Thus, the Problematization phase, proposed by [8], in order to be applied to health education activities, emerges from generating issues proposed by animators/researchers, leading to an immersion in the subject from the experiences of the group, full of personal and collective meanings intrinsic to the involvement of each member in the learning process. The teaching and learning in the Circles are indivisible, dialectical interactions, providing a unique and dynamic process. According to Freire [17], only authoritarian teachers and educators deny solidarity between the act of teaching and the act of being educated by the students.

For the construction of new knowledge, the Problematization phase does not end in itself. The animator must consider the characteristics of the groups participating in Circles and use teaching techniques such as educational games, videos, pictures, drawings and/or dramatization, providing a dynamic and enjoyable learning.

The application of a Culture Circle can provide an intense flow of critical, reflective and mobilizing knowledge committed to a renewed practice in Health education [16]. According to Paulo Freire, idealizer of the Culture Circles, the use of this pedagogical proposal is essential to the construction of health education strategies, enabling to assume that teenagers have knowledge, values, principles and feelings and, at the same time, understanding of their responsibility to transform reality [8].

The educational intervention, developed during the Culture Circles, included themes that addressed specific knowledge on epidemiological and physical characteristics, emotional factors and social and cultural aspects of leprosy, as well as diagnosis and treatment.

The proposed Culture Circles establish a partnership relation between multipliers and community groups with the understanding of health as a product of real social conditions and the commitment to health promotion actions [8]. The contextualized learning of the subject by teenagers consolidated an empowerment posture essential to elaborate a proposal for educational intervention as multipliers in health.

A key issue for educational activities on health awareness is not in perfecting techniques of sending a message or persuading people, but in rethinking the assumption according to which the existence of scientific information in the received messages is sufficient to increase the competence and/or the freedom of decision in order to incorporate, in everyday life, the appropriate or desired behavior in its autonomy to maintain the health or care of oneself [18] and one's community, thus leading to a change in behavior and perceiving educational activities as a process of forwarding information where the listener is a passive learner.

The feelings and anxieties associated with this ancient disease, such as fear, shame, guilt, social exclusion, rejection and anger, are internalized in individuals with leprosy. The prejudice remains rooted in our culture and society mainly due to the lack of access to information, causing a great suffering to individuals with the disease [19].

Some results evidences the prejudice of people against individuals under treatment or those who are already cured of leprosy due to a lack of knowledge. While there are no effective educational activities aiming to disseminate information about leprosy contagion means, the society will continue to create means to understand and protect themselves from it, symbolically repelling from its contagion [20].

To overcome the challenge of making health education activities more effective, it is necessary that such actions be based on concern for each other and one's individual needs, favoring care and not directing, but respecting the existence and the essence of the human being [18].

Health promotion activities using active methodologies contribute to a critical reflection of actions and strategies that could culminate in promoting and maintaining interventions regarding the quality of life of teenage students [21].

5. Conclusions

In the development of teaching and learning methods with teenagers, it is essential to consider the peculiar characteristics of growth, physical, psycho-emotional, social and cultural developments of this age group. In this sense, the Culture Circle embraced the universe of the teenager in its entirety, bringing together motivation and learning, joy and knowledge, reflection and commitment, challenges and concerns with a desire for change. This culminated in the full participation of teenagers in a process of construction and reconstruction of knowledge and attitudes related to leprosy.

The school scenario was an environment favorable to health education interventions from an intersectoral action, which integrates education and health in a proactive proposal for a comprehensive care towards the teenager in both its cognitive development and the good exercise of one's behavior. Thus, investment in educational prevention programs, supported by emancipatory paradigms, can promote the work of teenagers as protagonists in discussions of public health issues, and developing of coping strategies for the prevention of leprosy, allowing intervene in conditions of health, life and care in the community.

In this sense, health education knowledge about the leprosy was essential to face the stigma and prejudice by establishing a human look in caring for each other and the possibilities of formation of support networks to promote an early detection and the treatment of leprosy. The study also reveals the importance of strategic planning, at the management level, of actions promoting health that allow bringing health services closer to the school community when attending the needs of teenagers and their families in the context of neglected diseases such as the leprosy. In addition, it stresses the need for further research that uses the Culture Circle method with different age groups and with other themes.

6. Limitations

As this is a qualitative intervention study with the local development of a critical and awareness-educational action, involving a sample of adolescents with peculiar characteristics, the results allow not being generalized to the population.

References

[1]   Souza, V.B., Silva, M.R.F., Silva, L.M.S., Torres, R.A.M., Gomes, K.W.L., Fernandes, M.C. and Jereissati, J.M.C.L. (2013) Epidemiological Profile of Leprosy Cases in a Family Health Center. *Brazilian Journal in Health Promotion*, **26**, 110-116.

[2]   Magalhães, M.C.C. (2007) Diferenciação territorial da hanseníase no Brasil. *Epidemiol Serv Saude*, **16**, 75-84.

[3]   Fernandes, C., Beltrão, B.A., Chaves, D.B.R., Leandro, T.A., Silva, V.M. and Lopes, M.V.O. (2013) Assesment of the Resilience Level of Adolescents with Leprosy. *Revista Enfermagem UERJ*, **21**, 496-501. http://www.e-publicacoes.uerj.br/index.php/enfermagemuerj/article/view/10021/8133

[4]   Secretária de Saúde do estado de Pernambuco. Programa Estadual de Vigilância, Prevenção e Controle da Hanseníase (2013) Boletim Epidemiológico-Hanseníase. http://portal.saude.pe.gov.br/programa/secretaria-executiva-de-vigilancia-em-saude/programa-estadual-de-vigilancia-prevencao-e

[5]   Pereira, D.L., Brito, L.M., Nascimento, A.H., Ribeiro, E.L., Lemos, R.K.M., Alves, J.N. and Brandão, L.C.G. (2012) Estudo da prevalência das formas clínicas da hanseníase na cidade de Anápolis-GO. *Ensaios & Ciência*, **16**, 55-67. http://www.redalyc.org/articulo.oa?id=26025372004

[6]   Neto, G.X., Rosemiro, F., Dias, A., Rocha, M.S. and Cunha, I.C.K.O. (2007) Gravidez na adolescência: Motivos e percepções de adolescentes. *Revista Brasileira de Enfermagem*, **60**, 279-285. http://dx.doi.org/10.1590/S0034-71672007000300006

[7]   Ponte, K.M.A. and Ximenes Neto, F.R.G. (2005) Hanseníase: A realidade do ser adolescente. *Revista Brasileira de Enfermagem*, **58**, 296-301. http://dx.doi.org/10.1590/S0034-71672005000300008

[8]   Monteiro, E.M.L.M. and Vieira, N.F.C. (2010) Educação em saúde a partir de círculos de cultura. *Revista Brasileira de Enfermagem*, **63**, 397-403. http://dx.doi.org/10.1590/S0034-71672010000300008

[9]   Peroza, J., Silva, C.P. and Akkari, A. (2013) Paulo freire e a diversidade cultural: Um humanismo político-pedagógico para a transculturalidade na educação. *Reflexão e Ação*, **21**, 461-481.

[10]   Merriam, S. (2009) Qualitative Research: A Guide to Design and Implementation. Jossey-Bass, San Francisco.

[11]   Monteiro, E.M.L.M., Brandão Neto, W., Lima, L.S., Aquino, J.M., Gontijo, D.T. and Pereira, B.O. (2015) Culture

Circles in Adolescent Empowerment for the Prevention of Violence. *International Journal of Adolescence and Youth*, **20**, 167-184. http://dx.doi.org/10.1080/02673843.2014.992028

[12] Flick, U. (2014) An Introduction to Qualitative Research. 5th Edition, Sage Publications, London.

[13] Brazil (2012) Resolution 466, Issued on December 12th, 2012. Discusses the Guidelines and Regulatory Standards of Research Involving Human Beings. National Health Council, Ministry of Health, Brasilia, DF. http://conselho.saude.gov.br/resolucoes/2012/Reso466.pdf

[14] Brito, A.K.A., Silva, F.I.C. and França, N.M. (2012) Programas de intervenção nas escolas brasileiras: Uma contribuição da escola para a educação em saúde. *Saúde debate*, **36**, 624-632. http://dx.doi.org/10.1590/S0103-11042012000400014

[15] Freire, P. (2008) Education as the Practice of Freedom. 31th Edition, Paz e Terra, Rio de Janeiro.

[16] Linhares, F.M.P., Pontes, C.M. and Osório, M.M. (2014) Using the Theoretical Constructs of Paulo Freire to Guide Breastfeeding Promotion Strategies. *Revista Brasileira de Saúde Materno Infantil*, **14**, 433-439. http://dx.doi.org/10.1590/S1519-38292014000400013

[17] Freire, P. (2011) Pedagogy of the Oppressed. 50th Edition, Paz e Terra, Rio de Janeiro.

[18] Paz, E.P.A. and Silva, M.C.D. (2012) Educação em saúde no programa de controle da hanseníase: A vivência da equipe multiprofissional. *Escola Anna Nery*, **14**, 223-229. http://dx.doi.org/10.1590/S1414-81452010000200003

[19] Baialardi, K.S. (2007) O Estigma da Hanseníase: Relato de uma Experiência em Grupo com Pessoas Portadoras. *Hansenologia Internationalis*, **32**, 27-36. http://www.ilsl.br/revista/imageBank/301-862-1-PB.pdf

[20] Palmeira, I.P., Queiroz, A.B.A. and Ferreira, M.A. (2012) Quando o preconceito marca mais que a doença. *Tempus Actas de Saúde Coletiva*, **6**, 187-199.

[21] Moreira, R.M., Boery, E.M., Oliveira, D.C., Sales, Z.N., Boery, R.N.S.O., Teixeira, J.R.B., Ribeiro, I.J.S. and Mussi, F.C. (2015) Social Representations of Adolescents on Quality of Life: Structurally-Based Study. *Ciência & Saúde Coletiva*, **20**, 49-56. http://dx.doi.org/10.1590/1413-81232014201.20342013

13

Did You Sleep Well, Darling?—Link between Sleep Quality and Relationship Quality

Angelika Anita Schlarb[1*], Merle Claßen[1], E.-S. Schuster[2], Frank Neuner[1], Martin Hautzinger[2]

[1]Faculty of Psychology and Sports, University of Bielefeld, Bielefeld, Germany
[2]Faculty of Science, University of Tuebingen, Tuebingen, Germany
Email: *angelika.schlarb@uni-bielefeld.de

Abstract

Background: Relationship quality and sleep quality influenced physiological and psychological health. Therefore, the aim of the present study was to determine a possible connection between relationship satisfaction and sleep quality and to test a theoretical model of sleep quality as related to relationship and psychological well-being. Methods: Fifty-one heterosexual, cohabitating couples between 24 and 70 years old participated. The relationship quality was measured by the German short version of relationship questionnaire. To determine the sleep quality, the Pittsburgh Sleep Quality Index and a two-week sleep diary were implemented. To gather information about psychological well-being, especially depression and anxiety, the German Symptom Checklist was used. Results: Sleep quality was measured by the Pittsburgh Sleep Quality Index and relationship quality correlated significantly negative. In addition, the study found a positive correlation between sleep duration and relationship quality. In a multiple regression model, fighting and mental strain explained 38% of variance of sleep quality. Depression, anxiety and relationship quality showed no further improvement of the model. These findings suggested that relationship quality, constructive partnership behavior and mental strain played an essential role in sleep quality.

Keywords

Relationship Quality, Cohabitating Couples, Sleep Quality, Fighting, Mental Health

1. Introduction

Both relationships and sleep have a high impact on quality of life and well-being [1]. As sleep and relationships

---

*Corresponding author.

are connected with well-being [2] [3] and sleep is typically shared within close relationships [3], it is easily deduced that sleep, relationship quality and mental health are strongly associated. Sleep is commonly seen as a critical health behavior linked with much morbidity via various physiological and psychological mechanisms. Due to the subjective importance, relationships influence mental health. But mental health also has a high impact on relationship quality [4].

1.1. Sleep and Relationship Satisfaction

A large Korean longitudinal study showed a bidirectional association between sleep and relationship quality. Low marriage quality led to a higher risk of a clinically relevant sleep disorder. *Vice versa*, a low sleep quality in the early stages predicted lower marriage satisfaction four years later [5]. Sleep duration seemed to be influenced by relationship status, as singles and divorced people sleep less than married participants [2]. Furthermore, unmarried people were more at risk of sleep disturbances compared to married adults [6]. Haslers and Troxel assessed couples about sleep and relationship functioning [7]. In men, higher sleep efficiency (measured by sleep diary) had a predictive value on less negative interaction with the partner. *Vice versa*, positive interactions reported by women seemed to influence men's sleep efficiency positively.

Various mechanisms might explain the association between relationship quality and sleep. For example, attachment styles impacted sleep in married couples [8]. Individuals reporting higher scores in fear of attachment had a decreased sleep quality. Furthermore, couples being physically apart reported increased sleep problems in nights they spent without their partners [9]. In addition, women in happy relationships seemed to have no sleep difficulties, whereas women with sleep problems reported less satisfaction with their marriages [10]. Cacioppo and colleagues [11] investigated the influence of loneliness on sleep. They found a relationship between loneliness and sleep efficiency, stating that people who felt lonely had lower sleep efficiency (83%) than people who did not (90%). Relationship status seemed to influence sleep in women, especially [3]. Comparing 367 middle-aged women longitudinally for eight years in terms of relationship status and sleep quality measured by polysomnography, questionnaires and actigraphy, they found significant differences between women in a consistent marriage and women who had lost their partners. Married women had shorter phases of nightly awakenings than women who lost their partners or had never been married. Women who lost their partners had poorer sleep quality. Women who had never been married had longer sleep latency than married women. In men, no comparable studies were available.

Mental illnesses could influence the partner's sleep as well. For example, partners reported shorter sleep duration if their spouses suffered from anxiety. But depressive husbands led to longer sleep durations in women [12].

Intimate partner violence also influenced sleep quality [13] [14]. A bidirectional association of sleep on intimate partner violence and *vice versa* was found in couples living together and having at least one child [14]. Furthermore, psychological violence predicted sleep problems two years later, mediated by depression and anxiety [13].

1.2. Relationship Quality

Investigating long term influences on relationships Orbuch and colleagues found only ethnicity and educational status to be significant predictors on divorces over a duration of 14 years [15]. A lower educational level and African-American race tend to predict a divorce. Furthermore, with increasing age, satisfaction within the relationship decreases [1]. Conflict behavior seems to play an important role in relationship satisfaction [16]. Destructive behavior such as screaming, insulting and disdainfulness is associated with divorces one year after marriage. Even if one partner behaves constructively and the other's reaction is withdrawal, risk for divorce increases. Nevertheless, fighting alone does not account for relationship satisfaction. Tenderness seems to be more important than the absence of conflicts [1].

Beyond that, the regularity of sexual intercourse influences relationship satisfaction as reported in a multiple regression. Results suggest younger women are more satisfied with sexual intercourse than older women. Younger women tend to be slightly more satisfied with their relationships in general [17].

1.3. Sleep and Mental Health

Taylor and colleagues found a connection between sleep, depression and anxiety [18]. Participants with insomnia reported significant depression and anxiety scores. Furthermore, functional impairments such as reduced self-care, mobility, cognition, social functioning, time out of role and components of productive role functioning have been studied in people suffering from insomnia with comorbidities [19]. Neckelmann, Mykletun and Dahl surveyed participant's anxiety, depression and insomnia twice in 11 years [20]. Longitudinal data showed that participants with insomnia were at higher risk to develop depression and anxiety later on. Zawadzki and colleagues [21] investigated the influence of rumination and the feeling of loneliness on sleep. Their data suggests that loneliness and depression lead to poorer sleep quality. Supporting this, as soon as the feeling of loneliness decreases, symptoms of anxiety and rumination improve [21].

1.4. Other Variables Influencing Sleep

Stress negatively influences sleep as Vahtera and colleagues [22] showed in a longitudinal study performed. All stressful events were predictive for sleep disorders. Despite that, patients suffering from insomnia often report significantly more stressful and negative events than healthy sleepers [23]. Furthermore, arousal and coping strategies mediated the stress' influence on sleep, in patients with insomnia and healthy sleepers [23].

In addition age and gender influence sleep. Higher age seems to be associated with sleep disorders as more women over 60 suffered from disturbed sleep (31.4%) about twice as many as women between 18 and 39 (17.9%). For men the rate was even three times higher. Between the age of 18 and 39 years about 9.5% reported sleep disturbances, where as nearly one third of men above 60 years showed sleep disorder symptoms (29.0%) [24].

As relationships and sleep seem to influence quality of life and health, the present study's aim is to determine the link between sleep quality and relationship quality. Firstly, it is assumed that (1) women report subjectively poorer sleep quality than men. Women tend to suffer from more difficulties falling asleep and maintaining sleep. Secondly, (2) psychological well-being is associated with sleep quality in both sexes, since previous studies reported overall mental health, depression and anxiety to be associated with sleep disturbances. Thirdly, (3) sleep quality and relationship quality is correlated. Low relationship quality is associated with low sleep quality. Fourthly, (4) fighting in intimate relationships seems impact sleep negatively. Finally, (5) a theoretical model including relevant factors will be tested. The influence of partnership quality, fighting and mental health on sleep quality will be investigated.

2. Materials and Methods

2.1. Procedure

Participants were recruited in public presentations and hearings at Landau University. All participants were informed prior to their participation about the content and duration of the study and gave their written consent. Furthermore, the Ethics Committee University of Landau permitted the study. Participants took part voluntarily. The participants filled out three questionnaires and recorded on their sleep for one week. After filling out the questionnaire, participants mailed them back via postal sending. Inclusion criteria were that couples cohabitated and both partners filled out the questionnaires.

2.2. Questionnaires

2.2.1. Pittsburgh Sleep Quality Index (PSQI)
The Pittsburgh Sleep Quality Index (PSQI) was implemented to assess sleep problems. 18 items (ranging from 0 to 3) measure self-rated sleeping habits within the last four weeks. The items are divided into seven scales, sleep quality, sleep latency, sleep duration, habitual sleep efficiency, sleep disturbances, use of sleep medication and daytime dysfunction. A total sum score is built with a cut-off score above five indicating bad sleepers and a score above 10 suggesting severe sleep problems [25].

2.2.2. Sleep Diary
In addition, a standardized sleep-diary was used for diagnostics for 14 days. Every day, participants answered questions about the time they went to bed, when they got up and their latency to fall asleep. There were open questions about the amount of exercise, intake of medicine (type, dose and time), as well as consumption of alcohol, nicotine and caffeine. Subjective measures of mood, sleepiness and performance were rated in a scale from one (very good) to six (very bad). The diary compromised a morning and an evening component. The

morning section should be completed immediately after getting up and consists of 12 items. The nine items of the evening component should be done just before turning off the light. Additionally dichotome items (yes or no) about sexuality, tenderness and fights were generated.

2.2.3. Partnership

To evaluate partnership quality, a short version of a relationship questionnaire was used [26]. This German questionnaire (PFB-K) consists of nine items (ranging from 0 to 3), which are divided into three scales, fighting-behavior (coded inversely), tenderness and commonality. In a tenth item the happiness of the relationship was rated. A sum score is generated. A score lower than 17 means an unhappy relationship. Two additional items were generated, concerning sex and satisfaction with sex.

2.2.4. Symptom-Checklist (SCL-90-R)

For mental health the symptom-checklist (SCL-90-R) [27] measured subjective impairment by physiological and psychological symptoms. In 83 items aspects about somatization, obsessive behavior, social phobia, depression, anxiety, aggression, phobic anxiety, paranoid thoughts and psychoticism were quantified. There are seven additional items. Via a calculated sum score a comparison to a validation sample can be done. In the present study the sum score and the scales depression and anxiety have been used.

2.3. Data Analysis

The statistical analysis was calculated with IBM SPSS 21 for Windows. Pearson correlations were calculated to determine associations and t-tests were performed to test differences between genders. To investigate the influence of age, well-being and relationships on sleep parameters, a linear regression was performed. A multifactorial variance analysis was performed to identify different factors explaining sleep quality.

3. Results

3.1. Subjects

Seventy-one couples received questionnaires with 68% mailing them back. Data analysis included a total of 102 participants ($n = 102$), or 51 heterosexual couples. The couples' age ranged between 24 and 70 years (M = 42.37, SD = 14.18). For further information see **Table 1**.

All couples cohabited between 6 months and 44 years. Twenty-five (24.5%) participants had children living with them, whereas 35 (34.3%) had children, who were not living with the many more. Most of the participants had a fulltime job (54.9%). For further information see **Table 2**.

Table 1. Demographic data.

	Male M (SD)	Female M (SD)	Couples M (SD)
age	43.76 (14.52)	40.98 (13.82)	42.37 (14.18)
Time as a couple			16.02 (14.19)

Note: M = mean; SD = standard deviation.

Table 2. Descriptive statistics of the couples: number of children, medication intake, profession.

		Frequencies	Percent
Children	None	42	41.2
	Living at home	25	24.5
	Not living at home	35	34.3
Medication	Yes	35	34.3
	No	67	65.7
Profession	None	7	6.9
	Retirement	9	8.8
	Full-time	56	54.9
	Part-time	19	18.6
	University student	11	10.8

3.1.1. Sleep Characteristics

According to the PSQI, in mean the sample reported marginally poor sleep (M = 5.21; SD = 2.70). Overall, the participants (76.5%) needed up to 30 minutes to fall asleep (sleep latency PSQI-score; range 0 - 3: M = 0.98, SD = 0.89) and slept for more than seven hours in mean (sleep duration PSQI-score; range 0 - 3: M = 0.46, SD = 0.76).

In the morning participants rated their mood in the sleep diary and in mean their mood was fairly good (range 1 - 6, M = 2.55; SD = 0.64). Furthermore, participants felt fairly fresh in the mornings (range 1 - 6, M = 2.93; SD = 0.77). In mean, participants fell asleep after 14 minutes (M = 13.96; SD = 12.52). But sleep latency ranged between zero and 95 minutes. Only 4.9% needed more than 30 minutes to fall asleep and would therefore lie above clinical cut-off according to the DSM-5. Participants reported in mean 7.12 hours sleep with nightly awakenings occurring for 1.16 minutes on average. No participants experienced awakenings at night lasting longer than 30 minutes. Overall, participants were physically active for 67.73 minutes (SD = 73.53) per day. Couples reported close to no fights (M = 0.085; SD = 0.14). Zero to 10 (9.8%) reported a fight with the partner on any morning/evening protocol. Eight (7.8%) to 21 (20.6%) participants reported sexual intercourse per day. Forty (39.25%) to 82 (80.4%) reported tenderness.

3.1.2. Well-Being

Overall, the sample was mentally sane, as measured by the SCL-90-R (GSI t-transformed M = 50.51; SD = 9.44).

3.1.3. Relationship Characteristics

In mean the participants reported happy relationships above the cut-off (sum score > 17) for a satisfying relationship (M = 18.52; SD = 4.70). 26.5% of all participants showed a sum score of 16 or lower and seemed unhappy in their relationship. The mean for fighting behavior is M = 6.98 (SD = 1.95), for tenderness M = 5.76 (SD = 2.24) and for communality M = 5.80 (SD = 1.65). All above cut-off (<5.66), suggesting good relationships in all areas. Most couples considered sexual intercourse important in their relationship (range 0 - 3; M = 1.91; SD = 0.72), with higher scores indicating higher subjective importance. Furthermore, satisfaction with their inter course seemed common (range 0-3; M = 1.87; SD = 0.67).

3.1.4. Demographic Variables and Sleep

Age and sleep duration correlated significantly ($r = -0.402$, $p = 0.000$) as older people slept less and age explains 16% of the variance. In a regression of daytime sleepiness and age, 5% of daytime sleepiness variance was explained by higher age. No other variables of the PSQI showed an association with age.

Gender had a significant influence on sleep latency ($p = 0.037$) and sleep duration (p = 0.049) with woman needing more time to fall asleep (M = 16.55; SD = 15.76) than men (M = 11.38; SD = 7.47). Furthermore, women slept longer (M = 7.28; SD = 0.81) than men (M = 6.96; SD = 0.80).

3.1.5. Sleep and Mental Health

A significant relationship between sleep and mental health was found. The PSQI and SCL-90-R correlated significantly ($r = 0.592$; $p < 0.001$). In a linear regression 35% of variance was detected. The scales PSDI (Positive Symptom Distress Index), depression and anxiety correlated significantly with the PSQI sum score, but not with all subscales as seen in **Table 3**. Linear regression showed the Positive Symptom Distress Index subscale explained 26% of PSQI variance ($F(1, 100) = 35.942$), the depression subscale 22% of the PSQI variance ($F(1, 100) = 28.135$; $p = 0.000$) and anxiety 19% ($F(1, 100) = 22.898$; $p = 0.000$).

But no significant correlations have been found between the SCL-90-Rs subscales and the sleep diary (all $p > 0.05$).

3.1.6. Sleep and Relationship

A significant negative relationship between PSQI and PFB-K (Relationship satisfaction Questionnaire) was found ($r = -0.198$; $p = 0.047$). This indicates low relationship quality is connected with low sleep quality. Higher scores on PFB-K resulted in lower PSQI scores, but only 4% of the variance was accounted for. A significant negative correlation between sleep medication and PFB-K ($r = -0.219$; $p = 0.027$) was found, but none for other PSQI subscales. For further details, see **Table 4**.

Table 3. Correlations SCL-90-R (Sum score GSI, subscales PSDI, depression and anxiety) und PSQI.

	GSI		Positive Symptom Distress Index (PSDI)		Depression		Anxiety	
	r	p	r	p	r	p	r	p
PSQI total score	0.592	**0.000**	0.514	**0.000**	0.469	**0.000**	0.432	**0.000**
PSQI.1 sleep quality	0.504	**0.000**	0.468	**0.000**	0.353	**0.000**	0.306	**0.002**
PSQI.2 sleep latency	0.336	0.001	0.306	**0.002**	0.242	0.014	0.257	**0.009**
PSQI.3 sleep duration	0.208	**0.036**	0.140	0.163	0.142	0.157	0.167	0.094
PSQI.4 sleep efficiency	0.248	**0.013**	0.202	**0.043**	0.170	0.090	0.154	0.125
PSQI.5 sleep disturbances	0.515	**0.000**	0.517	**0.000**	0.418	**0.000**	0.393	**0.000**
PSQI.6 sleep medication	0.225	**0.023**	0.135	0.176	0.213	**0.032**	0.223	**0.024**
PSQI.7 daytime sleepiness	0.556	**0.000**	0.521	**0.000**	0.532	**0.000**	0.394	**0.000**

Marked results are based on $p < 0.05$.

Table 4. Correlations of PFB-K and PSQI subscales.

	PFB-K		Fighting		Tenderness		Comunality		Hapiness Item		Sex Importance		Sex Satisfaction	
	r	p	r	p	r	p	r	p	r	p	r	p	r	p
PSQI sum score	0.198	**0.047**	0.321	**0.001**	0.072	0.471	0.095	0.344	0.118	0.238	0.030	0.762	0.176	0.074
PSQI.1 sleep quality	0.102	0.310	0.128	0.203	0.028	0.783	0.101	0.317	0.057	0.569	0.029	0.777	0.164	0.100
PSQI.2 sleep latency	0.015	0.884	0.190	0.056	0.111	0.267	0.011	0.911	0.026	0.794	0.051	0.610	0.056	0.575
PSQI.3 sleep duration	0.155	0.120	0.178	0.075	0.117	0.244	0.083	0.407	0.148	0.139	0.066	0.513	0.052	0.603
PSQI.4 sleep efficiency	0.128	0.203	0.189	0.058	0.059	0.556	0.049	0.628	0.028	0.784	0.014	0.888	0.081	0.419
PSQI.5 sleep disturbances	0.172	0.084	0.144	0.148	0.139	0.162	0.135	0.176	0.078	0.438	0.102	0.305	0.275	**0.005**
PSQI.6 sleep medication	**0.219**	0.027	**0.312**	0.001	0.140	0.160	0.067	0.504	0.184	0.064	0.006	0.952	0.090	0.369
PSQI.7 daytime sleepiness	0.083	0.405	**0.237**	0.016	0.030	0.764	0.000	0.997	0.072	0.475	0.024	0.810	0.086	0.388

Marked results are based on $p < 0.05$.

Sleep duration based on the sleep diary correlated significantly with the PFB-K score ($r = 0.289$; $p = 0.003$). The PBF-K score explains 8% of the sleep durations variance, calculated by linear regression ($F(1, 99) = 9.020$, $p = .003$). No other sleep diary parameters correlated with the PBF-K. The effect of PFB-K score on sleep duration is mediated by the participant's age (see **Table 5**). Shorter sleep durations and lower relationship quality are associated with higher age.

The PFB-K subscale, fighting behavior, correlated significantly with the PSQI sum score ($r = =0.321$; $p = 0.001$), suggesting couples who were fighting more often slept worse. In a linear regression 10% of PSQIs variance was explained by fighting behavior.

Furthermore, fighting measured on basis of the sleep diary showed a negative correlation with sleep latency ($r = -0.286$, $p = 0.004$). Fighting during the night led to shorter sleep durations ($r = 0.202$; $p = 0.043$), whereas fighting during the day did not influence sleep duration ($r = 0.152$; $p = 0.129$).

No significant correlation was found between satisfaction with sexual intercourse and the PSQI sum score ($r = -0.176$; $p = 0.074$) but the PSQI subscale sleep disturbances correlated significantly with inter course satisfaction ($r = -0.275$; $p = 0.005$). The more satisfied the participants were with sex the less sleep disturbances they reported, in a linear regression with 8% of variance explained.

To prove the theoretical Partnership-Emotional wellbeing-Sleep model (PES), contained influences on sleep disturbances by relationship quality, fighting and well-being (as seen in **Figure 1**) were tested. All variables showing a significant correlation with the PSQI sum score were included in this theoretical model. Gender and age had no significant influence in this model. Fighting partnership-behavior and mental health, measured by the GSI, significantly influenced sleep ($F(2, 99) = 30.340$; $p = 0.000$, see **Table 6**). This model explains 38% of variance. But relationship satisfaction, anxiety and depression, failed to explain further variance within the model. This suggests that higher mental strain and dysfunctional fighting behavior impairs couple's sleep.

4. Discussion

In the present study a significant correlation of PSQI and PFB-K supports the association of sleep quality and relationship satisfaction. Previous studies showed that relationship quality predicted clinically relevant sleep disturbances. Women in a satisfying marriage experienced significantly fewer sleep problems than women in non-satisfying marriages [10]. In the present sample containing both men and women, similar findings suggest general mechanisms for both genders. Furthermore, the sample size in the present study is fairly good, compared to earlier studies in which sample sizes ranged between 46 couples [28] and 78 couples [8].

Sleep duration measured by the sleep diary correlated with relationship satisfaction. Age explains this link, as older people show shorter sleep durations and less relationship satisfaction [17] [24]. But in our sample with a wide range in age, subscales of either PSQI or PFB-K showed no correlations -except for sleep medication, which participants did not commonly take.

Table 5. Regression on relationship quality (PBF-K).

Variable	Standardized Coefficients Beta	t	Sig.
Age	−0.342	−3.432	0.001
Total sleep duration (sleep diary)	0.151	1.516	0.133

Regression coefficient B, standard deviation and β for variables in the model $^*p < 0.05.$ $^{**}p < 0.001.$

Table 6. Regression on sleep problems (PSQI sum score).

Variable	B	SE B	β
GSI	0.156	1.602	0.545**
PFB-K constructive fighting behavior	−0.248	0.114	−0.179*

Regression coefficient B, standard deviation and β for variables in the model $^*p < 0.05.$ $^{**}p< 0.001$

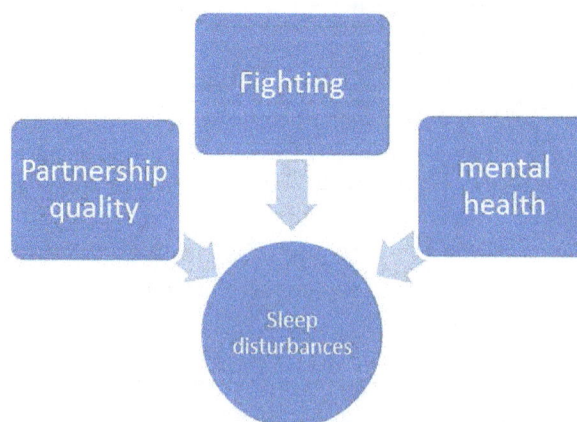

Figure 1. Theoretical model for sleep disturbances used for multiple regression. The Partnership-Emotional wellbeing-Sleep model (PES).

In addition, we found an association between destructive fighting behaviour and sleep quality. This result is in line with earlier studies [12]-[14] showing that sarcastic criticism, accusing the partner of something and aspersions are associated with less sleep quality and more daytime sleepiness. Birditt and colleagues reported that destructive fighting behaviour is related to a higher divorce rate [16]. Based on these findings one may suggest that constructive fighting behaviour and therefore a higher relationship satisfaction could lead to higher sleep quality. When participants reported a fight, longer sleep latencies and shorter sleep duration appeared. According to El-Sheikh and colleaguespsychological violence of women is correlated with more anxiety in their male partners [12]. Women showed longer sleep latency associated with the amount of psychological violence they used. Men's depression symptoms also lead to longer sleep latency in their partners. This association has also been shown vice versa: a poor night's sleep leads to more destructive fighting and less accurate empathetic reactions [29].

In our sample, satisfaction with sexual life correlated negatively with sleep disturbances. This suggests that couples who were satisfied with their sexual intercourse suffered from less sleep disturbances. Furthermore, participants reported a better mood when they had sex during the night. Supported is this finding by Ditzen and colleagues who stated intimacy alleviates stress [30]. Stress is known to have a negative impact on sleep [31] and might mediate the influence of sexual intercourses on sleep.

In a multiple regression model fighting and mental strain explained 38% of sleep quality variance. Depression, anxiety and relationship quality showed no further improvement of the model. Other factors—like attachment style—which were not considered in this study might improve the model, as Carmichael and Reisfound a higher fear of attachment to be associated with poor sleep quality in couples [8].

Consistent with findings by Schlack and colleagues we found a decrease in sleep duration with higher age [24]. Despite shorter sleep durations, daytime sleepiness decreased as well with higher age in the present sample. Studies suggest that older people take more daytime naps and therefore feel fitter [32]. Participants younger than—compared to those older than 40–did not report more trouble to fall or stay asleep. This finding contradicts Schlack and colleagues, suggesting that 40 years might not be an appropriate split point. But our sample does not provide a new split point, either.

In the present sample gender differences in sleep were only partly found. Women showed an equal number of sleep disturbances compared to men, contrary to earlier findings of more sleep disturbances in women [33] [34]. Nevertheless, sleep diary data showed a longer sleep onset latency of five minutes in mean for women. Furthermore, women slept longer than men. Van den Berg and colleagues found women slept 16 minutes longer than men. Women in the present sample slept 18 minutes longer [35]. Besides, sleep satisfaction did not differ in this sample, contrary to earlier studies [24] [35]. As another study consisted of people aged 68.4 in mean, age might be a possible explanation. Older women might be less satisfied with their sleep than men of the same age.

In addition, mental strain (measured by GSI) and sleep quality (measured by PSQI) correlated significantly positively, supporting earlier findings. Therefore, mental strains are associated with sleep disturbances and a lower sleep quality, like Taylor and colleagues stated [18]. Zawadzki and colleagues also found an association between sleep and mood [21]. Only depression and sleep onset latency were associated in our study, while no association of depression and sleep efficiency was found. Other studies suggest a general relationship between depression and sleeping problems [20] [36] [37]. Anxiety is linked to sleeping problems, in our sample as well as other studies [18] [20].

However, some limitations should be named. Intimate topics like sexuality and fighting in relationships might methodologically limit this study. Further anonymity–possibly through online questionnaires—might improve following studies about this topic. In addition, this sample did not show a continuous distribution of age. Longitudinal studies could determine causalities for underlying mechanisms. Additionally, intervention-studies concerning destructive fighting behaviour can give further information. Following studies should implement more couples which might help detect more underlying mechanisms.

5. Conclusions

In this study, subjective sleep quality and relationship satisfaction significantly correlated. In the theoretical Partnership-Emotional wellbeing-Sleep model (PES) higher relationship quality, better mental health and fewer conflicts in a relationship were associated with better sleep quality.

Conflicts often led to longer sleep latency and less sleep duration. Nevertheless the association of overall relationship quality and sleep quality was moderated by age, as older participants slept worse and were less satisfied with their relationships.

Sexual intercourses were another important factor influencing sleep quality. Intercourse at night led to a better mood in the morning.

These findings underlined that intimate relationships were important for sleep quality and *vice versa*. Therefore, relationship quality should always be taken into account and be asked for in adults suffering from sleep problems.

References

[1]   Hinz, A., Stöbel-Richter, Y. and Brähler, E. (2001) Der Partnerschaftsfragebogen (PFB). *Diagnostica*, **47**, 132-141. http://dx.doi.org/10.1026//0012-1924.47.3.132

[2]   Hale, L. (2005) Who Has Time to Sleep? *Journal of Public Health (Oxford, England)*, **27**, 205-211. http://dx.doi.org/10.1093/pubmed/fdi004

[3]   Troxel, W.M., Buysse, D.J., Matthews, K.A., Kravitz, H.M., Bromberger, J.T., Sowers, M. and Hall, M.H. (2010) Marital/Cohabitation Status and History in Relation to Sleep in Midlife Women. *Sleep*, **33**, 973-981.

[4]   Hamilton, N.A., Gallagher, M.W., Preacher, K.J., Stevens, N., Nelson, C.A., Karlson, C. and McCurdy, D. (2007) Insomnia and Well-Being. *Journal of Consulting and Clinical Psychology*, **75**, 939-946. http://dx.doi.org/10.1037/0022-006X.75.6.939

[5]   Yang, H, Suh, S., Kim, H., Cho, E.R., Lee, S.K. and Shin, C. (2013) Testing Bidirectional Relationships between Marital Quality and Sleep Disturbances: A 4-Year Follow-Up Study in a Korean Cohort. *Journal of Psychosomatic Research*, **74**, 401-406. http://dx.doi.org/10.1016/j.jpsychores.2013.01.005

[6]   Grandner, M.A., Patel, N.P., Gehrman, P.R., Xie, D., Sha, D., Weaver, T. and Gooneratne, N. (2010) Who Gets the Best Sleep? Ethnic and Socioeconomic Factors Related to Sleep Complaints. *Sleep Medicine*, **11**, 470-478. http://dx.doi.org/10.1016/j.sleep.2009.10.006

[7]   Hasler, B.P. and Troxel, W.M. (2010) Couples' Nighttime Sleep Efficiency and Concordance: Evidence for Bidirectional Associations with Daytime Relationship Functioning. *Psychosomatic Medicine*, **72**, 794-801. http://dx.doi.org/10.1097/PSY.0b013e3181ecd08a

[8]   Carmichael, C.L. and Reis, H.T. (2005) Attachment, Sleep Quality, and Depressed Affect. *Health Psychology Official Journal of the Division of Health Psychology, American Psychological Association*, **24**, 526-531.

[9]   Diamond, L.M., Hicks, A.M. and Otter-Henderson, K.D. (2008) Every Time You Go Away: changes in Affect, Behavior, and Physiology Associated with Travel-Related Separations from Romantic Partners. *Journal of Personality and Social Psychology*, **95**, 385-403. http://dx.doi.org/10.1037/0022-3514.95.2.385

[10]   Troxel, W.M., Buysse, D.J., Hall, M. and Matthews, K.A. (2009) Marital Happiness and Sleep Disturbances in a Multi-Ethnic Sample of Middle-Aged Women. *Behavioral Sleep Medicine*, **7**, 2-19. http://dx.doi.org/10.1080/15402000802577736

[11]   Cacioppo, J.T., Hawkley, L.C., Berntson, G.G., Ernst, J.M., Gibbs, A.C., Stickgold, R. and Hobson, J.A. (2002) Do Lonely Days Invade the Nights? Potential Social Modulation of Sleep Efficiency. *Psychological Science*, **13**, 384-387. http://dx.doi.org/10.1111/j.0956-7976.2002.00469.x

[12]   El-Sheikh, M., Kelly, R. and Rauer, A. (2013) Quick to Berate, Slow to Sleep: Interpartner Psychological Conflict, Mental Health, and Sleep. *Health Psychology*, **32**, 1057-1066. http://dx.doi.org/10.1037/a0031786

[13]   Rauer, A.J., Kelly, R.J., Buckhalt, J.A. and El-Sheikh, M. (2010) Sleeping with One Eye Open: Marital Abuse as an Antecedent of Poor Sleep. *Journal of Family Psychology*, **24**, 667-677. http://dx.doi.org/10.1037/a0021354

[14]   Rauer, A.J. and El-Sheikh, M. (2012) Reciprocal Pathways between Intimate Partner Violence and Sleep in Men and Women. *Journal of Family Psychology*, **26**, 470-477. http://dx.doi.org/10.1037/a0027828

[15]   Orbuch, T.L., Veroff, J., Hassan, H. and Horrocks, J. (2002) Who Will Divorce: A 14-Year Longitudinal Study of Black Couples and White Couples. *Journal of Social and Personal Relationships*, **19**, 179-202. http://dx.doi.org/10.1177/0265407502192002

[16]   Birditt, K.S., Brown, E., Orbuch, T.L. and McIlvane, J.M. (2010) Marital Conflict Behaviors and Implications for Divorce over 16 Years. *Journal of Marriage and the Family*, **72**, 1188-1204. http://dx.doi.org/10.1111/j.1741-3737.2010.00758.x

[17]   Klaiberg, A., Würz, J., Brähler, E. and Schumacher, J. (2001) Influences on Satisfaction with Sexuality and Partnership in Women. *Der Gynäkologe*, **34**, 259-269. http://dx.doi.org/10.1007/s001290050711

[18]   Taylor, D.J., Lichstein, K.L., Durrence, H.H., Reidel, B.W. and Bush, A.J. (2005) Epidemiology of Insomnia, Depres-

sion, and Anxiety. *Sleep*, **28**, 1457-1464.

[19] Soehner, A.M. and Harvey, A.G. (2012) Prevalence and Functional Consequences of Severe Insomnia Symptoms in Mood and Anxiety Disorders: Results from a Nationally Representative Sample. *Sleep*, **35**, 1367-1375. http://dx.doi.org/10.5665/sleep.2116

[20] Neckelmann, D., Mykletun, A. and Dahl, A.A. (2007) Chronic Insomnia as a Risk Factor for Developing Anxiety and Depression. *Sleep*, **30**, 873-880.

[21] Zawadzki, M.J., Graham, J.E. and Gerin, W. (2013) Rumination and Anxiety Mediate the Effect of Loneliness on Depressed Mood and Sleep Quality in College Students. *Health Psychology*, **32**, 212-222. http://dx.doi.org/10.1037/a0029007

[22] Vahtera, J., Kivimaki, M., Hublin, C., Korkeila, K., Suominen, S., Paunio, T. and Koskenvuo, M. (2007) Liability to Anxiety and Severe Life Events as Predictors of New-Onset Sleep Disturbances. *Sleep*, **30**, 1537-1546.

[23] Morin, C.M., Rodrigue, S. and Ivers, H. (2003) Role of Stress, Arousal, and Coping Skills in Primary Insomnia. *Psychosomatic Medicine*, **65**, 259-267. http://dx.doi.org/10.1097/01.PSY.0000030391.09558.A3

[24] Schlack, R., Hapke, U., Maske, U., Busch, M. and Cohrs, S. (2013) Häufigkeit und Verteilung von Schlafproblemen und Insomnie in der deutschen Erwachsenenbevölkerung: Ergebnisse der Studie zur Gesundheit Erwachsener in Deutschland (DEGS1). *Bundesgesundheitsblatt, Gesundheitsforschung, Gesundheitsschutz*, **56**, 740-748. http://dx.doi.org/10.1007/s00103-013-1689-2

[25] Buysse, D.J., Reynolds, C.F., Monk, T.H., Berman, S.R. and Kupfer, D.J. (1989) The Pittsburgh Sleep Quality Index: A New Instrument for Psychiatric Practice and Research. *Psychiatry Research*, **28**, 193-213. http://dx.doi.org/10.1016/0165-1781(89)90047-4

[26] Kliem, S., Job, A., Kröger, C., Bodenmann, G., Stöbel-Richter, Y., Hahlweg, K. and Brähler, E. (2012) Entwicklung und Normierung einer Kurzform des Partnerschaftsfragebogens (PFB-K) an einer repräsentativen deutschen Stichprobe. *Zeitschrift für Klinische Psychologie und Psychotherapie*, **41**, 81-89. http://dx.doi.org/10.1026/1616-3443/a000135

[27] Hessel, A., Schumacher, J., Geyer, M. and Brähler, E. (2001) Symptom-Checkliste SCL-90-R. *Diagnostica*, **47**, 27-39. http://dx.doi.org/10.1026//0012-1924.47.1.27

[28] Kane, H.S., Slatcher, R.B., Reynolds, B.M., Repetti, R.L. and Robles, T.F. (2014) Daily Self-Disclosure and Sleep in Couples. *Health Psychology*, **33**, 813-822. http://dx.doi.org/10.1037/hea0000077

[29] Gordon, A.M. and Chen, S. (2014) The Role of Sleep in Interpersonal Conflict: Do Sleepless Nights Mean Worse Fights? *Social Psychological and Personality Science*, **5**, 168-175. http://dx.doi.org/10.1177/1948550613488952

[30] Ditzen, B., Hoppmann, C. and Klumb, P. (2008) Positive Couple Interactions and Daily Cortisol: On the Stress-Protecting Role of Intimacy. *Psychosomatic Medicine*, **70**, 883-889. http://dx.doi.org/10.1097/PSY.0b013e318185c4fc

[31] Paulsen, V.M. and Shaver, J.L. (1991) Stress, Support, Psychological States and Sleep. *Social Science & Medicine*, **32**, 1237-1243.

[32] Neubauer, D.N. (1999) Sleep Problems in the Elderly. *American Family Physician*, **59**, 2551-2560.

[33] Zhang, B. and Wing, Y. (2006) Sex Differences in Insomnia: A Meta-Analysis. *Sleep*, **29**, 85-93.

[34] Ohayon, M.M. (2002) Epidemiology of Insomnia: What We Know and What We Still Need to Learn. *Sleep Medicine Reviews*, **6**, 97-111. http://dx.doi.org/10.1053/smrv.2002.0186

[35] van den Berg, J.F., Miedema, H.M.E., Tulen, J.H.M., Hofman, A., Neven, A.K. and Tiemeier, H. (2009) Sex Differences in Subjective and Actigraphic Sleep Measures: A Population-Based Study of Elderly Persons. *Sleep*, **32**, 1367-1375.

[36] Heilemann, M.V., Choudhury, S.M., Kury, F.S. and Lee, K.A. (2012) Factors Associated with Sleep Disturbance in Women of Mexican Descent. *Journal of Advanced Nursing*, **68**, 2256-2266. http://dx.doi.org/10.1111/j.1365-2648.2011.05918.x

[37] Brabbins, C.J., Dewey, M.E., Copeland, J.R.M., Davidson, I.A., McWilliam, C., Saunders, P., Sharma, V.K. and Sullivan, C. (1993) Insomnia in the Elderly: Prevalence, Gender Differences and Relationships with Morbidity and Mortality. *International Journal of Geriatric Psychiatry*, **8**, 473-480. http://dx.doi.org/10.1002/gps.930080604

14

Empirical Study on the Empowerment of Families Raising Children with Severe Motor and Intellectual Disabilities in Japan: The Association with Positive Feelings towards Child Rearing

Hiroshi Fujioka[1], Rie Wakimizu[2], Ryuta Tanaka[3], Tatsuyuki Ohto[3], Atsushi Ieshima[4], Akira Yoneyama[5], Kiyoko Kamibeppu[6*]

[1]Department of Nursing, Faculty of Health Sciences, Tsukuba International University, Tsuchiura-Shi, Japan
[2]Department of Child Health Care Nursing, Division of Health Innovation and Nursing, Faculty of Medicine, University of Tsukuba, Tsukuba-Shi, Japan
[3]Department of Child Health, Graduate School of Comprehensive Human Sciences, University of Tsukuba, Tsukuba-Shi, Japan
[4]Aiseikai Kinen Ibaraki Welfare & Medical Center, Mito-Shi, Japan
[5]National Rehabilitation Center for Children with Disabilities, Itabashi-Ku, Japan
[6]Department of Family Nursing, School of Health Sciences and Nursing, Graduate School of Medicine, The University of Tokyo, Bunkyo-Ku, Japan
Email: *kkamibeppu-tky@umin.ac.jp

Abstract

Background: "Children with severe motor and intellectual disabilities" refers to children with markedly limited activity due to severe overlapping of physical and intellectual disabilities. The physical and mental burden placed on families raising severely disabled children, particularly the primary caregivers, is great in home settings. For families to effectively utilize services and overcome child rearing problems, the families themselves need the "strength" to cooperate with others for the purpose of raising a severely disabled child. The ultimate goal of family support is to enable such families to achieve satisfaction and self-growth in child rearing. Methods: We used a questionnaire to survey 75 primary caregivers to empirically elucidate the empowerment and positive feelings towards child rearing of families raising children with severe motor and intellectual disabilities and the related factors. The t-test and Spearman's rank correlation coefficient

*Corresponding author.

were used to examine the association with bivariates. A multiple regression analysis was conducted for empowerment and positive feelings. Results: Results revealed that life events, livelihood, awareness of social support and the child's sleep problems were factors related to empowerment. Of these, awareness of social support from outside of the family was found to contribute the most to empowerment. Furthermore, improvement and maintenance of positive feelings towards child rearing reaffirmed the existence of empowerment in addition to reducing negative feelings towards child rearing and ensuring social support. Conclusions: Raising children with severe motor and intellectual disabilities requires specialist knowledge and skills. Support from professionals to empower the entire family is therefore important in order to strengthen positive feelings towards child rearing.

Keywords

Children with Severe Motor and Intellectual Disabilities, Family, Empowerment, Positive Feelings towards Child Rearing

1. Introduction

"Children with severe motor and intellectual disabilities" (SMID) is a term defined with reference to Japan's unique legislation and refers to "children with markedly limited activity due to severe overlapping of physical and intellectual disabilities" [1]. Globally, SMID is synonymous with "children with profound multiple disabilities," i.e. children who cannot use their hands and arms by themselves due to an IQ of less than 20 [2].

In Japan, approximately 70% of the estimated 40,000 severely disabled children live at home [1]. The physical and mental burden placed on the families raising severely disabled children, particularly the primary caregivers, is great in home settings [3] [4]. Factors that most influence the stress of families with disabled children include developmental problems of the child, health problems and difficulties with care [5]. Children with severe disabilities have markedly delayed development and low spare physical capacity, which makes them susceptible to complications when they are ill and leads them to require diverse and highly individualized care. This is why the stress of families with severely disabled children is very serious [6]. Social and economic problems have also been pointed out such as the financial hardship faced when family members have to quit their jobs in order to care for the child [6].

For families to effectively utilize services and overcome child rearing problems, the quantity and quality of services not only need to be enhanced, but families themselves also need the "strength" to cooperate with others for the purpose of raising a severely disabled child. Globally, services have changed from a model in which professionals are superior to a "family-oriented" service model in which the wishes of the parents are prioritized in cooperation between parents and professionals [7]. The strength of families to cooperate and get actively involved in various service organizations and communities, i.e. empowerment, is therefore an important indicator in family support [8]. The ultimate goal of family support is to enable families themselves to achieve satisfaction and self-growth in child rearing.

This study was designed to empirically elucidate the empowerment and positive feelings towards child rearing of families raising severely disabled children in Japan and the related factors.

2. Methods

2.1. Operational Definition: Empowerment

In this study, empowerment was defined as "the state or ability of families to cooperate with elements outside of their living scope by controlling their life for the purpose of raising a severely disabled child" with reference to definitions in previous studies [9] [10].

2.2. Subjects

Subjects comprised primary caregivers raising a severely disabled child at home. The inclusion criteria were as follows: aged 20 years or older; able to answer a questionnaire (good physical and mental state and good language proficiency); aware that they are the primary caregiver of the child; and caring for a "child with SMID" that is aged 5 to 18 years and has marked difficulty with everyday communication and is unable to maintain a standing position alone.

Care recipients were primarily restricted to school age children because families with children aged less than 5 years have only recently received a diagnosis and were assumed to be emotionally unstable. Moreover, the circumstances of children over 18 years of age were assumed to become more individualized as the child and family aged.

2.3. Procedure

The investigators asked primary caregivers (subjects) of severely disabled children who regularly visited one of three facilities (university hospitals and rehabilitation facilities for severely disabled children; hereinafter, research cooperation facilities) in the Tokyo metropolitan area on an outpatient basis to answer an anonymous self-administered questionnaire. Subjects were first given an explanation of the outline of this study using a briefing document. The attending physicians at the research cooperation facilities then selected subjects based on the inclusion criteria.

In addition to the briefing document, subjects were also handed a questionnaire, a 500-yen gratuity in the form of a bookstore gift card, and a return envelope. Subjects who agreed to cooperate in this research answered the questionnaire and returned it to the investigators in the enclosed return envelope. Returning the questionnaire was considered to indicate consent. The study period was from May 2012 to January 2013.

2.4. The Questionnaire

The following items were included in the questionnaire.

2.4.1. Empowerment

We used the Japanese version of the Family Empowerment Scale (FES) [11]. The original FES [9] was developed as a scale to measure the empowerment of caregivers of children with emotional and developmental disabilities and is the most versatile empowerment scale in the world [12]. The areas of child rearing in which caregivers are involved are divided into three domains: family (caregivers themselves), service system and community/political. The family domain primarily examines the internal awareness and beliefs of the caregiver themselves as well as the knowledge and abilities that they possess. The service system domain examines cooperation with service providers (professionals) when receiving services. The community/political domain examines cooperation with politicians and government personnel/staff to build a better system of services. The family domain is comprised of 12 items, the service system domain 12 items, and the community/political domain 10 items (total 34 items). Each item is rated with a 5-point scale (1 to 5 points). A higher score indicates a higher level of empowerment. Cronbach's alpha in this study was 0.88 for family, 0.87 for the service system and 0.83 for community/political.

2.4.2. Attributes of the Children with SMID

The following information was collected regarding the attributes of the severely disabled children. Items were created based on sex, age, disability onset, time of definitive diagnosis, time at which home care was started (home period), possession of a physical disability certificate and childcare handbook, activities of daily living, physical and mental function, problematic behavior or habits (hurting others or themselves, harassing those around them), sleep problems, and required care (score for profoundly severely disabled children) [13]. Respiratory, dietary and other forms of care were scored and a total score of 25 points or more indicated a profoundly severely disabled child, while a score of 10 to 24 points indicated a quasi-profoundly severely disabled child. The questionnaire also collected information about services used, including the location of the facility and the time required to visit each facility.

2.4.3. Attributes of the Primary Caregivers (Subjects Themselves) and Their Families

The following information was collected regarding the attributes of the family (including the subjects themselves): age, relationship to the child, marital status, occupation, educational background, sleep time, presence of chronic symptoms, household income, economic situation, and physical condition (the questionnaire on the physical condition of mothers of severely disabled children [14] was used). Higher scores indicated poorer physical condition. Cronbach's alpha in this study was 0.94, and life event items (10 yes-or-no questions) were created with reference to Natsume *et al.*'s life events scale [15].

2.4.4. Awareness of Social Support

The revised version of the Social Support Scale of Home Caregivers [16] was used. The scale is composed of 8 items on emotional support, 2 items on practical support, and 3 items on ineffective support (total 13 items). In this study, subjects answered questions regarding the perceived amount of support (how many individuals apply to each item) with "present" or "absent". Subjects were asked to answer with "within the family" or "outside of the family" to each item regarding the source of support (multiple answers were allowed from 11 options in the original version). In this study, the 3 ineffective support items and 10 other items were each treated as separate variables for negative and positive support during analysis. Cronbach's alpha in this study was 0.80 for "positive social support from within the family," 0.76 for "negative social support from within the family," 0.84 for "positive social support from outside of the family," and 0.56 for "negative social support from outside of the family" (hereafter, positive social support is treated as social support as long as there is no alternate notation).

2.4.5. Evaluation of Child Rearing

i) Positive feelings towards child rearing (positive evaluation)

The positive evaluation subscales of the Cognitive Caregiving Appraisal [17] were used. The scale is composed of 6 items for caregiving satisfaction, 4 items for positive feelings towards the care recipient, and 3 items for sense of self-growth (total 13 items) and is rated with a 4-point scale. A higher score indicates stronger positive feelings towards child rearing. Cronbach's alpha was 0.80, 0.82 and 0.75, respectively, for each of the above-mentioned subscales. Some of the notations were modified considering the care recipients in this study were children. Of the 4 items for positive feelings towards the care recipient, the caregivers of severely disabled children had marked difficulty regarding the following 3 items: determining whether "(the child was) thankful," "(the child) and the caregiver understood each other's feelings" and "(the child) thought positively of the caregiver;" therefore, these items were excluded from the analysis. Cronbach's alpha of the 10 items was 0.82.

ii) Negative feelings towards child rearing (negative evaluation)

The short, Japanese version of the Zarit Caregiver Burden Interview [18] was used. The scale is composed of a total of 8 items rated with a 5-point scale and divided into 2 factors: 5 personal burden items and 3 role burden items. Cronbach's alpha for all 8 items is 0.89 and Cronbach's alpha in this study was 0.83.

2.5. Analysis

The descriptive statistics (name, frequency and ratio for the ordinal scale, and mean and standard deviation for the interval scale) of each obtained variable were calculated.

The association of empowerment (family, service system, and community/political domains) and positive feelings towards child rearing with other variables (explanatory variables) was examined. The *t*-test or Spearman's rank correlation coefficient were used to examine the association with bivariates.

A multiple regression analysis was conducted with the three empowerment domains as objective variables. Variables (excluding positive feelings towards child rearing) that were found to be associated with empowerment in a univariate analysis were introduced as explanatory variables. Of the explanatory variables, variables for child and family attributes were introduced first, followed by variables for social support.

We conducted a multiple regression analysis with positive feelings towards child rearing as the objective variable. Variables for which an association with positive feelings towards child rearing and each empowerment domain was seen in a univariate analysis were introduced as explanatory variables.

IBM SPSS 21 statistical software was used for the analyses. The significance level was set at 5% on both sides. However, the significance level was set at 10% in the multiple regression analysis to enable a more exploratory interpretation of the results.

2.6. Ethical Considerations

The subjects were asked to cooperate after being given verbal and written explanations of the purpose of the study. Simple, easily understood expressions were used to explain the study purpose. Cooperation was voluntary for the subjects and returning the anonymous self-administered questionnaire was considered to indicate consent.

The ethics committees of the Faculty of Medicine, the University of Tokyo, University of Tsukuba Hospital, Ibaraki Disabled Children's Hospital, and National Rehabilitation Center for Children with Disabilities approved this study.

3. Results

A total of 122 questionnaires were distributed and 76 were returned (recovery rate 62.3%). Of these, one questionnaire was excluded due to noticeable deficits in each empowerment domain (5 of the 12 items in the family domain, 5 of the 12 items in the service system domain and 6 of the 10 items in the community/political domain). Responses from a total of 75 individuals were consequently included in the final analysis (valid response rate 61.5%).

3.1. Child, Subject and Family Attributes

The children of 66 of the 75 (88.0%) subjects had experienced disability onset at less than 1 year of age. The main diagnoses were cerebral palsy, sequelae of hypoxic encephalopathy in the perinatal period, chromosomal abnormalities, and congenital neurological disease. Those who had experienced disability onset at 1 year of age or older had diseases such as bacterial meningitis and post-measles encephalitis. Twenty-eight (37.3%) were profoundly severely disabled children or quasi-profoundly severely disabled children according to the score for severely disabled children. All children were visiting the facility on an outpatient basis and most visited at a frequency of once per month (60 subjects, 80%). The mean time required to visit outpatient facilities was 50.3 minutes. **Table 1** shows the child attributes. **Table 2** shows the subject and family attributes.

The score for empowerment was 37.02 ± 7.47 for the family domain, 39.09 ± 7.40 for the service system domain and 25.06 ± 6.18 for the community/political domain (mean ± standard deviation).

3.2. Association between Empowerment and Other Variables

3.2.1. Univariate Analysis

Subjects visiting facilities in Tokyo had higher empowerment scores for the family and service system domains than those visiting other facilities. The empowerment score for the service system domain was lower if the child had problematic behavior or habits and some kind of sleep problem. Moreover, subjects who had experienced life events and subjects who used at-home services had a higher level of empowerment. The level of empowerment also increased the more satisfied subjects were with their livelihood and the more aware they were of social support from within and outside of the family. These data are shown in **Table 3** and **Table 4**.

On examining the association between empowerment and each life event, the level of empowerment also tended to be higher in cases where there was "death of someone in the family" or "serious illness or accident of someone in the family". These data are shown in **Table 5**.

3.2.2. Multiple Regression Analysis

Variables (facilities, sleep problems, life events, livelihood) for which an association was seen in the univariate analysis were introduced as explanatory variables. Only 10 subjects responded with "present" to "problematic behavior and habits in the child". However, considering the mental and physical function of severely disabled children, it is unlikely that the children were deliberately exhibiting problematic behavior. This item was therefore not added to the explanatory variables.

Variables for child and family attributes were introduced first, followed by variables for social support. The results are shown in **Table 6**.

1) Facilities, sleep problems of the child, life events and livelihood

The model containing only the above 4 variables (model 1), excluding "facilities" in the community/political domain, contributed significantly to empowerment. Thereafter, on introducing variables for social support (model 2), the standard partial regression coefficient (β) of "facilities" was reduced and the contribution to empowerment was no longer seen.

Table 1. Child attributes.

		N	%	Mean ± SD	[range]
Facility	Outside of Tokyo	40	53.3		
	Tokyo	35	46.7		
Time required to go to facility from residence (minutes)	Outside of Tokyo	40		48.50 ± 30.74	[5 - 180]
	Tokyo	35		52.43 ± 35.68	[10 - 210]
	Total	75		50.33 ± 33.20	[5 - 210]
Sex of the child	Male	47	62.7		
	Female	28	37.3		
Age of the child (years)		75		11.95 ± 3.97	[5 - 18]
Age of disability onset	<1 year of age	64	85.3		
	≥1 year of age	9	12		
	No answer	2	2.7		
Physical disability certificate	Grade 1	69	92		
	Grade 2	6	8		
Rehabilitation handbook	Most severe	35	46.7		
	Severe	3	4		
	Do not have one	33	44		
	No answer	4	5.3		
Respiratory problems	Present	35	46.7		
	Absent	33	44		
	No answer	7	9.3		
Child disability classification	Severely disabled child	28	37.3		
	Other	47	62.7		
Gastroesophageal reflux	Present	20	26.7		
	Absent	52	69.3		
	No answer	3	4		
Problematic behavior and habits	Present	11	14.7		
	Absent	63	84		
	No answer	1	1.3		
Seizures more than once a week	Present	36	48		
	Absent	38	50.7		
	No answer	1	1.3		
Use of anticonvulsants	Present	63	84		
	Absent	12	16		
Sites of contracture	Present	59	78.7		
	Absent	15	20		
	No answer	1	1.3		
Sleep problems	Present	40	53.3		
	Absent	34	45.3		
	No answer	1	1.3		
Use of sleep-inducing drugs	Present	22	29.3		
	Absent	53	70.7		

Table 2. Subject and family attributes.

		N	%	Mean ± SD	[range]
Relationship to the child	Mother	74	98.7		
	Father	1	1.3		
Age of subject (years)		75		42.39 ± 5.85	[29 - 56]
Marital status	Married	66	88		
	Divorced	9	12		
Employment status	Employed	13	17.3		
	Unemployed	62	82.7		
Highest level of education	Middle school	1	1.3		
	High school	28	37.3		
	Junior college/vocational school	33	44		
	University or higher	13	17.3		
Sleep time (hours)		73		5.48 ± 0.84	[3 - 7]
Chronic symptoms	Present	31	41.3		
	Absent	44	58.7		
Family occupation	Self-employed	10	13.3		
	Other	65	86.7		
Number of cohabiting family members		75		4.01 ± 0.97	[2 - 6]
Living arrangements with grandparents	Living together	9	12		
	Living apart	66	88		
Number of siblings of the child	0	24	32		
	1	33	44		
	2	15	20		
	3	3	4		
Life events	Present	33	44		
	Absent	42	56		
Annual household income (million yen)	<3	11	14.7		
	3 to 5	18	24		
	5 to 7	31	41.3		
	7 to 10	6	8		
	≥10	11	14.7		
	No answer	3	4		
Livelihood	Dissatisfied	11	14.7		
	Slightly dissatisfied	18	24		
	Slightly satisfied	31	41.3		
	Satisfied	13	17.3		

Continued

	No answer	2	2.7		
Physical condition score		75		77.03 ± 18.44	[43 - 120]
Use of at-home services	Present	25	33.3		
	Absent	50	66.7		
Informal support	Yes	61	81.3		
	No	14	18.7		
Social support (positive, family)		75		7.31 ± 2.44	[0 - 10]
Social support (negative, family)		75		0.40 ± 0.84	[0 - 3]
Social support (positive, outside of the family)		75		6.55 ± 2.63	[0 - 10]
Social support (negative, outside of the family)		75		0.16 ± 0.49	[0 - 3]
Negative feelings towards child rearing		75		16.39 ± 5.71	[8 - 35]
Positive feelings towards child rearing		74		33.60 ± 4.12	[24 - 40]
Empowerment (family)		74		37.02 ± 7.47	[15 - 53]
Empowerment (services system)		73		39.09 ± 7.40	[17 - 60]
Empowerment (community/political)		75		25.06 ± 6.18	[12 - 40]

Table 3. Association of empowerment and positive feelings towards child rearing and explanatory variables.

		Empowerment (family)				Empowerment (service system)				Empowerment (community/political)				Positive feelings towards child rearing			
		N	Mean	SD	p	N	Mean	SD	p	N	Mean	SD	p	N	Mean	SD	p
Facility	Outside of Tokyo	39	34.85	7.34	**	39	37.20	6.80	*	40	24.16	6.13		39	32.69	3.98	*
	Tokyo	35	39.44	6.94		34	41.26	7.55		35	26.09	6.16		35	34.62	4.09	
Age of disability onset	>1 year of age	63	36.82	7.49		62	38.87	7.03		64	24.84	5.81		63	33.37	3.82	
	≥1 year of age	9	37.11	7.62		9	39.62	9.81		9	25.89	7.06		9	35.83	4.69	
Physical disability certificate	Grade 1	68	37.11	7.45		67	38.93	7.33		69	24.96	6.25		68	33.72	4.05	
	Grade 2	6	36.00	8.34		6	40.92	8.63		6	26.17	5.64		6	32.31	5.06	
Rehabilitation handbook	Present	37	35.40	8.11		36	38.00	6.93		38	24.91	6.64		38	32.61	4.04	*
	Absent	33	38.67	6.69		33	40.08	8.04		33	25.64	5.87		33	34.68	4.07	
Respiratory problems	Present	35	36.85	7.35		35	39.04	6.35		35	24.76	5.78		34	34.38	4.26	
	Absent	32	37.53	8.15		32	40.10	8.45		33	25.79	6.58		33	32.51	3.92	
Child disability classification	Severely disabled child	28	37.09	7.43		27	39.54	8.08		28	24.98	6.25		27	34.18	4.19	
	Other	46	36.98	7.57		46	38.83	7.04		47	25.11	6.20		47	33.27	4.09	
Gastroesophageal reflux	Present	20	38.66	6.32		19	41.11	6.31		20	25.50	4.36		19	34.21	4.48	
	Absent	52	36.60	7.86		51	38.74	7.68		52	25.22	6.77		52	33.15	3.99	
Problematic behavior and habits	Present	10	33.12	5.88		10	35.91	3.00	**	11	22.36	5.20		11	30.83	3.71	**
	Absent	63	37.83	7.43		62	39.80	7.66		63	25.64	6.22		62	34.22	3.92	
Seizures more than once a week	Present	36	38.07	6.94		36	40.06	6.59		36	25.03	5.47		35	33.87	4.29	
	Absent	37	35.92	7.98		37	38.15	8.09		38	25.09	6.93		38	33.26	4.01	

Continued

Variable	Category	n	Mean	SD		n	Mean	SD		n	Mean	SD		n	Mean	SD	
Use of anticonvulsants	Present	63	36.99	7.86		62	39.00	7.72		63	25.01	6.42		62	33.67	4.16	
	Absent	11	37.18	4.90		11	39.60	5.51		12	25.33	4.91		12	33.24	4.06	
Sites of contracture	Present	59	37.77	6.83		58	39.82	7.13		59	25.60	5.95		58	33.96	4.24	
	Absent	15	34.07	9.28		14	36.21	8.28		15	23.27	6.97		15	32.01	3.36	
Sleep problems	Present	39	35.54	6.83		39	37.46	6.62	*	40	23.81	5.65		40	33.17	4.04	
	Absent	34	38.75	7.99		33	40.96	8.01		34	26.62	6.56		34	34.11	4.22	
Use of sleep-inducing drugs	Present	22	35.00	7.20		21	38.48	7.78		22	23.34	5.30		21	33.48	3.79	
	Absent	52	37.88	7.48		52	39.34	7.30		53	25.77	6.41		53	33.65	4.28	
Marital status	Married	66	37.18	7.30		64	39.15	7.20		66	25.44	6.23		65	33.49	4.21	
	Divorced	8	35.75	9.22		9	38.68	9.14		9	22.27	5.23		9	34.44	3.54	
Employment status	Employed	13	35.55	5.69		13	37.08	5.31		13	24.31	5.42		13	33.77	4.80	
	Unemployed	61	37.34	7.80		60	39.53	7.74		62	25.22	6.35		61	33.57	4.01	
Chronic symptoms	Present	30	38.49	6.90		31	40.74	6.23		31	26.01	6.97		31	34.76	4.00	*
	Absent	44	36.02	7.75		42	37.87	8.01		44	24.39	5.53		43	32.77	4.05	
Family occupation	Self-employed	10	38.95	7.87		10	40.00	7.87		10	25.20	6.39		10	35.36	4.11	
	Other	64	36.72	7.42		63	38.95	7.37		65	25.04	6.19		64	33.33	4.09	
Living arrangements with grandparents	Living together	8	34.38	4.37		9	36.57	5.48		9	22.22	3.93		8	32.75	3.62	
	Living apart	66	37.34	7.72		64	39.45	7.59		66	25.45	6.34		66	33.71	4.19	
Life events	Present	32	39.50	5.53	**	33	41.00	6.21	*	33	26.76	6.19	*	32	33.99	3.50	
	Absent	42	35.13	8.23		40	37.51	7.98		42	23.72	5.90		42	33.31	4.56	
Use of at-home services	Present	24	40.06	6.77	*	24	42.30	7.52	**	25	27.04	6.39	*	25	35.56	2.55	**
	Absent	50	35.56	7.41		49	37.52	6.88		50	24.07	5.88		49	32.60	4.42	
Informal support	Present	14	38.64	4.97		13	40.38	5.20		14	27.79	5.21		14	34.72	3.66	
	Absent	60	36.64	7.92		60	38.81	7.80		61	24.43	6.25		60	33.34	4.21	

Unpaired t-test *p < 0.05, **p < 0.01.

2) Awareness of social support and usage of at-home services

Awareness of social support from within the family was not found to contribute to empowerment. On the other hand, awareness of social support from outside of the family was the variable that contributed the most to empowerment. In particular, the standard partial regression coefficient (β) increased further in the service system and community/political domains compared with the family domain. Use of at-home services was found to contribute to empowerment in the service system domain.

The increase in the rate of contribution from model 1 to model 2 greatly indicated that awareness of social support from outside of the family had a strong influence in each of the family, service system, and community/political domains.

3.3. Association between Positive Feelings towards Child Rearing and Other Variables

3.3.1. Univariate Analysis

Subjects visiting facilities in Tokyo had stronger positive feelings towards child rearing. These feelings were strong in subjects without a rehabilitation handbook and whose child exhibited no problematic behavior or habits. Subjects themselves with chronic symptoms and few cohabitating family members or siblings had stronger

Table 4. Correlation of empowerment and positive feelings towards child rearing and explanatory variables.

	Age of child	Age of subject	Highest level of education	Sleep time	Number of cohabitating family members	Number of siblings of the child	Annual household income	Livelihood	Physical condition	Social support (positive, family)	Social support (negative, family)	Social support (positive, outside of the family)	Social support (negative, outside of the family)	Negative feelings towards child rearing	Positive feelings towards child rearing	Empowerment (family)	Empowerment (service system)	Empowerment (community/political)
Age of child	1.00																	
Age of subject	0.57**	1.00																
Highest level of education	−0.20	0.03	1.00															
Sleep time	−0.18	−0.25*	0.13	1.00														
Number of cohabitating family members	−0.06	−0.01	0.06	0.01	1.00													
Number of siblings of the child	0.00	0.00	−0.06	0.05	0.86**	1.00												
Annual household income	0.13	0.45**	0.29*	−0.01	0.23*	0.17	1.00											
Livelihood	0.00	0.23	0.25*	0.08	0.10	0.12	0.58**	1.00										
Physical condition	0.18	0.01	−0.22	−0.39**	−0.04	−0.09	−0.10	−0.36**	1.00									
Social support (positive, family)	−0.07	0.06	0.04	−0.04	0.17	0.16	0.14	0.29*	−0.22	1.00								
Social support (negative, family)	−0.06	−0.13	0.21	0.02	0.20	0.03	0.14	0.10	0.19	0.04	1.00							
Social support (positive, outside of the family)	0.00	0.15	0.04	−0.14	0.04	0.01	0.12	0.12	−0.08	0.42**	0.08	1.00						
Social support (negative, outside of the family)	0.09	0.03	0.00	−0.14	−0.10	−0.11	−0.04	−0.01	0.17	0.05	0.34**	0.05	1.00					
Negative feelings towards child rearing	−0.13	−0.19	0.11	−0.15	0.15	0.13	−0.15	−0.25*	0.51**	−0.24*	0.35**	−0.27*	0.11	1.00				
Positive feelings towards child rearing	0.05	0.06	−0.02	−0.11	−0.35**	−0.31**	−0.01	0.15	−0.05	0.23	−0.17	0.29*	0.09	−0.34**	1.00			
Empowerment (family)	−0.15	0.01	0.09	−0.08	−0.10	−0.08	0.28*	0.29*	−0.20	0.33**	−0.04	0.41**	−0.04	−0.25*	0.38**	1.00		
Empowerment (service system)	−0.08	0.04	0.10	0.03	−0.11	−0.11	0.25*	0.38**	−0.11	0.27*	0.03	0.54**	0.05	−0.20	0.35**	0.80**	1.00	
Empowerment (community/political)	0.01	0.09	0.12	0.10	−0.04	−0.02	0.290*	0.34**	−0.03	0.28*	0.04	0.53**	0.06	−0.22	0.31**	0.55**	0.79**	1.00

Spearman's rank correlation coefficient. *$p < 0.05$, **$p < 0.01$.

Table 5. Association between empowerment and each life event.

		Empowerment (family)			Empowerment (service system)			Empowerment (community/political)		
		N	Mean	p	N	Mean	p	N	Mean	p
Death of someone in the family	Present	6	42.67	†	6	42.83		6	27.50	
	Absent	68	36.52		67	38.76		69	24.85	
Serious illness or accident of someone in the family	Present	8	41.63	†	9	40.68		9	27.00	
	Absent	66	36.46		64	38.87		66	24.79	
Major change to the living habits of someone in the family	Present	10	35.70		10	39.50		10	26.20	
	Absent	64	37.23		63	39.03		65	24.88	
Sudden deterioration of the household's financial situation	Present	9	38.44		9	38.00		9	23.56	
	Absent	65	36.83		64	39.24		66	25.26	
Starting to live together with grandparents	Present	3	37.67		3	42.33		3	25.00	
	Absent	71	36.99		70	38.95		72	25.06	
Trouble caused to others, and things going wrong	Present	2	41.50		2	45.00		2	28.00	
	Absent	72	36.90		71	38.92		73	24.98	
Relocation	Present	5	41.40		5	43.00		5	28.40	
	Absent	69	36.70		68	38.80		70	24.82	
Job transfer away from home without family	Present	2	38.50		2	43.00		2	24.50	
	Absent	72	36.98		71	38.98		73	25.07	

Unpaired *t*-test. †$p < 0.10$. No subjects responded present to "Job transfer or change of schools" or "Birth of a child".

Table 6. Results of the multiple regression analysis with empowerment.

	Empowerment (family)				Empowerment (service system)				Empowerment (community/political)			
	Model 1		Model 2		Model 1		Model 2		Model 1		Model 2	
	β	p	β	p	β	p	β	p	β	p	β	p
Facility (outside of Tokyo 1, Tokyo 0)	−0.27	*	−0.12		−0.23	*	−0.06		−0.09		−0.12	
Sleep problems (present 1, absent 0)	−0.33	**	−0.25	*	−0.29	**	−0.21	*	−0.28	*	−0.25	*
Life events (present 1, absent 0)	0.32	**	0.26	**	0.28	*	0.21	*	0.30	**	0.26	**
Livelihood	0.22	*	0.19	†	0.28	*	0.26	*	0.28	*	0.19	†
Awareness of social support (within the family)			0.00				−0.13				0.00	
Awareness of social support (outside of the family)			0.33	**			0.45	***			0.33	**
Use of at-home services (present 1, absent 0)			0.16				0.19	†			0.16	
Adjusted R-squared	0.29	***	0.38	***	0.26	***	0.44	***	0.21	**	0.39	***
Amount of R-squared change			0.11	**			0.19	***			0.20	***

†$p < 0.1$, *$p < 0.05$, **$p < 0.01$ ***$p < 0.001$. β: Standard partial regression coefficient.

positive feelings towards child rearing. Moreover, these feelings were stronger in those who were aware of social support from outside of the family and who used at-home services. Positive feelings towards child rearing were stronger if negative feelings towards child rearing were weak and empowerment (each domain) was high. These data are shown in **Table 3** and **Table 4**.

3.3.2. Multiple Regression Analysis

Of the variables for which an association with positive feelings towards child rearing was seen in the univariate analysis, empowerment and variables for negative feelings towards child rearing and social support were selected as explanatory variables. In this study, social support and empowerment were assumed to be variables directly associated with positive feelings towards child rearing. However, among the variables for other attributes, negative feelings towards child rearing in particular had thus far been treated as a contrast to positive feelings towards child rearing; thus, the control of negative feelings is an important factor when examining support to promote positive feelings towards child rearing.

As a result, social support from outside of the family was not found to contribute to positive feelings towards child rearing. On the other hand, use of at-home services was found to contribute. The most contribution was seen from negative feelings towards child rearing. It was revealed that positive feelings towards child rearing were enhanced when negative feelings towards child rearing were reduced. Contributions were seen in the family and community/political domains of empowerment. These data are shown in **Table 7**.

4. Discussion

4.1. Subject Attributes

In this study, profoundly severely disabled children and quasi-severely disabled children accounted for 37.3% of all severely disabled children. The number of profoundly severely disabled children and quasi-severely disabled children is estimated at 10,000 nationwide in Japan, and at least 6,000 of these children live at home [19]. Given that the number of severely disabled children living at home is estimated to be 28,000 [1], it is likely that profoundly severely disabled children and quasi-severely disabled children account for at least about 20% of these severely disabled children living at home. There may therefore have been a strong bias towards subjects with profoundly severely disabled children and quasi-severely disabled children in this study. This is thought to have been influenced by the fact that subjects were limited to those who made regular outpatient visits, since the subjects in this study were recruited during outpatient visits.

The mean score for "physical condition," which indicates the mental and physical state of the subjects in this study, was 77 points. This score is almost the same as that in a similar previous study of mothers of severely disabled children living at home [14]. The mean sleep time in previous studies [14] [20] was stated to be consistently 5 to 6 hours, which was the same as in this study. The sleep time of caregivers of severely disabled children is short when compared to the mean daily sleep time of 6 to 7 hours for adult women [21].

Table 7. Results of multiple regression analysis with positive feelings towards child rearing.

	β	p	β	p	β	p
Negative feelings towards child rearing	−0.27	*	−0.29	**	−0.29	**
Awareness of social support (outside of the family)	0.13		0.11		0.11	
Use of at-home services (present 1, absent 0)	0.25	*	0.26	*	0.28	**
Empowerment (family)	0.22	†				
Empowerment (service system)			0.18			
Empowerment (community/political)					0.20	†
Adjusted R-squared	0.27	***	0.25	***	0.38	***

†p < 0.1, *p < 0.05, **p < 0.01, ***p < 0.001. β: Standard partial regression coefficient.

In a study that examined the families of children with developmental disabilities in Japan [11], the empowerment score was 34.4 ± 9.0 for the family domain, 36.1 ± 9.2 for the service system domain and 21.2 ± 6.5 for the community/political domain (mean ± standard deviation). Meanwhile, the empowerment score in this study, which examined the families of severely disabled children, was 37.02 ± 7.47 for the family domain, 39.09 ± 7.40 for the service system domain and 25.06 ± 6.18 for the community/political domain (mean ± standard deviation). The score for each domain was significantly higher in this study, which examined the families of severely disabled children (family domain: $p < 0.05$, service system domain: $p < 0.01$, community/political domain: $p < 0.001$). Compared with children with developmental disabilities, the need for support of severely disabled children and their families is acknowledged as a long-term requirement and while support remains adequate, it has been provided by support systems and institutions [22]. No studies limited to the families of severely disabled children can be found overseas; the majority of studies examine the families of children with developmental disabilities. In a study by Koren et al., which examined the families of children with emotional and developmental disabilities [9], the mean score for each domain was 45.8 for the family domain, 48.6 for the service system domain and 31.4 for the community/political domain. A study that examined the families of children with developmental disabilities and normal children [23] showed markedly higher scores compared with families in Japan. This was likely due to differences in culture more than the type of disability. Japan has a culture in which modesty is emphasized, in which one step is taken back to value overall harmony, as opposed to the individual asserting oneself. This makes a simple comparison of Japanese and overseas scores for empowerment difficult. Further accumulation of empirical studies on empowerment will therefore be needed in Japan in the future.

4.2. Factors Related to Empowerment and Support Strategies

A hierarchical multiple regression analysis in this study revealed that three variables contributed to empowerment: sleep problems of the child, life events and livelihood. Facilities did not contribute to empowerment. In terms of variables related to support, awareness of social support from outside of the family contributed to empowerment.

4.2.1. Facilities, Sleep Problems of the Child, Life Events and Livelihood

A comparison of facilities in Tokyo with other facilities revealed that facilities in Tokyo scored higher for empowerment in the family and service system domains. A study that examined the families of children with developmental disabilities [11] also found that those visiting facilities in Tokyo scored higher for empowerment. On the other hand, no significant difference was seen in the community/political domain. It is thought that because the items in the community/political domain are regarding government and politics, and because the same laws (e.g. the Services and Supports for Persons with Disabilities Act and Child Welfare Act) apply irrespective of the facilities in this study, inter-facility differences did not have an impact. Furthermore, by introducing other variables in the multiple regression analysis, the differences that arose in the family and service system domain no longer affected empowerment. Thus, the inter-facility difference that emerged in this study can be interpreted as the difference between other variables, particularly awareness of social support from outside of the family and use of at-home services.

Therefore, when providing support to enhance empowerment, focusing on the family's usage of at-home support and awareness of support offered by other services is more effective than lumping facilities or the entire region where the facilities are located together.

The nighttime sleep situation of the child is of particular importance to the family in daily care at home. In addition to respiratory and nutritional management, care for severely disabled children involves control of seizures, muscle tone and other factors. This care essentially needs to be provided day and night. In such situations, the child obviously needs to rest at night, but the family providing the care also needs to rest at night. If anything hinders the child's nighttime sleep, the family providing care cannot rest and this has an impact on daytime activities [24]. In this study, the mean sleep time of subjects was 3 to 6 hours, which is short even when compared to typical adults, and suggests that the subjects were providing childcare with barely any attention to their own physical condition. Nurses must take corrective action by properly asking families about the nighttime situation of the child and taking measures by devising methods of using sleep-inducing drugs and embracing the child through consultations with the family.

The entire family may be deprived of their energy in situations where a family member requires care due to illness or an accident. Lifestyle changes such as relocation, job transfers away from home without family and changes in family members can also cause problems with child rearing. However, the results of this study revealed that those who had experienced lifestyle changes (life events) had higher levels of empowerment. A possible interpretation of this is that lifestyle changes acted as a driving force for the family itself to put effort into child rearing. Resilience is a similar concept to empowerment. Resilience is "the psychological trait and ability to adapt and recover from difficult situations despite experiencing previous hardship" [25] and indicates the strength to proactively overcome and thrive against so-called adversity. The process of triggering resilience is complicated and largely unclear, although support from within and outside of the family at least is considered an effective means of triggering such ability [25]. Nonetheless, life events are desirable for child rearing [26]. For example, families may relocate in order to offer an appropriate environment for child rearing, such as a barrier-free environment. Further study will be needed after elucidating how subjects perceive life events.

The multiple regression analysis revealed that sleep problems of the child and livelihood were variables that consistently affected empowerment. The child's sleep rhythm, usage situation of anticonvulsants and the family's financial situation therefore need to be assessed and continuous support needs to be provided based on an understanding of the family's support situation and awareness situation of child rearing.

4.2.2. Awareness of Social Support and Use of At-Home Services

The variable that contributed the most as the explanatory variable of empowerment was awareness of social support from outside of the family. Previous studies have suggested an association between empowerment and social support [23] [27], but the situation of receiving support is thought to be similarly important as awareness of the subject themselves and of feeling that they are being supported. In addition to providing practical support, it is important when providing support to understand how the subject perceives their situation and to provide support that works on awareness to alter the subject's perception to a proactive one.

As a source of support, support from both within and outside of the family is necessary for the formation of empowerment [23]. However, support from outside of the family showed a strong association in this study. Specialist knowledge and skills, such as ventilator and enteral nutrition management and coping with seizures, is required for raising a severely disabled child. Total support from professionals for the child, primary caregiver and other family members is therefore particularly important in order for the family to continue raising their child.

To enhance the service level for empowerment, *i.e.* to improve the ability of a family with a severely disabled child to continue to use services through cooperation with professionals, it is necessary to build a system together with families that allows the continuous use of services.

4.3. Support Strategies to Enhance Positive Feelings towards Child Rearing

This study revealed that to enhance positive feelings towards child rearing, negative feelings towards child rearing must first be reduced. Use of at-home services and improving the empowerment of the subject themselves (or family itself) were also found to enhance positive feelings towards child rearing.

Many services offer care, so negative feelings towards child rearing can be reduced by implementing services [3]. However, the fundamental goal of family support is to allow the family, commencing with the primary caregiver, to continue proactively raising their child with a sense of fulfillment. To improve and maintain these positive feelings towards child rearing, it is important during the provision of services to encourage the family to become empowered. For example, services should nurture proactive feelings towards child rearing in the family by focusing on small changes indicative of growth of the child and sharing these with the family. Traditional factors that contribute to positive feelings towards child rearing include social support and negative feelings towards child rearing [3] [23], but this study newly showed that empowerment is a contributing factor. However, the causal relationship between social support and empowerment is said to go both ways [28]. The interaction between variables will need to be examined in the future. Specifically, we propose qualitatively elucidating the process of enhancing positive feelings towards child rearing through social support from the perspective of empowerment and conducting a covariance structure analysis with a larger subject sample.

4.4. The Limitations and Novelty of This Study

The subjects of this study were the families of children who regularly visited one of three facilities in the Tokyo metropolitan area on an outpatient basis. It is conceivable that some severely disabled children living at home who require little medical care do not make regular visits to facilities. In this study, there may have therefore been a bias towards subjects with severely disabled children with high medical needs. A study with a wider subject sample in other regions and facilities (schools, day care facilities, etc.) will need to be conducted in the future.

The questionnaires used in this study took about 30 minutes to complete and approximately 60% of the questionnaires were recovered. Some subjects may not have answered their questionnaires due to a lack of time. There is a need for questionnaires that are further refined and a method of explanation that grasps the main points to encourage subjects who did not answer the questionnaire this time to respond in the future.

On the other hand, the findings of this study suggested that support from professionals for the entire family was important because awareness of social support from outside of the family contributed the most to the empowerment of families with severely disabled children with high medical needs. Moreover, this study newly showed that, in addition to the reduction of negative feelings towards child rearing and ensuring social support, empowerment was a factor involved in the improvement and maintenance of positive feelings towards child rearing, which was the fundamental goal of family support. Practical family support for the purpose of promoting empowerment and positive feelings towards child rearing may become possible in the future based on the results of this study.

Acknowledgements

We would like to express our deepest gratitude to all the subjects and staff of the facilities at which this research was conducted for their cooperation in this study. This study was supported by a Grant-in-Aid for Young Scientists (B) (No. 24792517).

Disclosure

The authors declare that they have no competing interests.

References

[1]   Okada, K. (2006) The History of Children with Severe Motor and Intellectual Disabilities. In: Asakura, T., Ed., *Total Care of Children with Severe Motor and Intellectual Disabilities*, Herusu Shuppan , Tokyo, 15-20. (In Japanese)

[2]   Geeter, K.I., Poppes, P. and Vlaskamp, C. (2002) Parents as Experts: The Position of Parents of Children with Profound Multiple Disabilities. *Child: Care, Health and Development*, **28**, 443-453.
http://dx.doi.org/10.1046/j.1365-2214.2002.00294.x

[3]   Kuno, N., Yamaguchi, K. and Morita, C. (2006) The Sense of Burden of Mothers with Severely Disabled Children at Home and the Related Factors. *Journal of Japanese Society of Nursing Research*, **29**, 59-69. (In Japanese)
http://www.jsnr.jp/test/search/docs/202905003.pdf

[4]   Sugimoto, A., Nakamura, Y., Umeda, H., Akahane, E., Naijo, E. and Shibutani, H. (2009) The Characteristics of Family Function in Families with a Child with Disabilities: Research in A Prefecture. *Journal of Japan Academy of Human Care Science*, **2**, 49-56. (In Japanese)

[5]   Harden, J. (2005) Parenting a Young Person with Mental Health Problems: Temporal Disruption and Reconstruction. *Sociology of Health & Illness*, **27**, 351-371. http://dx.doi.org/10.1111/j.1467-9566.2005.00446.x
http://onlinelibrary.wiley.com/doi/10.1111/j.1467-9566.2005.00446.x/epdf

[6]   Sloper, P. and Turner S. (1993) Risk and Resistance Factors in the Adaptation of Parents of Children with Severe Physical Disability. *Journal of Child Psychology and Psychiatry*, **34**, 167-188.
http://dx.doi.org/10.1111/j.1469-7610.1993.tb00978.x

[7]   King, G.A., Rosenbaum, P.L. and King, S.M. (1997) Evaluating Family-Centred Service Using a Measure of Parents' Perceptions. *Child: Care, Health and Development*, **23**, 47-62. http://dx.doi.org/10.1046/j.1365-2214.1997.840840.x

[8]   Walsh, T. and Lord, B. (2004) Client Satisfaction and Empowerment through Social Work Intervention. *Social Work in Health Care*, **38**, 37-56. http://dx.doi.org/10.1300/J010v38n04_03

[9]   Koren, P.E., DeChillo, N. and Friesen, B.J. (1992) Measuring Empowerment in Families Whose Children Have Emotional Disabilities: A Brief Questionnaire. *Rehabilitation Psychology*, **37**, 305-321. http://dx.doi.org/10.1037/h0079106

[10]   Segal, S.P., Silverman, C. and Temkin, T. (1995) Measuring Empowerment in Client-Run Self-Help Agencies. *Community Mental Health Journal*, **31**, 215-227. http://dx.doi.org/10.1007/BF02188748

[11]   Wakimizu, R., Fujioka, H., Furuya, K., Miyamoto, S., Ieshima, A. and Yoneyama, A. (2010) Development of the Jap-

anese Version of the Family Empowerment Scale. *Journal of Health and Welfare Statistics*, **11**, 33-41. (In Japanese)

[12] Herbert, R.J., Gagnon, A.J., Rennick, J.E. and O'Loughlin, J.L. (2009) A Systematic Review of Questionnaires Measuring Health-related Empowerment. *Research and Theory for Nursing Practice*, **23**, 107-132.

[13] Ministry of Health, Labour and Welfare (2010) The 3rd General Welfare Committee Documents.
http://www.mhlw.go.jp/bunya/shougaihoken/sougoufukusi/2010/06/dl/0601-1d.pdf

[14] Hase, M. (2010) Development of a Questionnaire Concerning the Condition of Mothers of Children with Severe Motor and Intellectual Disabilities Who Live at Home. *Journal of Severe Motor and Intellectual Disabilities*, **35**, 143-150. (In Japanese)

[15] Natsume, M., Ota, Y., Noda, T., Sato, T., Yamada, K, Hanatani, T., Kamata, M., Iwata, K., Inui, T. and Murata, H. (1999) The Social Readjustment Rating Scale for the Elderly. *The Japanese Journal of Stress Sciences*, **13**, 222-229. (In Japanese)

[16] Ishikawa, R. (2007) The Stress and Social Support of Home Caregivers: A Health and Psychological Study. Kazama-shobo, Tokyo. (In Japanese)

[17] Hirose, M., Okada, S. and Shirasawa, M. (2005) The Factors Related to Family Caregivers' Positive Appraisal of Care. *Journal of Health and Welfare Statistics*, **52**, 1-7. (In Japanese)

[18] Arai, Y., Tamiya, N. and Yano, E. (2003) The Short Version of the Japanese Version of the Zarit Caregiver Burden Interview (J-ZBI_8): Its Reliability and Validity. *Japanese Journal of Geriatrics*, **40**, 497-503. (In Japanese)
https://www.jstage.jst.go.jp/article/geriatrics1964/40/5/40_5_497/_pdf

[19] Kitazumi, E., Iwasaki, Y., Izumi, M. and Akiyama, K. (2007) The Role of Facilities for Children with Super Severe Motor and Intellectual Disabilities as a System of Support for Daily Living. *Ryoushin no Tsudoi*, **606**, 2-18. (In Japanese)

[20] Ozawa, H., Kato, I., Ozaki, H., Ishizuka, T., Arimoto, K. and Kimiya, S. (2007) The Present Situation of Children with Psycho-Motor Disabilities and Their Parents. *Official Journal of the Japanese Society of Child Neurology*, **39**, 279-282. (In Japanese)

[21] Ministry of Health, Labour and Welfare (2013) The 2011 Fiscal Year National Health and Nutrition Survey.
http://www.mhlw.go.jp/bunya/kenkou/eiyou/dl/h23-houkoku.pdf

[22] Hori, T. (2006) Lobbying Movements by Parents of Children with Severe Motor and Intellectual Disabilities during High Economic Growth and Their Background. *Japanese Journal of Social Welfare*, **47**, 31-44. (In Japanese)

[23] Nachshen, J.S. and Minnes, P. (2005) Empowerment in Parents of School-aged Children with and without Developmental Disabilities. *Journal of Intellectual Disability Research*, **49**, 889-904.
http://dx.doi.org/10.1111/j.1365-2788.2005.00721.x

[24] Ozawa, H., Kimiya, S., Funahashi, M., Miyaji, S., Kurata, K., Tanuma, N., Tomita, S., Miyama, S., Shikura, K., Yamada, N., Uchiyama, K., Kurihara, E., Nakamura, Y. and Sasaki, M. (2010) The Present Situation of Children with Severe Motor and Intellectual Disabilities: Medical care-dependent Children and Their Parents in the Tama Area of Tokyo. *The Journal of the Japan Pediatric Society*, **114**, 1892-1895. (In Japanese)

[25] Oshio, A., Nakaya, M., Kaneko, H. and Nagamine, S. (2002) Development and Validation of an Adolescent Resilience Scale. *Japanese Journal of Counseling Science*, **35**, 57-65. (In Japanese)

[26] Zensho, M. (2006) A Study of Children with Severe Motor and Intellectual Disabilities and Their Family's Home Care Needs and Social Supports. *The Bulletin of Saitama Prefectural University*, **7**, 51-58. (In Japanese)
http://ci.nii.ac.jp/els/110005001975.pdf?id=ART0008078095&type=pdf&lang=jp&host=cinii&order_no=&ppv_type=0&lang_sw=&no=1448194448&cp=

[27] Orr, R.R., Cameron, S.J. and Day, D.M. (1991) Coping with Stress in Families with Children Who Have Mental Retardation: An Evaluation of the Double ABCX Model. *American Journal of Mental Retardation*, **95**, 444-450.

[28] Zimmerman, M.A. and Warschausky, S. (1998) Empowerment Theory for Rehabilitation Research: Conceptual and Methodological Issues. *Rehabilitation Psychology*, **43**, 3-16. http://dx.doi.org/10.1037/0090-5550.43.1.3

Appendix

The questionnaire that was actually used in this study can be referred to in the following URL. (In Japanese)
https://researchmap.jp/musrndur8-2070545/?action=multidatabase_action_main_filedownload&download_flag=1&upload_id=99758&metadata_id=170582

15

Comparative Study on Management of Vitiligo with Psoralen plus Steroid (Oxabet Formula) Alone VS Psoralen Formula plus Narrow Band of Ultraviolet B 311 nm in Khartoum Teaching Hospital of Dermatology and Venereology (KTHDV)

Hussein Salman Mohammed[1], Jahelrasoul Abdalla Edriss[2]

[1]Dermatology and Venereology, OIU, Khartoum, Sudan
[2]Dermatology and Venereology, KTHDV, Khartoum, Sudan
Email: dardaka@gmail.com

Abstract

A comparative study and management has been conducted in (KTHDV). For some patients who attend the out patients clinic concern on treatment of the vitiligo with a new formula (Oxabet) alone VS Oxabet (oxpsolaren plus betamethasone) formula plus NB. UVB311 is during a period from (Jan 2011-Jan 2013). The study sample includes different age groups of both sexes. The study revealed that the formula alone gives good results. The localized vitiligo has a good response to the formula than generalized one. The early lesions have good responses than the old ones. The continuations of applying the treatment and the follow up of the patients enhance the efficacy of the treatment.

Keywords

Vitiligo, Oxabet Formula, L.V. (Localize Vitiligo), G.V. (Generalize Vitiligo), Leukoderma, Psoralen, NB UVB 311nm, PUVA

1. Introduction

Vitiligo is specific common, and often is a heritable or acquired disorder of the skin and mucous membranes, characterized by well circumscribed milky white cutanous macules and patches devoid of identifiable meleno-cytes [1]-[3]. The likely incidence is between 1% - 2% [4]-[6]. All races are affected. Both sexes are affected equally [7] [8]. Vitiligo may develop at any age, and the average age of onset is 20 years [9]-[11]. Extensive tri-als of treatment have been done, which are rarely successful [12]-[14].

Clinical types:
1) Localized:
a) Focal vitiligo
b) Segmental vitiligo [15]-[17]
2) Generalized:
a) Vulgaris vitiligo
b) Lip-tip vitiligo
c) Arcofacial vitiligo
d) Universal vitiligo [18]-[19]

2. Psoralean Compounds

Tricyclic furocoumarin-like molecules found naturally in a variety of plants throughout the world and also pro-duced synthetically [21] [22], radically increase the erythema response of skin to long-wave ultraviolet light (UVA) after either topical application or systemic administration [2]-[4] [23]-[25].

Types: 3-TMP, 5-MOP, 8-MOP yjey are used with phototherapy or heliotherapy or bulb [26] [27].

3. Management

Various options are available Topical phototherapy, Systemic therapy, Surgical, Depigmentation, Laser therapy (Excimer 308 nm) [28]-[30].

This study is conducted from a MD study: 8-MOP plus Betamethazone (Oxabet) topical alone or with UVB Narrow Band 311 nm [2]-[4] [31] [32].

4. Methodology

For the formula tests had been carried out on 20 volunteer patients. The study had been accomplished in Khar-toum teaching hospital of dermatology and venereology (KTHTV).

The study was done during a period of three months by evaluation the treatment of vitiligo with psoralen plus steroid alone and psoralen plus steroid with N.B UVB311 nm.

The patients were selected among the patients revising the outpatients clinic in Khartoum hospital of derma-tology.

The number for sampling were (100) patients.

The patients had been requested to sign a consent paper.

The patients had been divided in two groups, a psoralen plus steroid and B psoralen plus steroid plus NB UVB311 nm.

The result had been tabulated, analyzed and discussed according to the study.

Lastly the conclusion and recommendation had been added

The drug was composed of 8 methoxalen powder 0.3 g in 20 g betamethazone.

Both drugs were marketed in the Sudan, their effect in vitiligo is summative *i.e.* they increase the devision of melanocytes and enhance the number of melanocytes in leukodermic area, and increase synthesis of the melanin (melanogenesis). The steroid therapy acts against autoantibodies of melanocytes (immunomodulators). The treatment name we suggest for the formula is (Oxabet).

5. Results

38 of the adult patients had localized vitiligo (L.V.) and were treated with formula as group A, who gave results as follows:

35 of patients had complete healing and 3 of them had marked improvement. (See **Figures 1-13**).

35 of the adult patients had generalized vitiligo (G.V.) who were treated with formula as group B and gave results as follows:

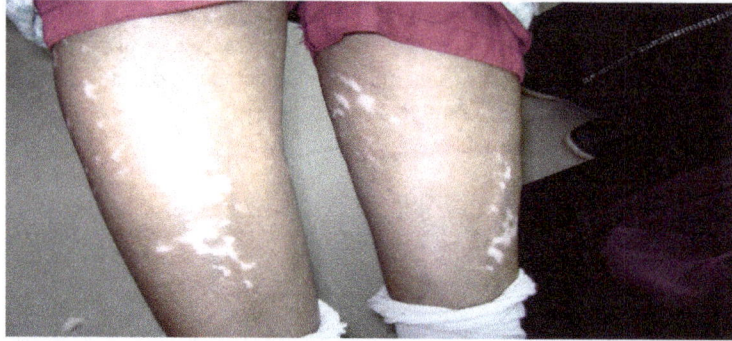

Figure 1. Lower limbs before treatment with Oxabet formula plus UVB NB 311 nm.

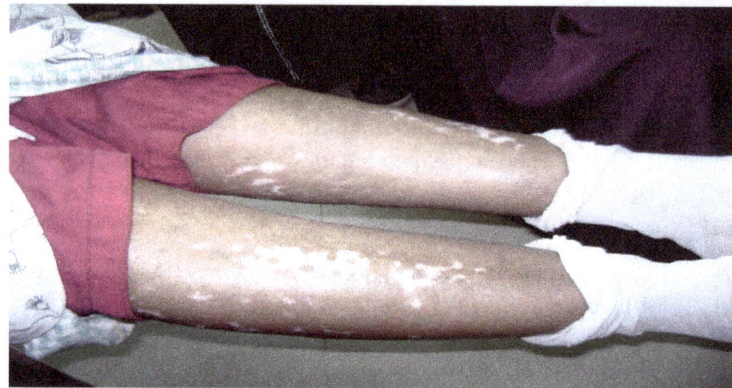

Figure 2. Lower limbs before treatment with Oxabet formula plus UVB NB 311 nm.

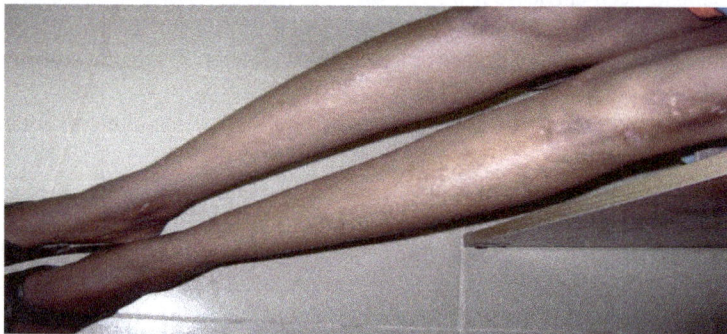

Figure 3. Lower limbs after three months of treatment with Oxabet formula plus UVB NB 311 nm had completely healing.

20 of them had complete healing, and 15 of them had good improvement (see **Figures 14-18**)).

The children treated with formula as group A and gave results as follows:

20 of patients had complete healing, 5 patients had good results and 2 patients had been resistance to the treatment. The (L.V.) patients gave good results rather than the (G.V.) (See **Figure 19** and **Figure 20**).

M.B. all patients are have no associated problems.

Patient not responding to treatment with a formula should anxiety.

Although the results are promising, yet we cannot guaranty to prevent the recurrence.

The lesions need 2 - 3 moths to heal.

Children have better results than adults.

The drug can cause contact eczema noticed in three children and two adults.

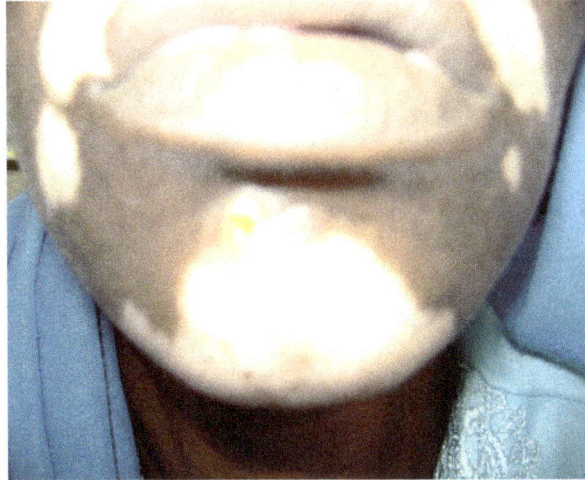

Figure 4. A child group A before treatment with Oxabet formula plus UVB NB 311 nm (acral lesion).

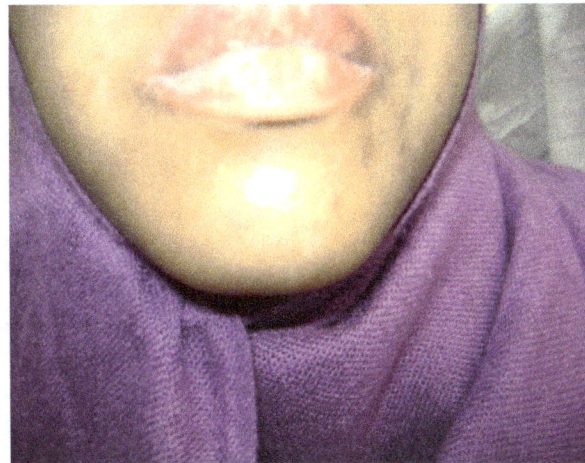

Figure 5. A child group A after three months of treatment with Oxabet formula plus UVB NB 311 nm had improvement.

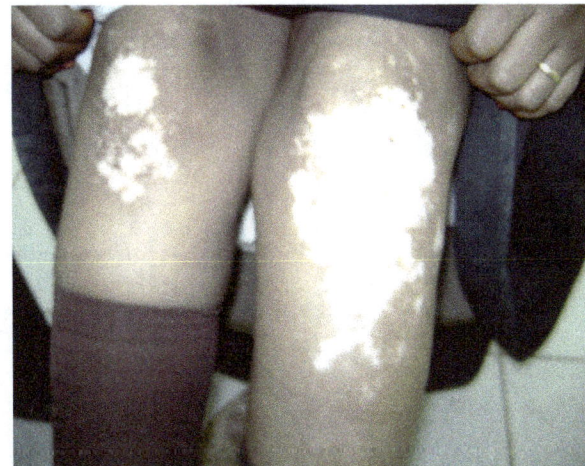

Figure 6. Adult female group A before treatment with Oxabet formula.

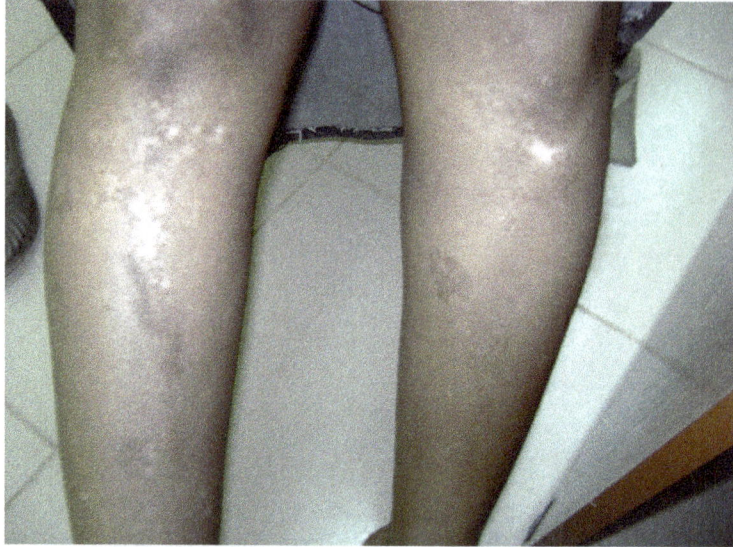

Figure 7. adult female group A after three months of treatment with Oxabet formula had completely healing.

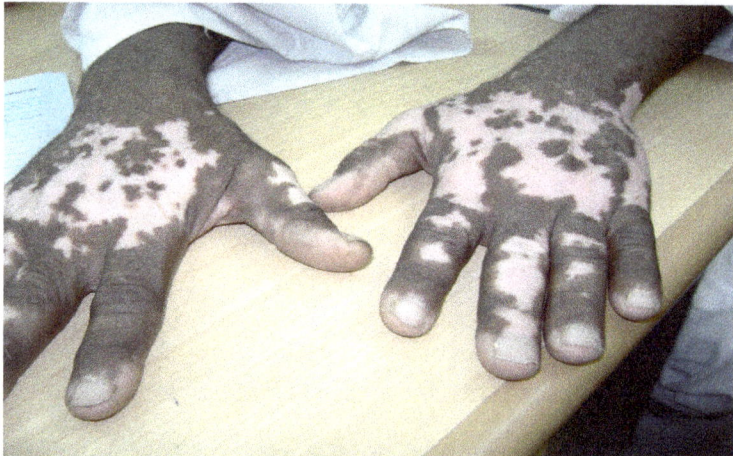

Figure 8. Acral vitiligo, adult male group A before treatment with Oxabet formula.

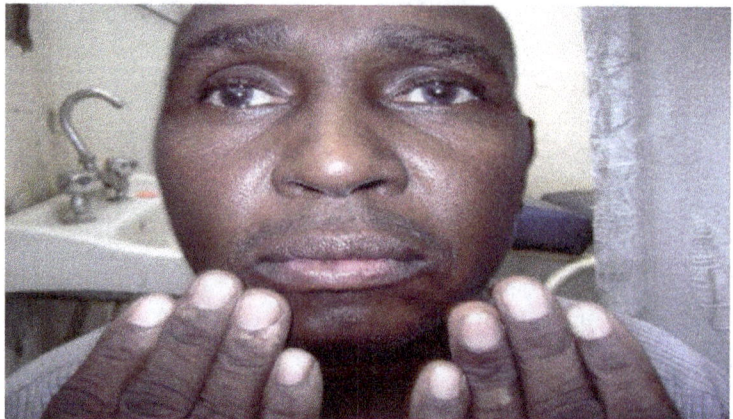

Figure 9. Acral vitiligo, adult male group A after three months of treatment with Oxabet formula had completely healing.

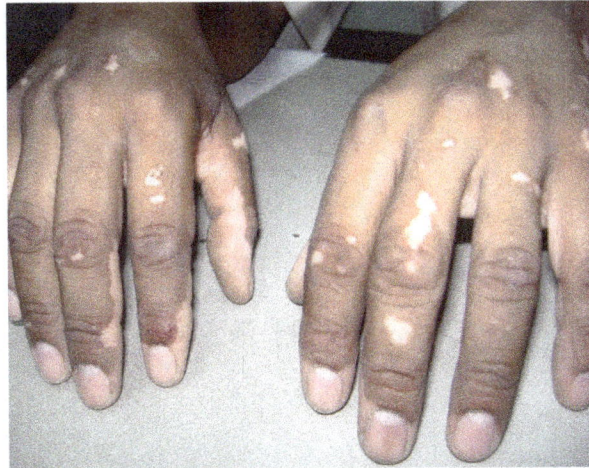

Figure 10. Acral Vitiligo, adult male group A before treatment with Oxabet formula.

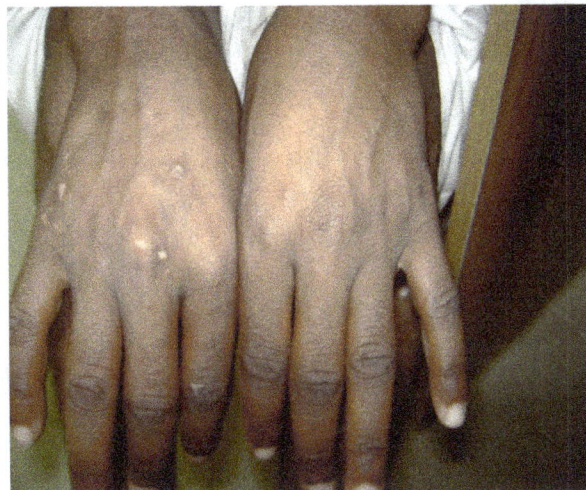

Figure 11. Acral Vitiligo, adult male group A after three months of treatment with Oxabet formula had complete healing.

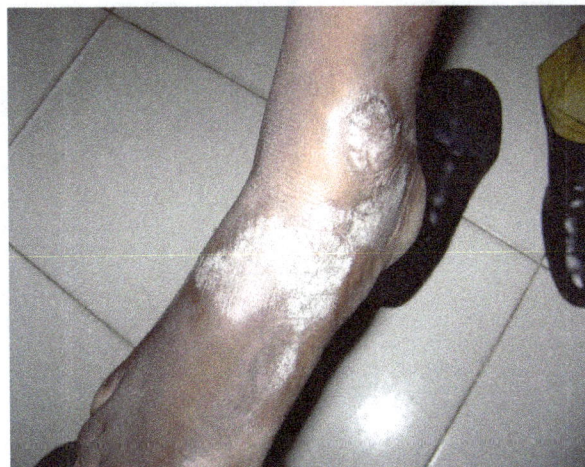

Figure 12. Acral vitiligo partially responding to Oxabet theraby.

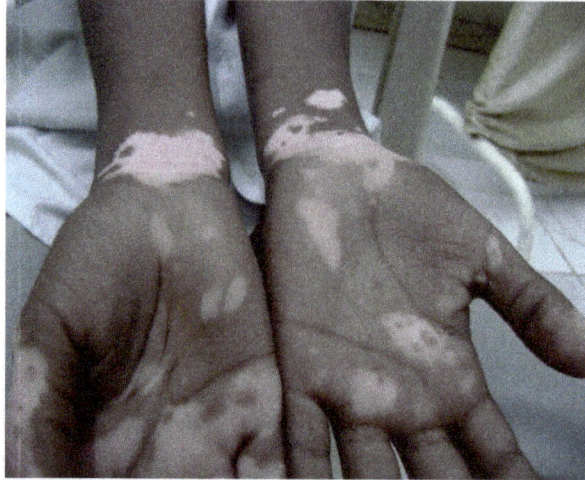

Figure 13. Acral vitiligo partially repigmented with Oxabet and UVB.

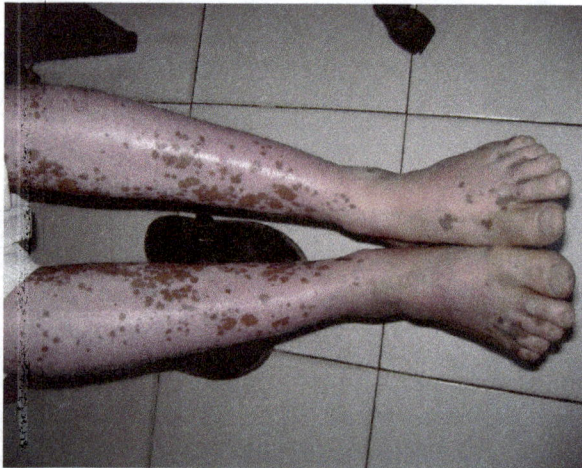

Figure 14. Acral vitiligo treated with Oxabet and UVB. Improvement in the legs but the feet are resistant to treatment.

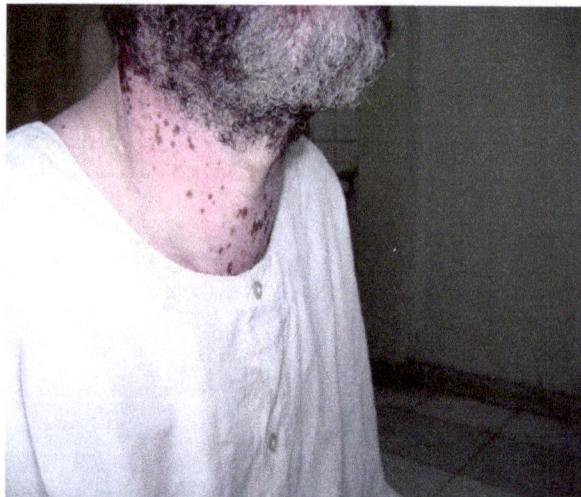

Figure 15. Slow response to treatment.

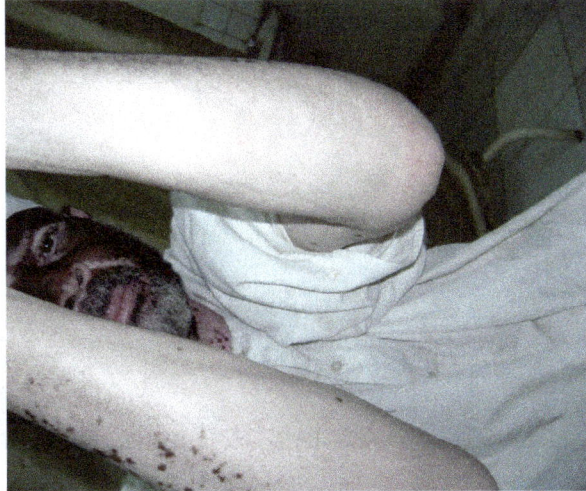

Figure 16. Generalised vitiligo before treatment.

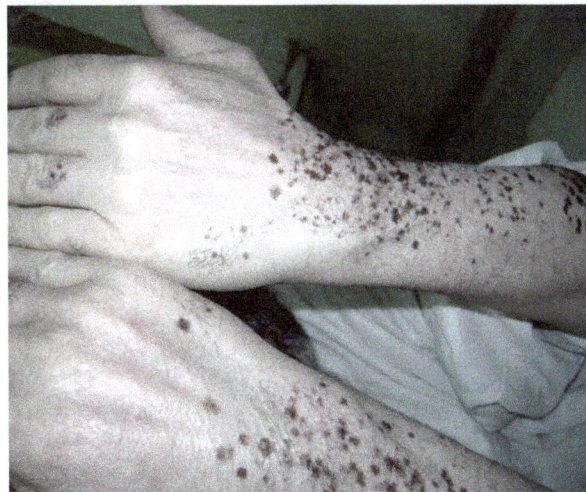

Figure 17. Generalised vitiligo after one month with Oxabet treatment.

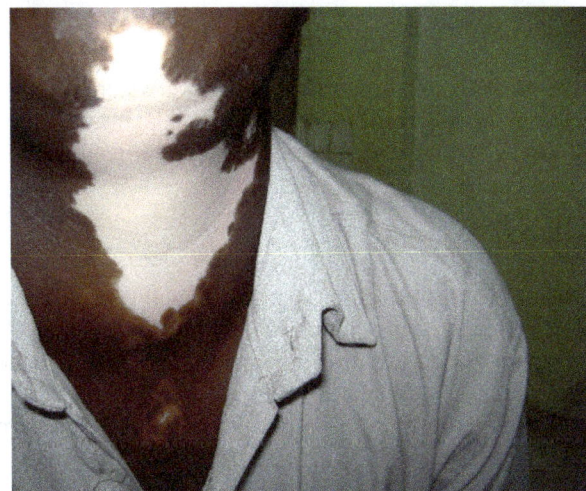

Figure 18. Focal vitiligo resistant to treatment with Oxabet.

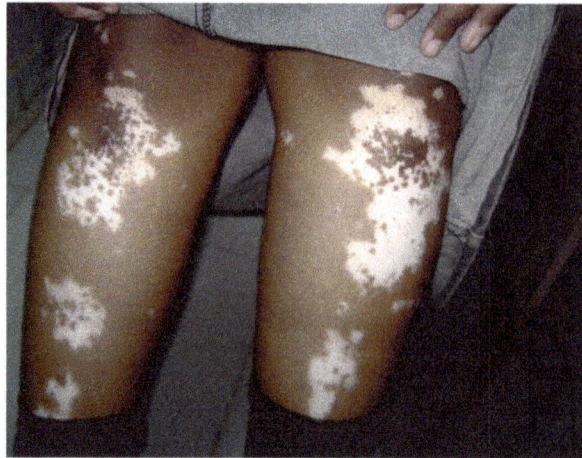

Figure 19. Adult female group A before treatment with Oxabet formula.

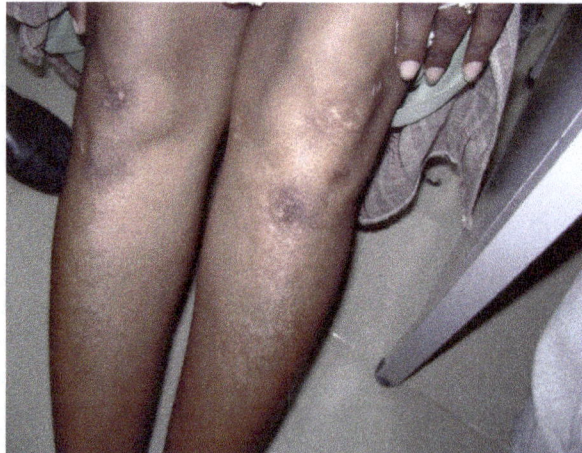

Figure 20. Adult female group A after three months of treatment with Oxabet formula had complete healing.

Acral vitiligo is difficult to heal.

6. Discussions

This study is a pilot one so far no recorded formula or study in a literature is found.

The formula gave a good result in the treatment of the (L. V.) than the G. V.

The children gave good results than the adult. The formula with combination of NB. UVB311 used in the treatment of G. V. and gave less degree than the formula alone.

7. Conclusions

The formula has a good promise for a future of treatment of vitiligo. It gives good results in shorter times around 3 months. It has an affordable price. It is easy to prepare apply with less side effect. The formula of Oxabet is stable up to six months at room temperature, but we prefer not to use it beyond three months.

As far as I know, there is no similar study in the literature, so it is considered as a pilot study.

The idea for the formula has been inspired from personal experience in dermatology. That is to say, both drugs are prescribed to treat vitiligo through:

a) Helping in division of melanocytes

b) Assisting in melanogensis

c) Transferring of melanin

d) Immunomodulators

So the reaction 8s is additive and summative.

Recommendations

The formula initially should be kept at 8 degree °C shouldn't be used after 3 months until the preserving time is reported. The patients should be followed up for recurrent or permanent healing. If the recurrent occurs the patients should repeat a fresh sample of drug.

References

[1] Lestery, M. and Alikhan, A. (2011) A Comprehensive Overview Part II Treatment Options and Approach to Treatment. *Journal of American Academy of Dermatology: Vitiligo*, 493-513.

[2] (1998) Rook/Willkinson/Ebiling Text Book of Dermatology. 6th Edition, Black Well Science Ltd., 1802-1805.

[3] Andrews Diseases of the Skin Clinical Dermatology, 10th Edition, El Sevier Inc., 7531-8734.

[4] Fitzpatricks (2007) Dermatology in General Medicine. 6th Edition, Wilkinson/Ebiling, 823-847.

[5] Khanaa, N. (2009) All Illustrate Synopsis of Dermatology and Sexually Transmitted Diseases. Elsevier, 129-135.

[6] Behi, P.N. Practice of Dermatology. 10th Edition, Salih Kummer, India, 204-304-310.

[7] Bowers, K.E. (2002) Manual of Dermatologic Therapeutics. 6th Edition, Luppinco William & Wikins, 118-120.

[8] Shelleg, W.B. and Shelley, E.D. (2002) Advance Dermatology Therapy. Luppinco William & Wikins, 1179-1186.

[9] Refael Fulabella and Marial, Borna Update an Skin Repigmentation Therapies in Vitiligo. Publication 17 November. refalabella@uniweb.net.co

[10] Magid, I. (2010) Vitiligo Management: An Update, British. *Journal of Medical Practioners*, **3**.

[11] Eldir, D.E. (2005) Lever's Histopathology of the Skin. 9th Edition, Lippincott Williams & Winkins, Philadelphia, 710-711.

[12] Harn, S.K. and Lee, H.J. (1996) Segmental Vitiligo: Clinical Findings in 208 Patients. *Journal of the American Academy of Dermatology*, **35**, 671-674. http://dx.doi.org/10.1016/S0190-9622(96)90718-5

[13] Schallreuter, K.U., Wood, J.M., Pielkow, M.R., Buttner, G., Swanson, N., Korner, C. and Ehrke, C. (1996) Increased Monoamine Oxidase A Activity in the Epidermis of Patients with Vitiligo. *Archives of Dermatological Research*, **288**, 14-18. http://dx.doi.org/10.1007/BF02505037

[14] Alkhateeb, A., Fain, P.R., Thody, A., Bennett, D.C. and Spirtz, R.A. (2003) Epidemiology of Vitiligo and Associated Autoimmune Diseases in Caucasian Probands and Their Families. *Pigment Cell Research*, **16**, 208-214. http://dx.doi.org/10.1034/j.1600-0749.2003.00032.x

[15] Nath, S.K., Majumder, P.P. and Van Nordlund, J.J. (1994) Genetic Epidemiology of Vitiligo: Multilocus Recessivity Cross-Validated. *American Journal of Human Genetics*, **55**, 981-990.

[16] Bystryn, J.C., Riget, D., Friedman, R.J. and Kopf, A. (1987) Prognostic Significance of Hypopigmentation in Malignant Melanoma. *Archives of Dermatology*, **123**, 1053-1055. http://dx.doi.org/10.1001/archderm.1987.01660320095019

[17] Naralond, J.J., Kirkwood, J.M., Forget, S.M., Milton, G., Albert, D.M. and Lerner, A.B. (1983) Viltiligo in Patients with Metastatic Melanoma: A Good Prognostic Sign. *Journal of the American Academy of Dermatology*, **9**, 689-696. http://dx.doi.org/10.1016/S0190-9622(83)70182-9

[18] Alajlan, A., Alfadley, A. and Pedersen, K.T. (2002) Transfer of Vitiligo after Allogeneic Bone Marrow Transplantation. *Journal of the American Academy of Dermatology*, **46**, 606-610. http://dx.doi.org/10.1067/mjd.2002.117215

[19] Aubin, F., Calm, J.Y., Ferrand, C., Angonmn, R., Humbert, P. and Tberghien, P. (2000) Extensive Vitiligo after Ganciclovir Treatment of GvHD in a Patient Who Had Received Donor T Cells Expressing Herpes Simplex Virus Thymidine Kinase. *Lancet*, **355**, 626-627. http://dx.doi.org/10.1016/S0140-6736(99)04215-4

[20] Bystryn, J.C. (1989) Serum Antibodies in Vitiligo Patients. *Clinics in Dermatology*, **7**, 136-145. http://dx.doi.org/10.1016/0738-081X(89)90063-1

[21] Cui, J., Harning, B., Henn, M. and Bystryn, J.C. (1992) Identification of Pigment Cell Antigens Defined by Vitiligo Antibodies. *Journal of Investigative Dermatology*, **98**, 162-165. http://dx.doi.org/10.1111/1523-1747.ep12555773

[22] Cui, J., Arita, Y. and Bystryn, I.C. (1995) Characterization of Vitiligo Antigens. *Pigment Cell Research*, **8**, 53-59. http://dx.doi.org/10.1111/j.1600-0749.1995.tb00774.x

[23] Norris, D.A., Capin, L., Muglia, I.I., Osborn, R.L., Zerbe, G.O., Bystrjn, C. and Tonneseni, M.G. (1988) Enhanced

Susceptibility of Melanocytes to Different Immunologic Effector Mechanisms *in Vitro*: Potential Mechanisms for Postinflammatory Hypopigmentation and Vitiligo. *Pigment Cell Research*, 1, 113-123. http://dx.doi.org/10.1111/j.1600-0749.1988.tb00801.x

[24] Song, Y.H., Connar, E., Li, Y., Zorovrich, B., Baidaccl, P. and Maclaren, N. (1994) The Role of Tyrosinase in Autoimmune Vitiligo. *Lancet*, **344**, L1049-L1052. http://dx.doi.org/10.1016/s0140-6736(94)91709-4

[25] Hedstrand, H., Ekwall, O., Olsson, M.J., Landgren, E., Kemp, E.H., Weetman, A.P., *et al.* (2001) The Transcription Factors SOX9 and SOX10 Are Vitiligo Autoantigens in Autoimmune Polyendocrine Syndrome Type I. *The Journal of Biological Chemistry*, **276**, 35390-35395. http://dx.doi.org/10.1074/jbc.M102391200

[26] Baharav, E., Merimski, O., Shoenfeld, Y., Zigelman, B., Gilbrud, B., Yechskl, G., *et al.* (1996) Tyrosinase as an Autoantigen in Patients with Vitiligo. *Clinical & Experimental Immunology*, **105**, 84-88. http://dx.doi.org/10.1046/j.1365-2249.1996.d01-727.x

[27] Cui, J., Arita, Y. and Bystryn, J.C. (1993) Cytolytic Antibodies to Melanocytes in Vitiligo. *Journal of Investigative Dermatology*, **100**, 812-815. http://dx.doi.org/10.1111/1523-1747.ep12476636

[28] Harning, R., Cui, J. and Bystryn, I.C. (1991) Relation between the Incidence and Level of Pigment Cell Antibodies and Disease Activity in Vitiligo. *Journal of Investigative Dermatology*, **97**, 1078-1080. http://dx.doi.org/10.1111/1523-1747.ep12492607

[29] Norris, D.A., Kissinger, R.M., Naughton, G.M. and Bystryn, J.C. (1988) Evidence for Immunologic Mechanisms in Human Vitiligo: Patients' Sera Induce Damage to Human Melanocytes *in Vitro* by Complement-Mediated Damage and Antibody-Dependent Cellular Cytotoxicity. *Journal of Investigative Dermatology*, **90**, 783-789. http://dx.doi.org/10.1111/1523-1747.ep12461505

[30] Schallreuter, K.U., Wood, J.M., Ziegler, I., Lemke, K.R., Pittelkow, M.R., Lindsey, N.J. and Gütlich, M. (1994) Defective Tetrahydrobiopterin and Catecholamine Biosynthesis in the Depigmentation Disorder Vitiligo. *Biochimica et Biophysica Acta*, **1226**, 181-192. http://dx.doi.org/10.1016/0925-4439(94)90027-2

[31] Thappa, D.M. (2008) Textbook of Dermatology, Leprology & Venereology. 3rd Edition, Elsevier, Amsterdam, 196-200.

[32] Arndt, K.A., Hsu, J.T.S., Alam, M., Bhatia, A. and Chilukuri, S. (2002) Manual of Dermatologic Therapeutics. 8th Edition, Lippincott Williams & Wilkins, Philadelphia, 119-123.

16

Using Teacher Goal Boards to Promote Healthy Eating and Physical Activity among Elementary Students

P. Cougar Hall, Josh H. West, Benjamin T. Crookston, Yvonne Allsop

Department of Health Science, Brigham Young University, Provo, UT, USA
Email: cougar_hall@byu.edu

Abstract

Background: The purpose of this study was to explore the feasibility and understand the potential impact on elementary students' perceptions of, and intentions related to, healthy eating and physical activity when their classroom teacher sets and shares goals related to these health behaviors. Methods: Participants in this study included 16 teachers and 229 students of grades 3 - 6 at a large elementary school in the Western United States. Participating students were surveyed before and after a six-week intervention conducted by classroom teachers that consisted of a weekly displaying of *Teacher Goal Boards* in a prominent classroom location and sharing of goals set for the week. Teacher reports of the previous week's goals occurred each Monday prior to sharing and posting of new goals for the new week. Results: Respondents reported significantly higher post-test values for over half of pre-post comparisons. Respondents were more likely to intend to be physically active (post = 52.6% vs. pre = 39.0%, p = 0.003), to eat nutritious foods (52.0% vs. 36.4%, p = 0.001), and to maintain a healthy body weight (62.8% vs. 52.2%, p = 0.022). Similar results were found for summary measures. Intention to be physically active, to eat healthy, to maintain a healthy weight, as well as descriptive norms for physical activity and perception and value of personal health behaviors were all significantly higher at post-test. Discussion: This study and its findings are significant because teacher participants were able to significantly and positively impact on students' behavioral intent, subjective norms, and perception and value of personal health behaviors amongst students without spending additional time on formal health promotion and education instruction. Conclusion: Schools should incentivize and encourage faculty and staff to engage in a variety of health behaviors to improve both personal health outcomes and role model health behaviors for students.

Keywords

Health Education, Health Behavior, School Health, Nutrition, Physical Activity, Elementary Students

1. Introduction

Healthy eating and regular physical activity play a substantial role in preventing chronic disease [1]-[3]. Poor diet and physical inactivity among children increase the risk for chronic health conditions, including high blood pressure, type-2 diabetes, and obesity [3]. The percentage of obese children aged 6 - 11 has tripled over the past 30 years [4]. Obese children have higher rates of social and psychological problems, such as discrimination and poor self-esteem [5]-[8]. Engaging children in healthy eating and regular physical activity can lower these risks and greatly decrease future burdens on health-care and education systems.

Schools play a particularly critical role in improving the physical activity and dietary behaviors of children. With greater than 95% of children enrolled in schools and in attendance for approximately 6 hours each day [8] schools have unmatched access to young people. School health programs and policies may be one of the most efficient and universal means to prevent or reduce risk behaviors and limit serious health problems among students. Nine guidelines outlining research-based best practices for specifically promoting healthy eating and physical activity have been established by the Centers for Disease Control and Prevention [9]. Each guideline is accompanied by a series of recommendations and strategies for schools to implement. The second guideline addresses the need to establish school environments that support healthy eating and physical activity. Included in this guideline is the recommendation that schools work to establish a psychosocial environment "that encourages and does not stigmatize healthy eating and physical activity" [9]. It is believed that faculty and staff can influence the school environment by working to establish social norms supportive of healthy eating and physical activity [10]. Similarly, the eighth guideline addresses the need for school employee wellness programs to include healthy eating and physical activity goals and services. Activities that promote healthy eating and physical activity among faculty and which emphasize behavioral skills are recommended [9]. Teachers modeling healthy behaviors and skills can help to create a psychosocial climate that encourages students to likewise be physically active and make healthy nutritional choices.

There is strong theoretical support backing the recommendation that schools create an environment supportive of healthy eating and physical activity. Multiple prominent health behavior change theories include constructs related to the example and influence of others. More specifically, several key theoretical constructs support the assertion that referents such as teachers and other school employees who model healthy behaviors can have a powerful influence on the attitudes and behaviors of students. For instance, *modeling* or *observational learning* included in Social Cognitive Theory express the impact and influence that observed behaviors have on an individual's decision-making [11]. In particular, the modeling of a desired skill or behavior by a credible role model provides an ideal learning opportunity for the observer who may acquire the targeted skill or behavior through watching the actions and outcomes of others. As Bandura noted, "A good example is therefore a much better teacher than the consequences of unguided actions" [12]. Observations greatly impact on behavior according to the Theory of Planned Behavior as well, where *descriptive* and *injunctive norms* included in the *subjective norm* construct emphasize the impact that an individual's perception of other' beliefs, attitudes and behavior has on his or her own decision-making [13]. Building upon the subjective norm construct, Cialdini, Kallgren, and Reno [14] developed the Focus Theory of Normative Conduct to describe how individuals implicitly juggle multiple behavioral expectations at once; expanding on conflicting prior beliefs about whether cultural, situational or personal norms motivate action, the researchers suggested the focus of an individual's attention will dictate what behavioral expectation they follow. They define a *descriptive norm* as people's perceptions of what is commonly done in specific situations; it signifies what most people do, without assigning judgment. The absence of trash on the ground in a parking lot, for example, transmits the descriptive norm that most people there do not litter [15] [16]. An *injunctive norm*, on the other hand, transmits group approval about a particular behavior; it dictates how an individual *should* behave [15]-[18]. Watching another person pick up trash off the ground and throw it out, a group member may pick up on the injunctive norm that she ought to not litter. Descriptive norms depict what happens while injunctive norms describe what should happen. Collectively, each of these theoretical constructs highlight the influence important referents, such as teachers, can have in shaping the beliefs, attitudes, and behaviors of school children with whom they enjoy a close proximity and regular contact. Despite the belief that modeling healthy behaviors by school personnel is an important factor for promoting health, relatively few studies have explored role-modeling of healthy eating and physical activity among teachers. One notable exception is a study conducted by Kubik, Lytle, Hannan, Story, and Perry [19], which examines the eating behaviors teachers model at school. While nearly all (97%) of the 490 middle school teachers in this study agreed that a healthy school environment was important, the majority did not model healthy eating behavior at school. Most teachers reported high-fat intakes and frequently purchased sweetened soft drinks and high-fat or high-sugar snack foods from school vending machines. A recent observational study of 140 teachers' dietary practices during the school day in Western Saudi Arabia concluded that positive teacher role modeling is necessary in reducing poor dietary behaviors and outcomes among children [20]. Arcan *et al.* [21] studied classroom food practices and food-related beliefs of 75 kindergarten and first grade teachers on a large American Indian reservation. Many teachers in this study sample did not model healthy eating behavior, yet more than half agreed that students' nutritional choices are influenced by what they see their teachers eat. Power, Bindler, Goetz, and Daratha [22] worked with student, parent, and teacher focus groups to understand how schools might best promote healthy eating and physical activity. Based on their qualitative data, the authors concluded that sending students consistent messages and establishing school-wide social norms supportive of healthy lifestyles is a key to school-based interventions. Hendy and Raudenbush [23] found teacher modeling to have a limited impact on preschoolers' acceptance of new foods. Silent modeling in particular had little sway whereas enthusiastic teacher modeling and peer modeling were of greater effect respectively. Finally, Rossiter, Glanville, Taylor, and Blum [24] examined the classroom food practices, personal health, fat intake, and nutritional knowledge of 103 preservice teachers in Canada. The authors concluded that unhealthy nutritional practices of prospective teachers may act as a barrier to promoting healthy eating and that teachers who fail to model healthy behaviors feel largely hypocritical taking a "Do as I say, not as I do" approach to health promotion in the classroom. While each of these previous studies aimed at understanding teacher modeling of healthy eating or physical activity, to date no study has examined the impact teacher role modeling of goal setting behaviors may have on students' behavioral intentions. The purpose of this study was to understand the potential impact on elementary students' perceptions of, and intentions related to, healthy eating and physical activity when their classroom teacher sets and shares goals related to these health behaviors. The following three research questions guided this study:

1) What impact does an elementary teacher modeling goal-setting behavior related to healthy eating and physical activity have on students' behavioral intentions to eat healthy and be physically active?

2) What impact does an elementary teacher modeling goal-setting behavior related to healthy eating and physical activity have on students' subjective norms related to these health-promoting behaviors?

3) What impact does an elementary teacher modeling goal-setting behavior related to healthy eating and physical activity have on students' perception and value of personal health behavior?

2. Methods

2.1. Participants

Participants in this study included teachers of grades 3 - 6 and their students at a large elementary school in the Western United States. Slightly more than half (53.9%) of the students were female whereas 84% were Caucasian, 5.2% were Hispanic, and 10.8% were "other". The largest proportion of students was in the 4th grade (42.1%) followed by 6th grade (22.8%), 5th grade (18.5%), and 3rd grade (16.7%). All teachers in grades 3 - 6 at the study school were invited to participate. Sixteen of the 23 eligible teachers (70%) agreed to participate in the study and completed a participant consent form. All students assigned to the classroom of a participating teacher were invited to participate. A combined 229 students of 408 possible student participants (56%) enrolled in the 16 participating classes agreed to participate in the study and qualified by returning signed child assent and parental/guardian consent forms.

2.2. Procedure

Upon approval from the University IRB and the school district Research and Evaluation Chair, researchers met with the principal of the study school to provide an overview of the project and establish a timeline for the intervention. The principal invited all teachers of grades 3 - 6 interested in the study to meet with the principal investigator during the lunch break of a teacher-preparation day prior to the 2013-2014 school year. The principal investigator provided the teachers in attendance an overview of the study, including basic requirements and study incentives. It was explained that participation was voluntary and that participants wanting to discontinue in the study at any time were free to do so with no questions asked. Potential participants were shown a *Teacher Goal Board* and provided information and a demonstration on setting S-M-A-R-T goals. The *Teacher Goal Board* was a 24" × 36" laminated poster with space to write with a dry-erase marker the teacher's weekly *physical activity*, *healthy eating*, and *life-long learning* goals (**Figure 1**). It was explained that teacher participants would be expected to set a S-M-A-R-T goal in each of these three areas (physical activity, healthy eating, and life-long learning) each week for six weeks and report to their students how well they accomplished their goals (**Figure 2**). Teachers were told that for their participation they would receive, and could keep, a *FitBit®* *Zip* accelerometer with a retail value of 60US dollars. All attendees were provided consent forms and instructed

---

TEACHER GOAL BOARD

★ **PHYSICAL ACTIVITY:**

★ **HEALTHY EATING:**

★ **LIFE-LONG LEARNING:**

Figure 1. Teacher goal board.

Use the S-M-A-R-T approach in setting each weekly goal:

<u>Specific</u> and <u>Measurable</u>: Make certain your goals are specific and can be measured. "*I will get in shape*" or "*I will eat better*" are both far too general and difficult to measure. "*I will walk for 30 minutes five days this week*" or "*I will eat at least one serving of fruit at breakfast, lunch, and dinner every day this week*" are more specific and measurable.

<u>Appropriate</u> and <u>Realistic</u>: On occasion individuals set ill-advised nutrition and exercise goals. Goals such as "*I will lose 10 pounds this week*" and "*I will work out four times a day this week*" are likely unsafe and unachievable. The following list includes behaviors recommended by the Centers for Disease Control and Prevention that may help you set appropriate and realistic goals: eat breakfast every day; eat healthy snacks; eat healthy foods when dining out; eat a variety of foods within each food group every day; eat an abundance of fruits and vegetables every day; choose to eat whole grain products and fat-free or low-fat milk; drink plenty of water every day; limit foods and beverages high in added sugars, solid fat, and sodium; engage in moderate to vigorous physical activity every day; engage in warm-up and cool-down activities.

<u>Timed</u>: Every goal needs an end date by which time it will be accomplished. This study includes just short-term goals lasting one week.

Please set your own goals based upon what you personally would like to achieve. The examples of goals in each area listed below are simply to help you begin this process. Challenge yourself with your own goals and have fun!

Physical Activity	Healthy Eating
• I will reach 10,000 steps on my *FitBit®* each day this week.	• I will eat breakfast every day this week.
• I will walk for 20 minutes during recess each day this week.	• I will not eat or snack after 8PM this week.
• I will go jogging 3 times this week.	• I will eat 5 servings of vegetables each day this week.
• I will ride my bike to and from work 4 times this week.	• I will not drink soda this week.
• I will go to my early morning aerobics class 2 times this week.	• I will not pass a drinking fountain this week without stopping for a drink.
• I will run 20 miles this week.	• I will replace ice cream with yogurt for dessert this week.
• I will do my Pilates workout 3 days this week.	• I will only use low-fat milk and dressings this week.
• I will park in the furthest parking spot from the store each time I shop this week.	

Figure 2. Hidden hollow goal board study guidelines.

to complete and turn them in to a selected teacher within two weeks if they desired to participate. Consent forms were collected two weeks later by the principal investigator and participating teachers were provided parental/guardian consent forms and child assent forms for each student enrolled in their class. Parents/Guardians and students were informed that participation was voluntary and would not impact class grades. Participating students would receive a healthy snack while completing both the pre- and post-intervention questionnaire. Participating teachers accepted and collected consent and assent forms for two weeks at which time enrollment in the study was closed. A week later the principal investigator administered the student questionnaire in each of the 16 participating classes. On Monday of the following week participating teachers began the day by displaying their individual *Teacher Goal Board* in a prominent location in the classroom and sharing the goals they had set for the week. The following Monday teachers reported on the previous week's goals before sharing and posting their new goals for the new week.

Teachers responded to student inquiries related to their goal progress as such inquiries arose naturally throughout the week. This weekly goal-setting and reporting routine continued for six weeks. Following the six-week intervention, the principal investigator returned to each participating classroom to administer both the student questionnaire and the teacher questionnaire.

2.3. Instrumentation

Student participants completed the same 20-item questionnaire before and after the six-week intervention. The questionnaire included two demographic questions (sex and race/ethnicity) and 18 questions designed to measure behavioral interventions, subjective norms, and perception and value of personal health behavior [25]. Nine items measured three specific behavioral intentions (healthy eating, physical activity, maintaining a healthy weight) with each behavioral intention addressed by three questions (*i.e., I expect to be physically active; I want to be physically active; I intend to be physically active)* answered using a 5-point Likert scale (*strongly disagree, disagree, neither agree or disagree, agree, strongly agree*). Six items measured subjective norms, with three questions specifically targeting descriptive norms (*i.e., I think my teacher is physically active; I think that being physically active is important to my teacher; I think that my teacher eats healthy and nutritious foods)* and three questions specifically targeting injunctive norms (*i.e., I think it is important to my teacher that I engage in physical activity every day; I think it is important to my teacher that I eat healthy and nutritious foods; I think it is important to my teacher that I maintain a healthy body weight)*. Finally, three items measured student perception and value of personal health behavior (*i.e., I am physically active; Physical activity is important to me; I eat healthy and nutritious meals)*.

Teacher participants completed a brief questionnaire at the conclusion of the six-week intervention which included the following first items: 1) *I was motivated to share my Goal Board with my students*; 2) *I was motivated to set and reach my Goal Board goals*; 3) *The six-week Goal Board activity was enjoyable for me*; 4) *I completed the Goal Board activity with my class*; and 5) *The six-week Goal Board activity was meaningful to my students*.

2.4. Data Analysis

Change scores were computed using pre- and post-intervention measures of participants' behavioral intent, subjective norms, and perception and value of personal health behavior. Individual measures were dichotomized as strongly agree vs. all other responses (strongly disagree, disagree, neither agree or disagree, and agree). Summary measures were constructed by averaging the Likert scores across sets of variables. For example, intention to be physically active was constructed by taking the average Likert score of *I expect to be physically active, I want to be physically active*, and *I intend to be physically active*. Analogous summary intention measures were constructed for ... *eat healthy and nutritious foods* and ... *maintain a healthy body weight*. Summary measures for descriptive and injunctive norms and perception and value of personal health behavior were similarly created using the questions targeting descriptive and injunctive norms and perception and value of personal health behavior described above. Percentages and Pearson chi-square tests were used to compare Likert score means.

3. Results

Students had significantly higher post-test responses for over half of pre-post comparisons (**Table 1**). Students were more likely to intend to be physically active (post = 52.6% vs. pre = 39.0%, $p < 0.003$), to eat nutritious foods (52.0% vs. 36.4%, p < 0.001), and to maintain a healthy body weight (62.8% vs. 52.2%, p < 0.002). There was a significant increase in the belief that the teacher was physically active (55.9% vs. 45.7%, p < 0.028) and that the teacher eats healthy and nutritious foods (53.0% vs. 43.3%, p < 0.036), but not in the belief that physical activity is important to the teacher (59.5% vs. 53.7%, p < 0.028). There was no significant improvement in the belief that the teacher felt the student's physical activity, diet, and body weight was important.

Pre-post comparisons for girls and boys differed considerably (**Table 2**, **Table 3**). Girls were more likely at

Table 1. Pre- and post-test comparisons of individual health measures, girls (n = 229).

	Pre	Post	p-value
I expect to be physically active	39.22	55.84	0.000
I want to be physically active	51.72	67.10	0.001
I intend to be physically active	38.96	52.61	0.003
I expect to eat healthy and nutritious foods	41.20	49.56	0.071
I want to eat healthy and nutritious foods	50.65	56.71	0.191
I intend to eat healthy and nutritious foods	36.36	51.95	0.001
I expect to maintain a healthy body weight	55.90	63.79	0.084
I want to maintain a healthy body weight	67.39	75.65	0.050
I intend to maintain a healthy body weight	52.19	62.77	0.022
I think my teacher is physically active	45.65	55.90	0.028
I think that being physically active is important to my teacher	53.68	59.48	0.208
I think that my teacher eats healthy and nutritious foods	43.29	53.02	0.036
I think it is important to my teacher that I engage in physical activity every day	45.69	47.41	0.710
I think it is important to my teacher that I eat healthy and nutritious foods	45.06	48.71	0.431
I think it is important to my teacher that I maintain a healthy body weight	38.53	46.52	0.083
I am physically active	49.13	58.87	0.036
Physical activity is important to me	57.52	68.26	0.018
I eat healthy and nutritious foods	26.29	37.72	0.009

Notes: Proportions reported are "strongly agree".

Table 2. Pre- and post-test comparisons of individual health measures, girls (n = 124).

	Pre	Post	p-value
I expect to be physically active	31.45	53.66	0.000
I want to be physically active	47.15	68.29	0.001
I intend to be physically active	33.06	50.41	0.006
I expect to eat healthy and nutritious foods	45.16	44.26	0.887
I want to eat healthy and nutritious foods	50.00	57.72	0.223
I intend to eat healthy and nutritious foods	37.10	47.15	0.109
I expect to maintain a healthy body weight	55.73	62.10	0.311
I want to maintain a healthy body weight	67.48	78.23	0.058
I intend to maintain a healthy body weight	48.36	62.60	0.025
I think my teacher is physically active	42.74	54.55	0.065
I think that being physically active is important to my teacher	54.03	61.29	0.247
I think that my teacher eats healthy and nutritious foods	40.65	52.42	0.064
I think it is important to my teacher that I engage in physical activity every day	43.55	47.58	0.524
I think it is important to my teacher that I eat healthy and nutritious foods	41.13	47.58	0.307
I think it is important to my teacher that I maintain a healthy body weight	34.96	44.72	0.118
I am physically active	48.78	52.85	0.524
Physical activity is important to me	49.58	63.41	0.030
I eat healthy and nutritious foods	25.00	36.88	0.044

Notes: Proportions reported are "strongly agree".

Table 3. Pre- and post-test comparisons of individual health measures, boys (n = 105).

	Pre	Post	p-value
I expect to be physically active	48.57	57.14	0.213
I want to be physically active	56.60	65.71	0.175
I intend to be physically active	46.15	55.77	0.165
I expect to eat healthy and nutritious foods	36.79	55.34	0.007
I want to eat healthy and nutritious foods	51.92	56.19	0.536
I intend to eat healthy and nutritious foods	35.58	57.14	0.002
I expect to maintain a healthy body weight	55.77	65.71	0.141
I want to maintain a healthy body weight	68.27	72.82	0.473
I intend to maintain a healthy body weight	57.28	62.86	0.412
I think my teacher is physically active	49.51	57.14	0.270
I think that being physically active is important to my teacher	53.85	56.19	0.733
I think that my teacher eats healthy and nutritious foods	45.71	53.33	0.270
I think it is important to my teacher that I engage in physical activity every day	48.57	47.62	0.890
I think it is important to my teacher that I eat healthy and nutritious foods	50.00	50.48	0.945
I think it is important to my teacher that I maintain a healthy body weight	52.86	49.04	0.370
I am physically active	49.04	65.71	0.015
Physical activity is important to me	66.35	74.04	0.225
I eat healthy and nutritious foods	28.57	36.89	0.117

Notes: Proportions reported are "strongly agree".

follow-up to expect, want, and intend to be physically active; to intend to maintain a healthy body weight; to indicate physical activity is important to them; and to report eating healthy and nutritious foods. Conversely, boys were more likely at follow-up to expect, want, and intend to eat healthy and nutritious foods, and to report being physically active. While a number of other comparisons for boys and girls from pre to post were not significant, all but one comparison for each group trended upwards.

Similar results were found for summary measures. Intention to be physically active, eat healthy, maintain a healthy weight, descriptive norms for physical activity, as well as perception and value of personal health behaviors were all significantly higher at post-test (**Table 4**). For example, the average summary score for intention to be physically active increased from 4.2 to 4.5 (p < 0.000). Only injunctive norms did not have a significant increase (pre = 4.1 vs. post = 4.2, p < 0.183). All summary measures for girls were statistically higher after the intervention (**Table 5**). Half of the summary measures for boys (intention to be physically active, intention to eat healthy, perception and value of personal health behavior) increased significantly (**Table 6**). Levels of intention to maintain a healthy weight (p < 0.066), descriptive norms (p < 0.083) and injunctive norms (p < 0.617) for boys were the same or higher, but were not significant.

4. Discussion

This study sought to answer the following research questions: 1) What impact does an elementary teacher modeling goal-setting behavior related to healthy eating and physical activity have on students' behavioral intentions to eat healthy and be physically active?; 2) What impact does an elementary teacher modeling goal-setting behavior related to healthy eating and physical activity have on students' subjective norms related to these health-promoting behaviors?; and 3) What impact does an elementary teacher modeling goal-setting behavior related to healthy eating and physical activity have on students' perception and value of personal health behavior?

Teacher modeling of goal-setting behavior related to healthy eating and physical activity significantly increased behavioral intentions related to physical activity, healthy eating, and maintenance of a healthy body weight. This finding is particularly encouraging as it provides a strong association between behavioral intentions and actual physical activity and healthy eating among boys and girls [26]-[28]. One unexpected finding

Table 4. Pre- and post-test comparison by summary measure of health (n = 229).

	Pre	Post	p-value
Behavioral intent to be physically active	4.2	4.5	0.000
Behavioral intent to eat healthy	4.1	4.4	0.000
Behavioral intent to maintain a healthy body weight	4.4	4.6	0.001
Descriptive norms for health	4.2	4.4	0.000
Injunctive norms for health	4.1	4.2	0.183
Perception and value of personal health behavior	4.2	4.4	0.000

Notes: Intention to be physically active is the average Likert score for "I expect to be physically active", "I want to be physically active", and "I intend to be physically active". Intention to eat healthy is the average Likert score for "I expect to eat healthy and nutritious foods", "I want to eat healthy and nutritious foods", and "I intend to eat healthy and nutritious foods". Intention to maintain a healthy body weight is the average Likert score for "I expect to maintain a healthy body weight", "I want to maintain a healthy body weight", and "I intend to maintain a healthy body weight". The summary measure for descriptive norms is the average Likert score for "I think my teacher is physically active", "I think that being physically active is important to my teacher", and "I think that my teacher eats healthy and nutritious foods". The summary measure for injunctive norms is the average Likert score for "I think it is important to my teacher that I engage in physical activity every day", "I think it is important to my teacher that I eat healthy and nutritious foods", and "I think it is important to my teacher that I maintain a healthy body weight". Student perception and value of personal health behavior is the average Likert score for "I am physically active", "Physical activity is important to me", and "I eat healthy and nutritious meals".

Table 5. Pre- and post-test comparison by summary measure of health, girls (n = 124).

	Pre	Post	p-value
Behavioral intent to be physically active	4.2	4.5	0.000
Behavioral intent to eat healthy	4.2	4.4	0.007
Behavioral intent to maintain a healthy body weight	4.5	4.6	0.001
Descriptive norms for health	4.3	4.5	0.000
Injunctive norms for health	4.1	4.3	0.008
Perception and value of personal health behavior	4.2	4.4	0.000

Notes: Intention to be physically active is the average Likert score for "I expect to be physically active", "I want to be physically active", and "I intend to be physically active". Intention to eat healthy is the average Likert score for "I expect to eat healthy and nutritious foods", "I want to eat healthy and nutritious foods", and "I intend to eat healthy and nutritious foods". Intention to maintain a healthy body weight is the average Likert score for "I expect to maintain a healthy body weight", "I want to maintain a healthy body weight", and "I intend to maintain a healthy body weight". The summary measure for descriptive norms is the average Likert score for "I think my teacher is physically active", "I think that being physically active is important to my teacher", and "I think that my teacher eats healthy and nutritious foods". The summary measure for injunctive norms is the average Likert score for "I think it is important to my teacher that I engage in physical activity every day", "I think it is important to my teacher that I eat healthy and nutritious foods", and "I think it is important to my teacher that I maintain a healthy body weight". Student perception and value of personal health behavior is the average Likert score for "I am physically active", "Physical activity is important to me", and "I eat healthy and nutritious meals".

Table 6. Pre- and post-test comparison by summary measure of health, boys (n = 105).

	Pre	Post	p-value
Behavioral intent to be physically active	4.3	4.5	0.009
Behavioral intent to eat healthy	4.1	4.4	0.000
Behavioral intent to maintain a healthy body weight	4.4	4.6	0.066
Descriptive norms for health	4.2	4.3	0.083
Injunctive norms for health	4.2	4.2	0.617
Perception and value of personal health behavior	4.2	4.4	0.001

Notes: Intention to be physically active is the average Likert score for "I expect to be physically active", "I want to be physically active", and "I intend to be physically active". Intention to eat healthy is the average Likert score for "I expect to eat healthy and nutritious foods", "I want to eat healthy and nutritious foods", and "I intend to eat healthy and nutritious foods". Intention to maintain a healthy body weight is the average Likert score for "I expect to maintain a healthy body weight", "I want to maintain a healthy body weight", and "I intend to maintain a healthy body weight". The summary measure for descriptive norms is the average Likert score for "I think my teacher is physically active", "I think that being physically active is important to my teacher", and "I think that my teacher eats healthy and nutritious foods". The summary measure for injunctive norms is the average Likert score for "I think it is important to my teacher that I engage in physical activity every day", "I think it is important to my teacher that I eat healthy and nutritious foods", and "I think it is important to my teacher that I maintain a healthy body weight". Student perception and value of personal health behavior is the average Likert score for "I am physically active", "Physical activity is important to me", and "I eat healthy and nutritious meals".

from this particular research question relates to a difference in behavioral intentions between girls and boys. Girls reported significantly higher intentions to be physically active compared to boys in the current study. This is promising as both middle and high school-aged females report engaging in significantly less physical activity than their male peers [29]. The current study intervention appears to impact girls' behavioral intent related to physical activity most appropriately. Despite having similar reports at pre-test, girls also reported significantly higher intentions to maintain a healthy body weight compared to boys in the current study. The reason for this difference is unknown yet may relate to dynamics between teachers' sex and students' sex. For example, most of the teachers in this pilot study were female and girls may be more responsive to a female teacher's report of her own health behavior. With only three male teacher participants, exploring such a hypothesis was beyond the scope of the current study, yet could be the focus of a future, larger study of this nature. The current study did not measure students' perceptions of their own weight status, but it is plausible that teachers' reports of their own health-related behaviors were more influential among girls for this reason. It is noted that middle school female students nationally are more likely to describe themselves as slightly or very overweight and report trying to lose weight at a significantly higher rate than male students despite boys being slightly more obese than girls nationally (18.6% vs. 15.0%) [29] [30]. Finally, boys' intentions to eat healthy were significantly different at post-test. The current study intervention impacted boys' behavioral intent related to healthy eating most appropriately as female students consume more fruits and vegetables, and less soda or pop than their male counterparts [31]. Summary measures clearly demonstrate the significant and positive impact the current intervention had on students' behavioral intentions related to physical activity, healthy eating, and maintenance of a healthy body weight.

Results of the impact teacher modeling of goal-setting behavior related to healthy eating and physical activity had on subjective norms were mixed. The intervention significantly impacted the descriptive norm, yet did not significantly impact the injunctive norm. Teachers sharing physical activity and healthy eating goals with students increased students' perception of the teacher's physical activity and healthy eating as well as their belief that each of these health-promoting behaviors is important to the teacher. However, teacher modeling did not significantly communicate to students that the teacher felt it important for students to be physically active, eat healthy, and maintain a healthy body weight. It may be that modeling alone is insufficient to significantly impact injunctive norms. It is also possible that students in this study felt valued and accepted unconditionally by teachers, thus buffering the potential impact of modeling on injunctive norms. It is noted that teacher participants were specifically instructed not to directly promote health behaviors to students. It is possible that when combined with classroom health promotion and education efforts, teacher modeling may significantly influence injunctive norms.

Teacher modeling of goal-setting behavior related to healthy eating and physical activity significantly increased student perception and value of personal health behavior. This finding is encouraging in that teacher modeling alone significantly impacted the value students place on physical activity. Teachers are powerful referents in the eyes of young students and when a teacher values a particular health-related behavior, that value can be adopted by students. While the intervention increased perceptions and values related to health behaviors in a positive direction for both girls and boys, only girls showed significant changes on the *Physical activity is important to me* and *I eat healthy and nutritious foods* items. Conversely, only boys showed significant changes on the *I am physically active* item.

This study and its findings are significant because teacher participants were able to significantly and positively impact students' behavioral intent, subjective norms, and perception and value of personal health behaviors amongst students without spending additional time on formal health promotion and education instruction. This is not to say that formal health promotion and education instruction should not occur in elementary classrooms. On the contrary, the authors of this study are adamant supporters of comprehensive pre K-12 school health education and advocate for Coordinated School Health, including increased health education instructional time at the elementary school level. Indeed, this intervention did not address the development of content knowledge or skills related to healthy eating or physical activity that students clearly need to adopt and maintain important health behaviors. Yet with minimal financial cost, minimal classroom time, a short intervention period, and no instructional time or materials, teacher role-modeling of health-related goal-setting had a positive impact on students.

These study results have health promotion implications for school policies and practices. *Faculty and staff health promotion*, commonly known as *employee wellness programs* outside of school settings, is an important component of Coordinated School Health [32]. *Faculty and staff health promotion* has been shown to be cost-effective and associated with reduced staff absenteeism [33], improved teacher morale [34], increased physical activity, weight loss, lowered blood pressure, and higher levels of general well-being [35]. While immunizations and flu vaccines are common inclusions in school-based employee wellness programs, less than 50% of school districts in the US provide physical activity programs for faculty and staff [36]. Policies designed to increase support for, and participation in, school-based faculty and staff physical activity health promotion are both necessary and feasible given the expertise of school district personnel and the health-related resources and facilities found in most school buildings [36]. Health promotion and education practice should be more consistent with theoretical constructs emphasizing the influence of modeling and subjective norms. For example, appropriately sharing the details of faculty and staff health promotion programs, their objectives, and subsequent outcomes with students may improve student health outcomes as well. School health educators may borrow a page form literacy educators who have encouraged teachers to display or discuss the current book or books they are reading in an effort to promote literacy and encourage students to read [37]. Such practices communicate to students that adults read, reading is a normal behavior, and reading is a behavior that the people students look up to enjoy. A similar approach with health-promoting behaviors should be encouraged by policy makers and school administrators. Allowing students to see behind the curtain so to speak, and realize the health-promotion efforts that faculty and staff are engaged in may impact their own behavioral intentions, subjective norms, and perceptions and values of personal health behaviors.

The findings from this study should be interpreted in the context of its limitations. First, study measures may have been difficult for respondents to differentiate. For example, the difference among *want*, *expect*, and *intend* to engage in a health related behavior may have caused some respondents to feel confusion about the questions, provided they each seem similar. This potential limitation is not limited to this study alone, but using recommended analysis methods of creating composite variables to represent prominent theoretical constructs may have minimized the impact [25]. Second, data for this study came from students' self-report, which may be influenced by social desirability to appear conscientious about one's health. It is plausible that some students at post-test remembered their pre-test responses and then intentionally reported higher values at post-test. The principal investigator clearly communicated to the respondents at the administration of both the pre- and post-test that all responses would remain confidential and disassociated from their names with the use of unique identifiers. Lastly, the effects of the brief intervention presented here are measured using pre- and post-test comparisons, without a control group. It is possible that other school-wide initiatives related to physical activity and healthy eating could have also contributed to higher post-test scores. Future research efforts using this brief intervention may benefit from a more rigorous methodology involving randomization of classrooms and a control group.

5. Conclusion

This study applied research-based best practices for promoting healthy eating and physical activity in schools as outlined by the Centers for Disease Control and Prevention. Teacher role modeling and sharing of goal setting behaviors related to healthy eating and physical activity had significant positive effects on students' behavioral intentions related to these important behaviors. Ideally schools will incentivize and encourage faculty and staff to engage in a variety of health behaviors to both benefit their own health and set an example for those they teach. A combination of role modeling, deliberately communicating care and concern for students' health behaviors, and providing quality formal classroom health instruction, helps teachers send a clear and consistent health-promoting message to students.

Acknowledgements

This study was funded by Brigham Young University through a Mentoring Environment Grant.

Human Subjects Approval Statement

All procedures were approved by the Brigham Young University Institutional Review Board and the Alpine School District Director of Research and Evaluation. Ethical guidelines were strictly followed including participant consent, parental consent, and child assent in English and Spanish.

References

[1] Lichtenstein, A.H., Appel, L.J., Brands, M., Carnethon, M., Daniels, S., Franch, H.A., *et al.* (2006) Diet and Lifestyle Recommendations Revisions 2006: A Scientific Statement from the American Heart Association Nutrition Committee. *Circulation*, **114**, 82-96. http://dx.doi.org/10.1161/CIRCULATIONAHA.106.176158

[2] US Department of Agriculture, Dietary Guidelines Advisory Committee (2010) Report of the Dietary Guidelines Advisory Committee on the Dietary guidelines for Americans, 2010, to the Secretary of Agriculture and the Secretary of Health and Human Services. US Department of Agriculture, Agriculture Research Service, Washington DC.

[3] US Department of Health and Human Services, Physical Activity Guidelines Advisory Committee (2008) Physical Activity Guidelines Advisory Committee Report, 2008. US Department of Health and Human Services, Washington DC.

[4] Ogden, C.L., Carroll, M.D., Curtin, L.R., Lamb, M.M. and Flegal, K.M. (2010) Prevalence of High Body Mass Index in U.S. Children and Adolescents, 2007-2008. *Journal of the American Medical Association*, **303**, 242-249. http://dx.doi.org/10.1001/jama.2009.2012

[5] Daniels, S., Arnett, D., Eckel, R., Gidding, S., Hayman, L., Kumanyika, S., *et al.* (2005) Overweight in Children and Adolescents: Pathophysiology, Consequences, Prevention, and Treatment. *Circulation*, **111**, 1999-2012. http://dx.doi.org/10.1161/01.CIR.0000161369.71722.10

[6] Dietz, W.H. (2004) Overweight in Childhood and Adolescence. *The New England Journal of Medicine*, **350**, 855-857. http://dx.doi.org/10.1056/NEJMp048008

[7] Institute of Medicine (2004) Preventing Childhood Obesity: Health in the Balance. The National Academies Press, Washington DC.

[8] National Center for Education Statistics (2005) Digest of Education Statistics: 2004. National Center for Education Statistics, Washington DC. http://nces.ed.gov/programs/digest/d04/

[9] Centers for Disease Control and Prevention (2011) School Health Guidelines to Promote Healthy Eating and Physical Activity. Morbidity and Mortality Weekly Report, 60(No. RR-5).

[10] Wechsler, H., Devereaux, R.S., Davis, M. and Collins, J. (2000) Using the School Environment to Promote Physical Activity and Healthy Eating. *Preventative Medicine*, **31**, S121-S137. http://dx.doi.org/10.1006/pmed.2000.0649

[11] Bandura, A. (1977) Social Learning Theory. Prentice Hall, Englewood Cliffs, NJ.

[12] Bandura, A. (1971) Social Learning Theory. General Learning Press, New York.

[13] Ajzen, I. and Fishbein, M. (1980) Understanding Attitudes and Predicting Social Behavior. Prentice Hall, Englewood Cliffs, NJ.

[14] Cialdini, R.B., Kallgren, C.A. and Reno, R.R. (1991) A Focus Theory of Normative Conduct: A Theoretical Refinement and Reevaluation of the Role of Norms in Human Behavior. In: Berkowitz, L., Ed., *Advances in Experimental Social Psychology*, Academic Press, San Diego, Vol. 24, 201-234.

[15] Cialdini, R.B. (2007) Descriptive Social Norms as Underappreciated Sources of Social Control. *Psychometrika*, **72**, 263-268. http://dx.doi.org/10.1007/s11336-006-1560-6

[16] Cialdini, R.B., Reno, R.R. and Kallgren, C.A. (1990) A Focus Theory of Normative Conduct: Recycling the Concept of Norms to Reduce Littering in Public Places. *Journal of Personality and Social Psychology*, **58**, 1015-1026. http://dx.doi.org/10.1037/0022-3514.58.6.1015

[17] Schultz, P.W., Nolan, J.M., Cialdini, R.B., Goldstein, N.J. and Griskevicius, V. (2007) The Constructive, Destructive, and Reconstructive Power of Social Norms. *Psychological Science*, **18**, 429-434. http://dx.doi.org/10.1111/j.1467-9280.2007.01917.x

[18] Rivis, A. and Sheeran, P. (2003) Descriptive Norms as an Additional Predictor in the Theory of Planned Behaviour: A Meta-Analysis. *Current Psychology*, **22**, 218-233. http://dx.doi.org/10.1007/s12144-003-1018-2

[19] Kubik, M. Leslie, A., Hannan, P., Story, M. and Perry, C. (2002) Food-Related Beliefs, Eating Behavior, and Classroom Food Practices of Middle School Teachers. *Journal of School Health*, **72**, 339-345. http://dx.doi.org/10.1111/j.1746-1561.2002.tb07921.x

[20] Bakhotmah, B. (2012) Teachers Dietary Practices During the School Day in Jeddah, Western Saudi Arabia. *Food and Nutritional Sciences*, **3**, 1553-1560. http://dx.doi.org/10.4236/fns.2012.311203

[21] Aracan, C., Hannan, P., Himes, J., Fulkerson, J., Rock, B., Smyth, M. and Story, M. (2013) Intervention Effects on Kindergarten and First-Grade Teachers' Classroom Food Practices and Food-Related Beliefs in American Indian Reservation Schools. *Journal of the Academy of Nutrition and Dietetics*, **113**, 1076-1083. http://dx.doi.org/10.1016/j.jand.2013.04.019

[22] Power, T.G., Bindler, R.C., Goetz, S. and Daratha, K.B. (2010) Obesity Prevention in Early Adolescence: Student, Parent, and Teacher Views. *Journal of School Health*, **80**, 13-19. http://dx.doi.org/10.1111/j.1746-1561.2009.00461.x

[23] Hendy, H.M. and Raudenbush, B. (2000) Effectiveness of Teacher Modeling to Encourage Food Acceptance in Pre-school Children. *Appetite*, **34**, 61-76. http://dx.doi.org/10.1006/appe.1999.0286

[24] Rossiter, M., Glanville, T., Taylor, J. and Blum, I. (2007) School Food Practices of Prospective Teachers. *Journal of School Health*, **77**, 694-700. http://dx.doi.org/10.1111/j.1746-1561.2007.00253.x

[25] Francis, J.J., Eccles, M.P., Johnston, M., Walker, A., Grimshaw, J., Foy, R., *et al.* (2004) Constructing Questionnaires Based on the Theory of Planned Behaviour: A Manual for Health Services Researchers. Centre for Health Services Research, University of Newcastle, Newcastle upon Tyne, UK.
http://openaccess.city.ac.uk/1735/1/TPB%20Manual%20FINAL%20May2004.pdf

[26] Blanchard, C.M., Kupperman, J., Sparling, P.B., Nehl, E., Rhodes, R.E., Courneya, K.S. and Baker, F. (2009) Do Ethnicity and Gender Matter When Using the Theory of Planned Behavior to Understand Fruit and Vegetable Consumption? *Appetite*, **52**, 15-20. http://dx.doi.org/10.1016/j.appet.2008.07.001

[27] Hagger, M.S., Chatzisarantis, N.L.D. and Biddle, S.J.H. (2002) The Influence of Autonomous and Controlling Motives on Physical Activity Intentions Within the Theory of Planned Behaviour. *British Journal of Health Psychology*, **7**, 283-298. http://dx.doi.org/10.1348/135910702760213689

[28] Lien, N., Lytle, L.A. and Komro, K. (2002) Applying Theory of Planned Behavior to Fruit and Vegetable Consumption of Young Adolescents. *American Journal of Health Promotion*, **16**, 189-197.
http://dx.doi.org/10.4278/0890-1171-16.4.189

[29] Centers for Disease Control and Prevention (2013) Youth Risk Behavior Survey. www.cdc.gov/yrbs

[30] Ogden, C.L., Carroll, M.D., Kit, B.K. and Flegal, K.M. (2012) Prevalence of Obesity in the United States, 2009-2010. NCHS Data Brief, No. 82. National Center for Health Statistics, Hyattsville, MD.
http://www.cdc.gov/nchs/data/databriefs/db82.pdf

[31] Centers for Disease Control and Prevention (2011) Youth Risk Behavior Survey. www.cdc.gov/yrbs

[32] Allegrante, J.P. (1998) School-Site Health Promotion for Faculty and Staff: A Key Component of the Coordinated School Health Program. *Journal of School Health*, **68**, 190-195. http://dx.doi.org/10.1111/j.1746-1561.1998.tb01299.x

[33] Aldana, S.G., Merrill, R.M., Price, K., Hardy, A. and Hager, R. (2005) Financial Impact of a Comprehensive Multisite Workplace Health Promotion Program. *Preventive Medicine*, **40**, 131-137.
http://dx.doi.org/10.1016/j.ypmed.2004.05.008

[34] Allegrante, J.P. and Michela, J. (1990) Impact of a School-Based Workplace Health Promotion Program on Morale of Inner-City Teachers. *Journal of School Health*, **60**, 25-28. http://dx.doi.org/10.1111/j.1746-1561.1990.tb04772.x

[35] Blair, S.N., Collingwood, T.R., Reynolds, R., Smith, M., Hagan, D. and Sterling, C.L. (1984) Health Promotion for Educators: Impact on Health Behaviors, Satisfaction, and General Well-Being. *American Journal of Public Health*, **74**, 147-149. http://dx.doi.org/10.2105/AJPH.74.2.147

[36] Centers for Disease Control and Prevention (2013) Results from the School Health Policies and Practices Study, 2012. US Department of Health and Human Services, Atlanta, GA. http://www.cdc.gov/HealthyYouth/shpps/index.htm

[37] Campbell, R. (1989) The Teacher as a Role Model during Sustained Silent Reading (SSR). *Literacy*, **23**, 179-183.
http://dx.doi.org/10.1111/j.1467-9345.1989.tb00364.x

17

Personality Styles, Psychological Adjustment and Gender Differences in Parents of Children with Congenital Disabilities

Rosa M. Limiñana-Gras[1,2], María del Pilar Sánchez-López[3,4], María Teresa Calvo-Llena[2], Francisco Javier Corbalán[2]

[1]Research Group Personality and Health: A Intercultural and Gender Perspective, Murcia, Spain
[2]Universidad de Murcia, Murcia, Spain
[3]Universidad Complutense de Madrid, Madrid, Spain
[4]Red Hygeia (Health & Gender International Alliance), Madrid, Spain
Email: liminana@um.es

Abstract

The present study analyzes the psychological adaptation of parents with children having congenital disabilities. The study included 83 men and 96 women, who were parents of children with severe spina bifida, cerebral palsy, cleft lip and cleft palate. The Millon Index of Personality Styles was used to identify the most distinctive personality styles of parents caring for a child with a chronic disability and parental psychological adjustment. We also investigated if personality profiles differ by gender, and educational and socioeconomic level. The personality styles identified may serve as indicators of the way parents adapt to the child with a congenital disability. The results also suggest that a child's disability has a differential impact on men and women. Gender issues are evaluated, as well as any repercussions these may have on women.

Keywords

Personality Styles, Congenital Disability, Parental Psychological Adjustment, Gender Differences

1. Introduction

The physical and psychological health of parents with children suffering from congenital malformations or diseases has become a topic of increasing interest. A review of the literature shows that most studies focus on the risks and vulnerabilities most frequently observed in this group [1]-[3], and particularly among mothers since they are the main caregivers [4] [5]. Most studies describe the presence of anxiety, stress, economic problems and family conflicts [6]-[10].

Practically every study confirms that the birth of a child with a chronic disease or disability involves painful long-term experiences and that parents are at increased risk of developing psychosocial problems [11]-[15].

Other studies have investigated the process of adaptation to chronic stress induced by caring for a child with a disability [16]-[19]. They report that the management or coping strategies used, continuously change over time, which increases the complexity of measuring such adaptation processes.

In the context of caring for disabled children, personality variables also have been identified as powerful factors that could explain individual differences in how parents face chronic stress. Most of these studies have identified personality traits using factorial models [5] [20]-[22].

Less frequent in this context are studies in which personality has been regarded as a mediating variable or as a predictor of coping [23]-[25].

The present study used Millon's Personality Model [26]-[28] to investigate and analyze the process of adaptation to chronic stress. This model allows us to use relatively stable variables, while still showing how parents cope with the situation and adapt to the child's disability. In the Millon Index of Personality Styles (MIPS), the concept of style is understood from an evolutionary perspective, whereby personality is organized into stable sets of adaptive functioning. This instrument has some advantages over other personality questionnaires because it has a dynamic perspective of human behavior, which enables the evaluation of styles rather than fixed or static personality traits. It focuses on the normal personality and includes three main areas: Motivating Styles, with a theoretical basis that derives from ecological and evolutionary theories; Thinking Styles, that are based on evolutionary perspectives, and the contributions of Jung and Myers; and Behaving Styles, are influenced by Sullivan, Leary, and the Five Factors Model.

Thus, a personality style is regarded as a set of traits derived from biological tendencies and experiential learning that characterizes a relatively stable way of behaving. The personality styles have proved more susceptible to environmental changes than traditional traits (more stable and definitive), and sufficiently sensitive to evaluate the adaptive functioning with more consistency and stability than other variables more situationally determined [26]. Models that have mainly focused on health have identified traits such as optimism, self-esteem, parental competence, resilience, the rewards and satisfaction of caring for the child, and problem-resolution skills as personality resources that have a positive effect on the stress management involved in caring for a child with disabilities [13] [29]-[31]. However, these are isolated variables that do not include all the personality dimensions that modulate the behavior of the individual.

In contrast to factorial models or multi-trait concepts, the Millon model involves a multidimensional approach to normal personality, and is based on integrating bio-psychosocial, evolutionary, and ecological viewpoints. Millon's concept of normal personality and his comprehensive approach to the person as a whole means that the MIPS (MIPS-Millon) [27] [28] includes a set of variables that are sufficiently broad to cover the range of behaviors found in parental adaptation to disability. On the other hand, the variables are simple enough to provide clear and accurate information that may contribute to future research and intervention. Another relevant point is that they provide a non-dysfunctional personality model that helps to identify parents' psychological resources.

The MIPS also includes a Clinical Index [27] that measures the degree to which a person adapts to your environment, compared to their reference group. Other studies incorporated the Clinical Index as an overall measure or indicator of psychological adjustment [24] [32], showing their relationship to psychological health in the health context [25] [33], and confirming the utility of this measure as an indicator of more adaptation to the environment and therefore as indicator of psychological adjustment.

Within the framework of this model, we studied the medium- and long-term impact on parental psychological organization and functioning, of having a child with a disability. The study aims were as follows: To identify stable adaptive functioning styles in these mothers and fathers, and their differences with normative population; to evaluate parental psychological adjustment and adaptability by using the Clinical Index; and to analyze the modulating effect of gender, educational and the socioeconomic level, on parent's personality styles and psychological adjustment.

The study included parents of children with severe spina bifida or Myelomeningocele (MM), cerebral palsy, and cleft lip and cleft palate. MM is the most common and severe form of spina bifida and the most common of the neural tube defects, a congenital medical condition in which the neural tube fails to close completely during early gestation, and is associated with sensory, motor and cognitive impairments [34]. Cerebral palsy is a group of permanent neurological disorders of the development of movement and posture that are caused by to no progressive disturbances that occurred in the development in fetal or infant brain. The motor disorders of cerebral palsy are often accompanied by disturbances of sensation, perception, cognition, communication, and behavior, epilepsy, and secondary musculoskeletal problems [35]. Cleft lip or cleft palate is an embryonic syndrome which accounts for 65% of all the congenital malformations of the head and the neck [36]. Cleft lip and cleft palate in newborns have implications for feeding, the child's psychosocial adjustment and growth is affected by factors including reactions to surgeries, and parents needed support beyond information about feeding after birth.

Taking into account the literature and the study aims, we formed three hypotheses: firstly, parents of children with disabilities will present personality styles significantly different from the normative population revealing a differential adaptive functioning; secondly, since mothers normally carry the main workload of caring for the child, mothers in this group will show a psychological adjustment (Clinical Index) significantly lower than women in the normative population, and also lower than the parents in this group; thirdly, the gender, the educational and the socioeconomic level of the parents, will moderate the differences observed in personality styles and psychological adjustment.

2. Method

2.1. Participants

The study included 83 men (46.4%) and 96 women (53.6%), both of Spanish nationality, who were parents of children with severe spina bifida (MM), cerebral palsy, and cleft lip and cleft palate. Of these, 87.2% (78 couples) belong to the same family, that is, they are fathers and mothers of the same child; and 12.8% not belonging to the same family, that is, only one parent has participated (5 fathers and 18 mothers). The age of the parents ranged from 22 years to 72 years M = 39.81, SD = 8.27). There were no statistically significant differences between the age of fathers and mothers [t (177) = 1.43; $p < 0.15$].

In total, 88.8% of the participants were married, 2.8% were separated or divorced, 1.1% were widows or widowers, and approximately 7.3% were single. The educational level was evenly distributed in the sample (35.2% had completed primary education, 34.6% secondary education, and 30.2% higher education). A significantly greater percentage of participants were working at the time of the study (74.9%); 18.2% were housewives, 3.4% were unemployed, and the remaining 2.8% were retired. Around 57% of participants had a low to medium socioeconomic level, whereas 43% had a medium to high level.

The mean age of the children was 8.04 (SD = 7.88), 12.3% are one year old or younger, 30.2% (1 thru 4) 36.3% (4 thru 12) and 21.2% are o are twelve year old or greater (to 28) ranging from 4 months to 28 years. Of these, 67 (66.3%) were diagnosed with severe spina bifida (myelomeningocele), 20 (19.8%) with cleft lip and cleft palate, and 14 (13.9%) with cerebral palsy. As an indicator of the severity of the child's disability, functional limitation was calculated and expressed in percentages using Spanish instruments that followed the WHO international guidelines [37] [38]. The mean percentage in our study group was 52.50 (SD = 21.05) ranging from 20% to 91%. The mean percentage in group diagnosed with myelomeningocele was 53.91 (SD = 20.65), in group diagnosed with cleft palate 33.84 (SD = 19.42), and in group diagnosed with cerebral palsy 58.31 (SD = 19.42).

2.2. Instruments

Questionnaire on socio-demographic data and the child's disease:

The parents completed a socio-demographic and clinical questionnaire, designed for this study. The first questionnaire collected basic demographic data of participants as the age, number of children, sex, marital status, place of residence, educational level, socioeconomic status and employment status or occupation. Socioeconomic status was measured as a combination of economic status, education and employment status or occupation.

The secondly collected child's clinical data: the child's diagnosis and severity of the disability; number of surgeries and hospitalizations; physical and neurological complications such as phonatory alterations, alterations of deglutition, paralysis, poor renal function, Arnold Chiari II malformation, scoliosis, back pain, and worsening bowel and/or bladder function, etc.; as well other difficulties, e.g. executive functions, selective attention or focused attention.

Millon Index of Personality Styles (MIPS):

This instrument adapted and validated for use in the Spanish population by Sánchez-López, Díaz, and Aparicio [39], assesses the normal personality. The MIPS [27] [28] provides a measure of personality styles organized according to tree key dimensions: Motivating styles, Thinking styles, and Behaving styles. It includes 24 scales, plus three validity control indexes. The scales are organized in bipolarities, 12 pairs of scales that are opposites from a theoretical viewpoint, although not in the psychometric sense, since each scale was designed in such a way that it could be measured independently from its opposite. First, three pairs of scales in the Motivating styles dimension: Pleasure/Enhancing and Pain/Avoiding, Actively Modifying and Passively Accommodating, Self-Indulging and Other Nurturing. Secondly, four pairs of scales in the Thinking Styles dimension: Externally Focused and Internally Focused, Realistic/Sensing and Imaginative/Intuiting, Thought-Guided and Feeling-Guided, Conservation-Seeking and Innovation-Seeking. And finally, five pairs of scales in the Behaving styles dimension: Asocial/withdrawing and Gregarious/outgoing, Anxious/hesitating and Confident/asserting, Unconventional/dissenting and Dutiful/conforming, Submissive/yielding and Dominant/controlling, Dissatisfied/complaining and Cooperative/agreeing.

The MIPS also incorporates an adjustment index (Clinical Index-Millon) [27] to measure the degree to which a person adapts to your environment, compared to their reference group. This index is obtained by weighting the scores on the scales "Pleasure/Enhancing and Pain/Avoiding" (Motivating styles) and the five pairs of scales in the Behaving styles dimension. This index was developed from theoretical and empirical foundations. The construct validity has been proven through its relationship with measures of psychological well-being or mental health [40] [24] [33] [39]. The internal consistency of the scale in the Spanish population is satisfactory (0.72), and the mean for all scales was 0.73 in the study sample. Details on the psychometric properties of the MIPS (*i.e.* internal consistency, temporal stability, and convergent and discriminant validity) in the Spanish population [39] and the American population [27] [28] have been previously published.

2.3. Procedure

The selection of participants was performed with the collaboration of Spanish parent associations of children with spina bifida, cerebral palsy, cleft lip and palate. The selection criterion used to recruit participants was having a child with a chronic physical illness.

The tests were administered by the clinical psychologist leading the study. The study protocol was approved by the Bioethics Committee of the University of Murcia and all participants gave their informed consent after the purpose of the research was explained and participation was voluntary. The anonymity of the data was also ensured. Parent associations provided space in their own centres, sent out the invitations by post, and scheduled the interviews and test administration sessions with both parents, who filled in the tests independently.

2.4. Data Analysis

Data were analyzed using the statistical software package SPSS 19.0 for Windows. Pearson's correlation coefficient was used to analyze the linear relationship between the psychological and demographic variables. Differences between the sample mean and the normative mean were analyzed using the Student t-test, (95% confidence interval) and the mean scores for the Spanish population were used as the test value [27] (Spanish adaptation). The Spanish normative sample was made up of 1184 adults, consisting of 643 women (54.3%) and 541 men (45.7%), with a mean age of 37.60 years. The Spanish adaptation of the Millon test provides basic statistics for the total adult normative population used in the study, and for women and men; thus, the study sample can be compared to the normative group according to gender. The effect sizes were calculated using Cohen's d based on sample size (Hedges Adjustment) to control for size differences in the 2 study groups.

A Multiple Analysis of Covariance (MANOVA) was performed to investigate the moderating effect of gender and sociodemographic variables on the differences in personality styles and psychological adjustment. We have followed a process of statistical modeling in which as a first step we tested the significance of the more complete model. The independent variables or factors to control for the differences between groups were gender, educational level and socioeconomic level. The covariates were age (age of parents and child) and the severity of the disability. However we have found no relationship between these covariates and dependent variables, so we have chosen not to include it. Before performing the MANOVA, normality and homogeneity of variance were verified (Box Test, Levene's test) as well as the correlation between the dependent variables (Bartlett's test of sphericity). The indexes for the effect size were also calculated using Partial Eta Squared (η^2), which indicates the proportion of variance explained by each variation source [41].

3. Results

Analysis of the MIPS indexes indicates that, in general, the parents did not attempt to give either a very positive image (*M* score IP = 3.3; *SD* = 2.1) or a very negative image of themselves (*M* score IN = 2.7; *SD* = 2.2). Furthermore, the mean value obtained for Consistency (*M* score C = 3.5; *SD* = 1.1), and the analysis of minimum values (range = 2 - 5), confirmed that the parents were consistent in their responses. There no statistically significant correlations were between the personality scales and the age of parents and children.

Table 1 shows the means, standard deviations, and the results of the Student t-test and Cohen's d on the MIPS scales and the Clinical Index for men and women (Hypothesis 1 and 2). The results show statistically significant differences in the personality styles of the men and women of our sample compared to the normative group.

Table 1. Means, standards deviations, Student t and effect sizes (d) in men and women on the MIPS scales.

MIPS scales	MIPS *Personality Styles* (N = 179)							
	Men (n = 83)				Women (n = 96)			
	M (SD)	*t*(82)	*p*	*d*	*M (SD)*	*t*(95)	*p*	*d*
Motivating Styles								
1A. Pleasure-Enhancing	25.95 (6.33)	3.27	0.002	0.33 (mod.)	22.65 (7.32)	−0.57	0.572	
1B. Pain-Avoiding	12.47 (8.43)	−5.21	0.000	−0.49 (mod.)	18.54 (10.52)	−0.15	0.883	
2A. Actively Modifying	26.52 (8.66)	−0.71	0.482		24.91 (8.41)	−1.19	0.236	
2B. Passively Accommodating	20.75 (8.98)	−1.60	0.115		23.84 (8.88)	1.17	0.243	
3A. Self-Indulging	17.54 (7.30)	−4.28	0.000	−0.46 (mod.)	14.51 (5.90)	−4.28***	0.000	−0.34 (mod.)
3B. Other Nurturing	29.20 (8.15)	1.45	0.152		34.15 (6.54)	3.93***	0.000	0.35 (mod.)
Thinking Styles								
4A. Externally Focused	24.76 (8.58)	1.77	0.080		23.64 (8.19)	−1.36	0.178	
4B. Internally Focused	10.42 (6.97)	−3.66	0.000	−0.39 (mod.)	11.61 (6.99)	0.26	0.796	
5A. Realistic/Sensing	21.45 (5.67)	2.76	0.007	0.29 (low)	20.98 (5.09)	2.46*	0.016	0.22 (low)
5B. Imaginative/Intuiting	15.33 (6.65)	−5.12	0.000	−0.45 (mod.)	17.15 (6.90)	−2.19*	0.031	−0.19 (low)
6A. Thought-Guided	22.25 (8.13)	−0.88	0.380		14.67 (8.06)	−3.76***	0.000	−0.38 (mod.)
6B. Feeling-Guided	24.02 (7.97)	−2.05	0.043	−0.21 (low)	30.59 (7.99)	1.78	0.078	
7A. Conservation-Seeking	36.42 (10.69)	0.85	0.400		34.98 (9.92)	−1.42	0.158	
7B. Innovation-Seeking	20.80 (7.72)	−3.89	0.000	−0.37 (mod.)	20.65 (8.25)	−2.36*	0.021	−0.22 (low)
Behaving Styles								
8A. Asocial/withdrawing	19.84 (8.70)	1.93	0.057	−0.20 (low)	19.82 (8.11)	0.31	0.761	
8B. Gregarious/outgoing	31.19 (12.19)	0.33	0.742		26.05 (9.68)	−3.37***	0.001	−0.32 (mod.)
9A. Anxious/hesitating	14.31 (8.83)	−4.39	0.000	−0.42 (mod.)	19.81 (10.44)	0.97	0.335	
9B. Confident/asserting	34.81 (11.36)	1.42	0.160		26.34 (8.96)	−4.01***	0.000	−0.35 (mod.)
10A. Unconventional/dissenting	17.67 (8.28)	−5.33	0.000	−0.57 (high)	17.18 (6.97)	−3.34***	0.001	−0.27 (low)
10B. Dutiful/conforming	40.99 (9.08)	1.05	0.296		40.09 (8.58)	0.95	0.343	
11A. Submissive/yielding	13.76 (6.51)	−3.92	0.000	−3.36 (mod.)	17.03 (8.00)	0.17	0.863	
11B. Dominant/controlling	24.06 (8.19)	−0.70	0.486		19.06 (−2.39)	−3.68***	0.000	−0.32 (mod.)
12A. Dissatisfed/complaining	18.35 (8.75)	−6.00	0.000	−0.63 (high)	8.70 (9.59)	−3.92***	0.000	−0.39 (mod.)
12B. Cooperative/agreeing	36.11 (9.05)	2.78	0.007	0.33 (mod.)	41.45 (8.18)	4.00***	0.000	0.36 (mod.)
Iaj.t. Clinical Index	51.50 (12.30)	0.85	0.339		43.45 (13.45)	−4.56***	0.000	−0.59 (high)

*p < 0.05; **p < 0.01; ***p < 0.001.

There were statistically significant differences between the fathers and the men from the normative population on 14 scales. According to the MIPS guidelines, statistically significant differences in a given bipolarity enhance the meaning of the scales regarding personality traits. Thus, the statistically significant differences in 3 bipolarities (Pleasure/Enhancing and Pain/Avoiding, Realistic/Sensing and Imaginative/Intuiting, Dissatisfied/complaining and Cooperative/agreeing), indicate that the personality style of the fathers in our sample is more motivated towards finding pleasure and enhancing in their lives (pleasure/enhancing), more oriented towards concrete and observable information (sensation), as well as more agreeableness in interpersonal relationships.

There were statistically significant differences between the mothers and the women from the normative population on 12 scales. Statistically significant differences in 3 bipolarities (Self-Indulging and Other Nurturing, Realistic/Sensing and Imaginative/Intuiting, Dissatisfied/complaining and Cooperative/agreeing) suggest that the mothers of the sample favor a style which is strongly protective, oriented to sensation (concrete and observable information) and more agreeable and acquiescent. Finally, the Clinical Index indicated a significantly lower level of psychological adjustment in the mothers' sample than in the normative group, the size of the effect was high ((Hypotheses 2)

Before performing the MANOVA (Hypothesis 3), the inclusion in the model of the covariates parental age (age of parents and child) and disability level was analyzed. We found no relationship between these covariates and the dependent variables.

The multivariate analysis Pillai's Trace show a statistically significant effect for gender [Pillai's (25, 150) = 0.55; $p < 0.000$] and educational level (Pillai's (50, 302) = 0.38; $p < 0.035$); but not for socioeconomic level (Pillai's (25, 150) = 0.18, $p < 0.171$), so we can say that the differences are explained by the gender of the subjects and their level of education. Therefore, we can state that multivariate differences are explained by the gender of the subjects and their level of education.

The univariate tests (see **Table 2**) showed a statistically significant effect of the variable gender in 19 of the 24 scales and in the Clinical Index, with moderate and high sizes of the effect. The fathers group differ significantly of the mothers group in: Self-Indulging, Externally Focused, Realistic/Sensing, Conservation-Seeking, Gregarious/outgoing scales ($p < 0.05$); Actively Modifying and Cooperative/agreeing scales ($p < 0.01$); and finally, highly significant differences in Passively Accommodating, Other Nurturing, Internally Focused, Imaginative/Intuiting, Thought-Guided, Feeling-Guided, Anxious/hesitating, Confident/asserting, Submissive/yielding and Dominant/controlling scales, and the Clinical Index($p < 0.001$). Educational level was significant on three scales: the Primary Education group obtained significantly higher scores than the Secondary Education group in Other Nurturing scale ($p < 0.01$); significantly higher scores than the Secondary and Higher Education groups in Conservation-Seeking scale ($p < 0.01$); and also significantly higher scores than the Higher Education group in Dutiful/conforming scale ($p < 0.05$).

Economic level also was significant in 10 of the 24 scales and in the Clinical Index, with small and moderate sizes of the effect. The medium-low group obtained significantly higher scores than the medium-high group in: Passively Accommodating, Asocial/withdrawing, Anxious/hesitating and Submissive/yielding scales ($p < 0.05$). On the contrary, this group obtained significantly lower scores than the medium-high group in: Actively Modifying scale ($p < 0.01$), Externally Focused and Conservation-Seeking scales ($p < 0.05$), Gregarious/outgoing and Confident/asserting scales ($p < 0.01$) and in the Clinical Index ($p < 0.01$).

4. Discussion

As stated in the first hypothesis, personality styles are a proven source of information on the psychological organization/pattern and adaptive behavior of parents with a disabled child. We have identified personality profiles which are significantly different from those in the normative population.

Taking these differences into account, we can provide a characteristic profile of personality for fathers and mothers in the three dimensions mentioned above: motivating styles, thinking styles, and behaving styles.

In the group of men, the differences suggest a motivating style characterized by vitality, energy, optimism, and the search for positive reinforcement in the light of misfortune (pleasure-enhancing); less tendency towards preservation, pessimism and avoidance, than the normative population; and less individuality than men from the normative population. This motivating style suggests the presence of a strong protective factor, given that the decreased use of coping strategies based on escape-avoidance has been associated with greater psychological adjustment [23]-[25] [42]-[44].

Table 2. MANCOVA results from the MIPS scales and Clinical Index: Effects of the variables gender, educational level and socioeconomic level.

MIPS scales	GENDER			EDUCATIONAL LEVEL			SOCIOECONOMIC LEVEL		
	Father[a] (n = 83) Mother[b] (n = 96)			Primary education[1] (n = 63) Secondary education[2] (n = 62) Higher education[3] (n = 54)			Medium-Low[a] (n = 102) Medium-High[b] (n = 77)		
	$F(1, 174)$	η^2	Contrast	$F(2, 164)$	η^2	Contrast	$F(1, 164)$	η^2	Contrast
Motivating Styles									
1A. Pleasure-Enhancing	12.15***	0.065	a > b	0.14	0.002		7.75**	0.043	a < b
1B. Pain–Avoiding	24.82***	0.125	a < b	1.01	0.011		3.50	0.020	
2A. Actively Modifying	6.10**	0.034	a > b	1.50	0.017		6.95**	0.038	a < b
2B. Passively Accommodating	19.99***	0.103	a < b	0.32	0.004		5.71*	0.032	a > b
3A. Self-Indulging	5.34*	0.030	a > b	0.54	0.006		0.09	0.000	
3B. Other Nurturing	22.09***	0.113	a < b	5.31**	0.057	1 > 2	1.36	0.008	
Thinking Styles									
4A. Externally Focused	4.10*	0.023	a > b	0.62	0.007		5.67*	0.032	a < b
4B. Internally Focused	14.53***	0.077	a < b	1.52	0.017		0.76	0.004	
5A. Realistic/Sensing	4.90*	0.027	a > b	1.40	0.016		1.68	0.004	
5B. Imaginative/Intuiting	13.98***	0.074	a < b	0.08	0.001		0.39	0.002	
6A. Thought-Guided	43.05***	0.198	a > b	1.70	0.019		1.07	0.006	
6B. Feeling-Guided	53.82***	0.236	a < b	1.51	0.017		0.01	0.000	
7A. Conservation-Seeking	5.10*	0.028	a > b	5.87**	0.063	1 > 3, 2 > 3	5.43*	0.030	a < b
7B. Innovation-Seeking	0.32	0.002		0.31	0.004		0.14	0.001	
Behaving Styles									
8A. Asocial/withdrawing	3.33	0.019		0.10	0.001		4.93*	0.028	a > b
8B. Gregarious/outgoing	4.46*	0.025	a > b	0.22	0.003		13.907***	0.074	a < b
9A. Anxious/ hesitating	25.79***	0.129	a < b	1.25	0.014		4.44*	0.025	a > b
9B. Confident/asserting	44.41***	0.203	a > b	0.36	0.004		7.82**	0.043	a < b
10A. Unconventional/dissenting	2.07	0.012		2.28	0.025		0.04	0.000	
10B. Dutiful/conforming	0.34	0.002		3.74*	0.041	1 > 3	2.02	0.011	
11A. Submissive/yielding	12.29***	0.066	a < b	0.34	0.004		4.37*	0.024	a > b
11B. Dominant/controlling	23.84***	0.120	a > b	0.26	0.003		3.51	0.020	
12A. Dissatisfed/complaining	3.54	0.020		1.96	0.022		1.79	0.010	
12B. Cooperative/agreeing	8.32**	0.046	a < b	0.78	0.009		0.38	0.002	
Iaj.t. Clinical Index	17.72***	0.092	a > b	0.06	0.001		7.61**	0.042	a < b

*$p < 0.05$; **$p < 0.01$; ***$p < 0.001$.

The presence of a markedly pleasure-enhancing and motivating style is also related to the impulse to improve their own and other people's lives, and to reinforce their survival ability. This style would explain the great capacity to adapt to stress reported in other studies [24] [31] [45]-[47]. It has also been reported that concerns over the precise cause of the problem can drive these fathers into a long pilgrimage from one specialist to another due to their need to relieve feelings of impotence or guilt, rather than to dissatisfaction with the answers received. In this sense, the chronic character of the child's disease becomes a need to repair something that is irreparable [48]. This could be interpreted as a basic compensatory mechanism in humans, *i.e.*, the drive to improve life, and to seek gratifying and pleasant experiences in the face of the pain and the sense of impotence and frustration generated by having a child with a severe disability [36].

On the other hand, mothers of children with chronic disabilities have a motivating style characterized by a strong predisposition toward caring for others, at the expense of oneself. Their style of being oriented to caring for others at the expense of themselves is closely related to caring for the child that mainly falls to mothers, and is also related to demands involved in taking care of a disabled child [4] [49]-[51]. This supports the findings of other studies that report increased levels of overprotection and receptivity towards children with disabilities [50]-[52], and positive assessments of the burden of care, as a way to adapt to a difficult situation such as the one these parents are experiencing [29] [30] [45] [53].

Secondly, the differences found in the cognitive dimension suggest that both fathers and mothers have a greater cognitive orientation toward direct experience, observable phenomena, and practical, real and objective information; they also indicate an extremely low predisposition to handle abstract and ambiguous information, such an abstract reasoning with a symbolic character. This cognitive style is related to a pragmatic coping strategy that shows a clear preference for the specific aspects of the present and the need to plan day-by-day. This propensity has been identified by other studies as an important factor of psychological adjustment that helps parents to face the daily stressors associated with taking care of children, protecting themselves from pain, and improving self-esteem and efficiency [25] [31] [48]. Together with this pragmatic style, the mothers in our sample showed less tendency to the logical and objective analysis of reality; and the fathers, showed less predisposition to handle feelings. Originality and innovation are not among their strengths.

Regarding behaving styles, that encompass the way people relate with each other, the parents in our sample appear maintain good control in their interpersonal relationships, are not submissive, are not submissive, and show good adjustment to social norms (conventional behavior). Both, although more accentuated in mothers, show an interpersonal style in which cooperation, harmony and engagement has priority over any individual interest.

No significant effects of the age and severity of child's disability. Although some studies associate the severity of a chronic condition in children with the psychological health of their mothers [7] [15], the majority of the empirical studies do not support such a hypothesis [2] [5] [54]. Usually it is difficult to reach a consensus on this issue due to the variability of the criteria used as a indicators of severity in different studies [55].

Despite the wide age range of children in our study, child age was not a particularly influential variable on families of children with chronic disability. Results agree with those of Wiegner and Donders [2], but contradict the findings of Ulus and collaborators [55].

The second hypothesis was also confirmed. As predicted, the different levels of psychological adjustment found between fathers and mothers indicate lower psychological adjustment among mothers and therefore, the existence of cognitive, affective or interpersonal behaviors that are not positive for their health and well-being. Our results are consistent with many other studies that suggest that mothers are at increased risk due to being the main caregiver [4] [7] [13] [22] [46] [56] [57].

The third hypothesis suggested that the gender, educational level and socioeconomic level would modulate the differences found in personality.

Concerning the moderating role of gender, the results are consistent with studies previous [24] [58]. The differences between fathers and mothers show a division along opposite personality dimensions which suggest a marked asymmetry in gender roles. The traditional masculine and feminine roles seem to be more accentuated among fathers and mothers of children with a chronic disability. The more common profile for the father matches the traditional stereotype of the external provider: a greater pleasure-enhancing style, cognitively more reflexive, and sociable, assertive and dominating. The mother's profile is associated with the traditional stereotype of caring for the child and being a housewife: they are more conservative and oriented to caregiving, more receptive to emotional information, and more indecisive, submissive and acquiescent than their partners.

In this regard, it is commonly agreed that the level of stress and psychological maladjustment among mothers is higher, and this is mainly due to the differences in the caregiving and work roles within the relationship [2] [56]. The role of the mother as the primary caregiver has also been associated with greater uncertainty among these women in relation to their image as mothers and with an increased tendency to being more conventional [57] [58]. Complying to a gender stereotype may help to justify, rationalize, and understand painful events, and provide a model when external and internal demands overpower available resources, as occurs among these parents [25]. Future studies could confirm these hypotheses by evaluating the different responses of parents, not only according to being a man or a woman, but also to specific gender variables and prevailing social norms that might lead to inequality and disadvantage among these women.

On the other hand, educational and socioeconomic levels, independently of being a man or a woman, seem to moderate to some extent the differences found in personality variables and psychological adjustment.

In this sense, taking into account that some styles may be more effective than others regarding satisfactory adaptation to the environment [26]-[28] [40], the least adaptive personality styles, such as Pain-Avoidance, Passively accommodating, anxious/hesitating, Unconventional/Dissenting and Dissatisfied/Complaining styles, appear to be related to a low-to-medium socioeconomic level. Similarly, a medium-to-high socioeconomic level is associated with a more pleasure-enhancing, active, and transforming personality style, higher levels of extraversion, decisiveness and control, and, therefore with greater capacity for adaptation. However, low-to-medium educational level of the parents appears associated with more protective styles, cognitively more systematic and more conformist at the interpersonal level.

Regarding these findings, the economic level of the family has been associated with coping and psychological discomfort among parents in previous studies [51] [59] however, the educational level of parents has not been regarded as an important moderator of personal resources in parents with disabled children.

5. Conclusions

The present study analyzes the psychological adaptation of parents with children with congenital disabilities based on a model that focuses on the identification of adaptive resources, rather than on dysfunctional aspects. The personality styles evaluated provide a measure of the stability of the processes involved in parents' psychological adaptation, independently of the developmental stage of the child or the disease, and account for a wide range of psychologically relevant behavior, which may be of use to future research and intervention.

The results show significant behavioral tendencies that identify certain areas of vulnerability where parents may be putting their psychological health at risk, and at the same time, indicate behavioral resources that may act as protective factors.

Being a man or a woman has a differential impact that appears to be related to the adopting traditional gender roles by parents, as a way of facing and adapting to the situation. This would place mothers in a situation of greater vulnerability, as they show less psychological adjustment and adaptive personality styles than fathers. Therefore, gender issues may be acting in concert to differentiate how such mothers and fathers adapt psychologically. The educational and socioeconomic levels of parents could also act as risk factors in their adaptive functioning. Researchers and clinicians should explore these sociodemographic factors as they may contribute to the psychological adjustment of parents.

The present study has some limitations. The sample is comprised exclusively by parents belonging to parents' associations of children with chronic physical illness. To further our understanding of psychological adaptation of parents of children with a congenital disability, it would be relevant to study a more diverse sample. Finally, it underlines the limit of the use of self-report questionnaires. Although this study goes beyond the use of self-report measures, and provides a psychometrically standardized measure, to further our understanding of parental adaptation to chronic stress, future studies should include information gathered via multiple methods and from multiple sources.

Although these profiles may not always account for the great diversity of parental responses, they may serve as indicators of the way parents face to child's disability. Gaining a deeper understanding of the motivational, cognitive and behavioral dimensions involved in the adaptive functioning of these parents, and identifying those variables that are relevant to their well-being and psychological adjustment—as well as the educational and socioeconomic level of the family—could be of great use to the professional teams who provide these families with help and counselling, and may help them to design better intervention strategies to optimize personal resources.

Acknowledgements

We thank all fathers and mothers of children with spina bifida, cerebral palsy, cleft lip and palate, and their respective associations, for their commitment and involvement in the project.

References

[1]   Wallander, J.L. and Noojin, A.B. (1995) Mothers' Report of Stressful Experiences Related to Having a Child with a Physical Disability. *Children's Health Care*, **24**, 245-256. http://dx.doi.org/10.1207/s15326888chc2404_4

[2]   Wiegner, S. and Donders, J. (2000) Predictors of Parental Distress after Congenital Disabilities. *Journal Developmental Behavioral Pediatrics*, **21**, 271-274. http://dx.doi.org/10.1097/00004703-200008000-00003

[3]   Ki, Y.W. and Joanne, C.C.Y. (2014) Stress and Marital Satisfaction of Parents with Children with Disabilities in Hong Kong. *Psychology*, **5**, 349-357. http://dx.doi.org/10.4236/psych.2014.55045

[4]   Vermaes, I.P.R., Janssens, J.M.A.M., Bosman, A.M.T. and Gerris, J.R.M. (2005) Parents' Psychological Adjustment in Families of Children with Spina Bifida: A Meta-Analysis. *BMC Pediatrics*, **32**, 1-13.

[5]   Tifferet, S., Manor, O., Elizur, Y., Friedman, O. and Constantini, S. (2010) Maternal Adaptation to Pediatric Illness: A Personal Vulnerability Model. *Children's Health Care*, **39**, 91-107. http://dx.doi.org/10.1080/02739611003679840

[6]   Macias, M.M., Clifford, S.C., Saylor, C.F. and Kreh, S.M. (2001) Predictors of Parenting Stress in Families of Children with Spina Bifida. *Children's Health Care*, **30**, 57-65. http://dx.doi.org/10.1207/S15326888CHC3001_5

[7]   Uguz, S., Toros, F., Inanc, B.Y. and Colakkadioglu, O. (2004) Assessment of Anxiety, Depression and Stress Levels of Mothers of Handicapped Children. *Klinik Psikiyatri Dergisi*, **7**, 42-47. http://www.klinikpsikiyatri.org/files/journals/1/185.pdf

[8]   Weigl, V., Rudolph, M., Eysholdt, U. and Rosanowski, F. (2005) Anxiety, Depression, and Quality of Life in Mothers of Children with Cleft Lip/Palate. *Folia Phoniatricaet Logopaedica*, **57**, 20-27. http://dx.doi.org/10.1159/000081958

[9]   Macias, M.M., Roberts, K.M., Saylor, C.F. and Fussell, J.J. (2006) Toileting Concerns, Parenting Stress, and Behavior Problems in Children with Special Health Care Needs. *Clinical Pediatrics*, **45**, 415-422. http://dx.doi.org/10.1177/0009922806289616

[10] Glenn, S., Cunningham, C., Poole, H., Reeves, D. and Weindling, M. (2009) Maternal Parenting Stress and Its Correlates in Families with a Young Child with Cerebral Palsy. *Child: Care, Health and Development*, **35**, 71-78. http://dx.doi.org/10.1111/j.1365-2214.2008.00891.x

[11] Drotar, D., Baskiewicz, A., Irvin, N.A., Kennell, J.H. and Klaus, M.H. (1975) The Adaptation of Parents to the Birth of an Infant with a Congenital Malformation: A Hypothetical Model. *Pediatrics*, **56**, 710-717.

[12] Koomen, H.M.Y. and Hoeksma, J.B. (1992) Maternal Interactive Behaviour towards Children with and Children without Cleft Lip and Palate. *Early Development and Parenting*, **1**, 169-181. http://dx.doi.org/10.1002/edp.2430010306

[13] Holmbeck, G.N, Gorey-Ferguson, L., Hudson, T., Seefeldt, T., Shapera, W., Turner, T. and Uhler, J. (1997) Maternal, Paternal, and Marital Functioning in Families of Preadolescents with Spina Bifida. *Journal of Pediatric Psychology*, **22**, 167-181. http://dx.doi.org/10.1093/jpepsy/22.2.167

[14] Barlow, J.H. and Ellard, D.R. (2006) The Psychosocial Well-Being of Children with Chronic Disease, Their Parents and Siblings: An Overview of the Research Evidence Base. *Child: Care, Health and Development*, **32**, 19-31. http://dx.doi.org/10.1111/j.1365-2214.2006.00591.x

[15] Berge, J.M., Patterson, J.M. and Rueter, M. (2006) Marital Satisfaction and Mental Health of Couples with Children with Chronic Health Conditions. *Families Systems & Health*, **24**, 267-285. http://dx.doi.org/10.1037/1091-7527.24.3.267

[16] Aldwin, C.M. and Brustrom, J. (1997) Theories of Coping with Chronic Stress: Illustrations from the Health Psychology and Aging Literatures. In: Gottlieb, B.H., Ed., *Coping with Chronic Stress*, Plenum Press, New York, 75-99. http://dx.doi.org/10.1007/978-1-4757-9862-3_3

[17] Lazarus, R.S. (2006) Stress and Emotion: A New Synthesis. Springer Publishing Company, New York.

[18] Cousino, M.K. and Hazen, R.A. (2013) Parenting Stress among Caregivers of Children with Chronic Illness: A Systematic Review. *Journal of Pediatric Psychology*, **38**, 809-828. http://dx.doi.org/10.1093/jpepsy/jst049

[19] Cuzzocrea, F., Larcan, R. and Westh, F. (2014) Family and Parental Functioning in Parents of Disabled Children. *Nordic Psychology*, **65**, 271-287. http://dx.doi.org/10.1080/19012276.2013.824201

[20] Boll, T.J., Dimino, E. and Mattsson, A.E. (1978) Parenting Attitudes: The Role of Personality Style and Childhood Long-Term Illness. *Journal of Psychosomatic Research*, **22**, 209-213. http://dx.doi.org/10.1016/0022-3999(78)90026-0

[21] Dean, R.S. and Jacobson, B.P. (1982) MMPI Characteristics for Parents of Emotionally Disturbed and Learning-Disabled Children. *Journal of Consulting and Clinical Psychology*, **50**, 775-777. http://dx.doi.org/10.1037/0022-006X.50.5.775

[22] Vermaes, I.P.R., Janssens, J.M.A.M., Mullaart, R.A., Vinck, A. and Gerris, J.R.M. (2008) Parents' Personality and Parenting Stress in Families of Children with Spina Bifida. *Child: Care, Health and Development*, **34**, 665-674. http://dx.doi.org/10.1111/j.1365-2214.2008.00868.x

[23] Glidden, L.M., Billings, F.J. and Jobe, B.M. (2006) Personality, Coping Style and Well-Being of Parents Rearing Children with Developmental Disabilities. *Journal of Intellectual Disability Research*, **50**, 949-962. http://dx.doi.org/10.1111/j.1365-2788.2006.00929.x

[24] Limiñana-Gras, R.M. (2006) Personalidad y Adaptación Psicológica Parental en Discapacidad [Personality and Parental Psychological Adjustment in Disability]. Doctoral Thesis, University of Murcia, Murcia. http://www.tdx.cat/handle/10803/283282

[25] Limiñana Gras, R., Corbalán, F.J. and Sánchez-López, M.P. (2009) Thinking Styles and Coping When Caring for a Child with Severe Spina Bifida. *Journal of Developmental and Physical Disabilities*, **19**, 125-134. http://dx.doi.org/10.1007/s10882-009-9133-0

[26] Millon, T. (1990) Toward a New Personality: An Evolutionary Model. Wiley, New York.

[27] Millon, T. (1994) Millon Index of Personality Styles, Manual. The Psychological Corporation, San Antonio.

[28] Millon, T. (2004) Millon Index of Personality Styles, Manual Revised. Pearson Assessments, Minneapolis.

[29] Schwartz, C. (2003) Parent of Children with Chronic Disabilities: The Gratification of Caregiving. *Families in Society*, **84**, 576-584. http://dx.doi.org/10.1606/1044-3894.143

[30] Kearney, P.M. and Griffin, T. (2001) Between Joy and Sorrow: Being a Parent of a Child with Developmental Disability. *Journal of Advanced Nursing*, **34**, 582-592. http://dx.doi.org/10.1046/j.1365-2648.2001.01787.x

[31] Barakat, L.P. and Linney, J.A. (1995) Optimism, Appraisals and Coping in the Adjustment of Mothers and Their Children with Spina Bifida. *Journal of Child and Family Studies*, **4**, 303-320. http://dx.doi.org/10.1007/BF02233965

[32] Limiñana Gras, R.M., CorbalánBerná, F.J. and Patró Hernández, R.M. (2007) Coping and Psychological Adaptation in Parents of Children with Cleft Palate. *Anales de Psicología*, **23**, 201-206. http://www.um.es/analesps/v23/v23_2/04-23_2.pdf

[33] Cuéllar-Flores, I. and Sánchez-López, M.P. (2012) Adaptaciónpsicológicaen personas cuidadoras de familiaresensituación de dependencia [Psychological Adaptation in Caregivers of Relatives in a Situation of Dependence]. *Clínica y Salud*, **23**, 141-152. http://dx.doi.org/10.5093/cl2012a9

[34] Sandler, A.D. (2010) Children with Spina Bifida: Key Clinical Issues. *Pediatric Clinics of North America*, **57**, 879-892. http://dx.doi.org/10.1016/j.pcl.2010.07.009

[35] Rosenbaum, P., Paneth, N., Leviton, A., Goldstein, M., Bax, M., Damiano, D., Dan, B. and Jacobsson, B. (2007) A Report: The Definition and Classification of Cerebral Palsy April 2006. *Developmental Medicine and Child Neurology. Supplement*, **109**, 8-14.

[36] Gorlin, R.J., Cohen, M.M. and Hennekam, R.C.M. (2001) Syndromes of the Head and Neck. Oxford University Press, New York.

[37] World Health Organization (1980) International Classification of Impairments, Disabilities and Handicaps. A Manual of Classification Relating to the Consequences of Disease. WHO, Geneva.

[38] World Health Organization (2001) International Classification of Functioning, Disability and Health (ICF). WHO, Geneva.

[39] Millon, T. (2001) Inventario de Estilos de Personalidad de Millon, Manual. [Millon Index of Personality Styles, Manual]. Adaptación de M.P. Sánchez-López, J.F. Díaz-Morales and M.E. Aparicio-García. TEA Ediciones, Madrid.

[40] Cardenal, V. and Fierro, A. (2001) Sexo y edadenestilos de personalidad, bienestar personal y adaptación social. *Psicothema*, **13**, 118-126. http://www.psicothema.com/psicothema.asp?id=422

[41] Keppel, G. (1991) Design and Analysis: A Researcher's Handbook. 3rd Edition, Prentice Hall, Englewood Clifts, New York.

[42] Judge, S.L. (1998) Parental Coping Strategies and Strengths in Families of Young Children with Disabilities. *Family Relations*, **47**, 263-268. http://dx.doi.org/10.2307/584976

[43] Abbeduto, L., Seltzer, M., Shattuck, P., Krauss, M., Orsmond, G. and Murphy, M. (2004) Psychological Well-Being and Coping in Mothers of Youths with Autism, Down Syndrome, or Fragile X Syndrome. *American Journal on Mental Retardation*, **109**, 237-254. http://dx.doi.org/10.1352/0895-8017(2004)109<237;PWACIM>2.0.CO;2

[44] Stoneman, Z. and Gavidia-Payne, S.T. (2006) Marital Adjustment in Families of Young Children with Disabilities: Associations with Daily Hassles and Problem-Focused Coping. *American Journal on Mental Retardation*, **111**, 1-14. http://dx.doi.org/10.1352/0895-8017(2006)111[1:MAIFOY]2.0.CO;2

[45] Lemanek, K.L., Jones, M.L. and Lieberman, B. (2000) Mothers of Children with Spina Bifida: Adaptational and Stress Processing. *Children's Health Care*, **29**, 19-35. http://dx.doi.org/10.1207/S15326888CHC2901_2

[46] Limiñana Gras, R., Corbalán Berná, F.J. and Calvo Llena, M.T. (2009) Resiliencia y discapacidad: unaaproximaciónpositiva al estudio de la adaptación parental enfamilias de niños con espinabífida [Resilience and Disability: A Positive Approach to Parental Adaptation in Families of Children with Spina Bifida]. Editorial Universidad de Murcia (EDITUM), Murcia.

[47] Hall, H.R., Neely-Barnes, S.L., Graff, J.C., Krcek, T.E., Roberts, R.J. and Hankins, J.S. (2012) Parental Stress in Families of Children with a Genetic Disorder/Disability and the Resiliency Model of Family Stress, Adjustment, and Adaptation. *Issues in Comprehensive Pediatric Nursing*, **35**, 24-44. http://dx.doi.org/10.3109/01460862.2012.646479

[48] Irvin, N.A., Kennell, J.H. and Klaus, M.H. (1976) Caring for Parents of an Infant with a Congenital Malformation. In: Klaus, M.H. and Kennell, J.H., Eds., *Maternal-Infant Bonding*, CV Mosby, St. Louis, 167-208.

[49] Dorner, S. (1973) Psychological and Social Problems of Families of Adolescent Spina Bifida Patients: A Preliminary Report. *Developmental Medicine and Child Neurology*, **15**, 24-26. http://dx.doi.org/10.1111/j.1469-8749.1973.tb04937.x

[50] Erickson, M. and Upshur, C.C. (1989) Caretaking Burden and Social Support: Comparison of Mothers of Infants with and without Disabilities. *American Journal on Mental Retardation*, **94**, 250-258.

[51] Wallander, J.L. and Venters, T.L. (1995) Perceived Role Restriction and Adjustment of Mothers of Children with Chronic Physical Disability. *Journal of Pediatric Psychology*, **20**, 619-632. http://dx.doi.org/10.1093/jpepsy/20.5.619

[52] Holmbeck, G.N., Coakley, R.M., Hommeyer, J.S., Shapera, W.E. and Westhoven, V.C. (2002) Observed and Perceived Dyadic and Systemic Functioning in Families of Preadolescents with Spina Bifida. *Journal of Pediatric Psychology*, **27**, 177-189. http://dx.doi.org/10.1093/jpepsy/27.2.177

[53] Noojin, A.B. and Wallander, J.L. (1997) Perceived Problem-Solving Ability, Stress, and Coping in Mothers of Children with Physical Disabilities: Potential Cognitive Influences on Adjustment. *International Journal of Behavioral Medicine*, **4**, 415-432. http://dx.doi.org/10.1207/s15327558ijbm0404_10

[54] Manuel, J., Naughton, M.J., Balkrishnan, R., Paterson Smith, B. and Koman, L.A. (2003) Stress and Adaptation in Mothers of Children with Cerebral Palsy. *Journal of Pediatric Psychology*, **28**, 197-201. http://dx.doi.org/10.1093/jpepsy/jsg007

[55] Ulus, Y., Tander, B., Akyol, Y., Ulus, A., Tander, B., Bilgici, A., Kuru, O. and Akbas, S. (2012) Functional Disability of Children with Spina Bifida: Its Impact on Parents' Psychological Status and Family Functioning. *Developmental Neurorehabilitation*, **15**, 322-328. http://dx.doi.org/10.3109/17518423.2012.691119

[56] Kazak, A.E. and Marvin, R.S. (1984) Differences, Difficulties and Adaptation: Stress and Social Network in Families with a Handicapped Child. *Family Relations*, **33**, 67-77. http://dx.doi.org/10.2307/584591

[57] Vermaes, I.P.R., Gerris, J.R.M. and Janssens, J.M.A.M. (2007) Parents' Social Adjustment in Families of Children with Spina Bifida: A Theory-Driven Review. *Journal of Pediatric Psychology*, **32**, 1214-1226. http://dx.doi.org/10.1093/jpepsy/jsm054

[58] Limiñana Gras, R.M. and Patró Hernández, R.M. (2004) Mujer y Salud: Trauma y cronificaciónenmadres de discapacitados [Women and Health: Trauma and Chronification in Mothers of Disabled Children]. *Anales de Psicología*, **20**, 47-54.

[59] Cleve, L.V. (1989) Parental Coping in Response to Their Child's Spina Bifida. *Journal of Pediatric Nursing*, **4**, 172-176.

SOCIODEMOGRAPHIC AND HEALTH HISTORY QUESTIONNAIRE

CODE: [   ]

Completedby:_____

DATA:_____

PERSONAL DATA OF THE CHILD:

NAMES AND SURNAMES: _____

NATIONALITY: _____

DATE AND PLACE OF BIRTH: _____

ADDRESS: _____

MEDICAL DIAGNOSIS: _____

DATE OF FIRST DIAGNOSIS: _____

PERCENTAGE OF DISABILITY AND DATE OF ISSUE: _____

ASSOCIATION TO WHICH BELONGS: _____

NUMBER OF SURGERIES: _____ NUMBER OF HOSPITALIZATIONS: _____

PHYSICAL AND NEUROLOGICAL COMPLICATIONS, MALFORMATIONS, OR DISEASESASSOCIATED:

_____

_____

OTHER ALTERATIONS ASSOCIATED: _____

_____

PERSONAL DATA OF THE FATHER:

NATIONALITY: _____

DATE OF BIRTH AND AGE: _____

PROFESSION: _____

MARITAL STATUS:

Single _____ 1		Married _____ 2	
Separated/divorced _____ 3		Widowed _____ 4	

LEVEL OF STUDIES COMPLETED:

Withoutstudies _____ 1		Primaryeducation _____ 2	
Secondaryeducation _____ 3		Highereducation _____ 4	

CURRENT EMPLOYMENT SITUATION

Employed _____ 1		Household chores _____ 2	
Employed _____ 3		Unemployed _____ 4	
Retiredorpensioner _____ 5		Others _____ 6	

SOCIOECONOMIC LEVEL:

Level upper-middle _____ 1   Level lower-middle _____ 2

PERSONAL DATA OF THE MATHER:

NATIONALITY: _____

DATE OF BIRTH AND AGE: _____

PROFESSION: _____

MARITAL STATUS:

Single _____ 1   Married _____ 2

Separated/divorced _____ 3   Widowed _____ 4

LEVEL OF STUDIES COMPLETED:

Withoutstudies _____ 1   Primaryeducation _____ 2

Secondaryeducation _____ 3   Highereducation _____ 4

CURRENT EMPLOYMENT SITUATION

Employed _____ 1   Household chores _____ 2

Employed _____ 3   Unemployed _____ 4

Retiredorpensioner _____ 5   Others _____ 6

SOCIOECONOMIC LEVEL:

Level upper-middle _____ 1   Level lower-middle _____ 2

18

Dimensions of Access to Antihypertensive Medications in Ceilândia, Distrito Federal, Brazil

Fabiana Xavier Cartaxo Salgado[1], Dayani Galato[1], Gislane Ferreira de Melo[2],
Marileusa Dosolina Chiarello[2], Aline Gomes de Oliveira[1], Letícia Farias Gerlack[1],
Micheline Marie Milward de Azevedo Meiners[3], Margô Gomes de Oliveira Karnikowski[1]

[1]Graduate Program in Health Sciences and Technology, Campus of Ceilândia, University of Brasília (FCE/UnB), Brasília, Brazil
[2]Graduate Program in Gerontology, Catholic University of Brasília (UCB), Brasília, Brazil
[3]Graduate Program in Public Health, University of Brasília (UnB), Brasília, Brazil
Email: fabianacartaxo@yahoo.com.br, dayanigalato@unb.br, gmelo@ucb.br, mdc@pos.ucb.br,
alinegoma1@gmail.com, leticiafg@yahoo.com.br, michelinemeiners@gmail.com, margo@unb.br

Abstract

Access can be understood as the sum of a number of elements of the interface between patients and the health care system. This study took a comprehensive approach to the dimensions of access to medications, employing indicators to evaluate the dimensions of access to antihypertensive medications in Ceilândia, DF, Brazil. This was a cross-sectional epidemiological study, administering questionnaires during home visits. The survey covered epidemiological and socioeconomic profiles, behavioral habits and the dimensions of access to antihypertensive medications comprising physical, financial, and geographic availability and accept ability according to the hypertensive population of Ceilândia. The total sample comprised 400 individuals and the hypertensive subset numbered 140 (35%). Indicators of physical availability of medications revealed that users found it difficult to acquire their drugs on almost one third of occasions and in some cases were unable to access any of these products. The greatest barriers to access were reported by users of pharmacies belonging to the Brazilian National Health Service (SUS) and on the "People's Pharmacies" network. More than one third of the hypertensive sample spent their own money on medications they could not find at these pharmacies. The majority of the hypertensive subsets were overweight/obese, a minority engaged in physical activity and 40% were smokers/ex-smokers. More women reduced their salt intake. Men had higher incomes, educational level, and socioeconomic status. Failure to keep the public health care system supplied has prejudiced access to essential medications for hypertension treatment, transferring the costs onto users. This population has lifestyle habits that increase the risk of exacerbation of hypertension. These results reveal a need for effective public policies to ensure access to antihypertensive medications and involve users of the health care system in changing their habits and behaviors in order to achieve adequate and lasting control of systemic arterial hypertension.

Keywords

Health Care Access, Systemic Arterial Hypertension, Drug Treatments

---

1. Introduction

Systemic arterial hypertension (SAH) is a multifactorial clinical condition characterized by consistently high blood pressure that is often associated with increased risk of fatal and non-fatal cardiovascular events [1]. The prevalence of hypertension is high, while the proportion of cases that are controlled is low, and it is considered one of the most important modifiable risk factors. Population-based studies conducted in Brazilian cities over the last 20 years have detected SAH prevalence rates exceeding 30% [2] [3].

Treatment with drugs is prescribed with the objective of protecting target organs, reducing the impact of elevated blood pressure and its associated risk factors and combatting progression of the atherosclerotic process [4]. Lack of the medications used to treat SAH has countless consequences, both individual and collective, since the social and economic costs of the possible sequelae and mortality that result when there are barriers impeding access to these products must be borne by the people affected and by society.

There is evidence that the control of arterial hypertension achieved in the United States of America over recent decades is a result of increased availability of drug-based treatment [5]. Access to medications can be understood as "[the relationship between the need for medications and their availability, by which this need is met at the time and place of patient need, while ensuring quality and sufficient information for correct use]" [6], or, alternatively, as the user's ability to obtain the medication prescribed them, with or without direct payment [7]. These conceptualizations imply recognition that access is only achieved when the medication is used.

Notwithstanding, access is not limited to the availability of a product or resource, but is part of a complex network and encompasses several different interrelated aspects and constructs. Access to health care includes the provision of medications to guarantee the right to health and, as a consequence, to the basic right to life, requiring proactive actions from the State, actions through which the State guarantees to its citizens provision of the medications indispensable for their treatment [8]. Access to medications can be understood as the sum of a number of more specific elements of the interface between the patient and the health care system. Literature on the subject deals with a number of specific dimensions, expanding the concept of access to medications and to health services [9].

The first of these is related to the physical availability of the product and is defined as the relationship between the type and quantity of the product or service that is needed and the type and quantity of the product that is provided. The second dimension is the ability to acquire care, related to the magnitude of the prices of products and the costs of services and to people's ability to pay. A third dimension is geographic accessibility, which covers the relationship between the location of products and services and the locations of the users of these products and services, taking into account user's resources and the distances to be travelled and the time taken to do so. The last of these is the dimension of acceptability or satisfaction and is the relationship between users' attitudes and expectations with respect to products and services and the actual characteristics of those products and services [9].

This study was conducted in the city of Ceilândia, which is in Brazil's Distrito Federal (DF), against a background of growing recognition of the importance of the production of information through scientific research to provide a foundation for strategic planning of public policies for promotion of the health, and improvement of the quality of life, of the population of Ceilândia. The town has the largest population in the DF and is home to one of the campuses of the University of Brasília.

To date there are no epidemiological studies describing the current scenario of the population of Ceilândia's access to drug-based treatment for SAH, which is prejudicial to redirecting and formulating policies and to planning of health care strategies.

From this perspective, it is important to assess access to antihypertensive medications, in order to contribute to public policies for pharmaceutical care and to improving the quality of health services. The objective of this study is to describe the profile of the hypertensive population of Ceilândia and to assess the dimensions of this population's access to medications for treatment of Systemic Arterial Hypertension.

2. Methods

This is an epidemiological study with a cross-sectional design investigating access to medications for treatment of SAH with surveys conducted during home visits.

The study target population comprised people aged 18 years or older living in households chosen by lots in the city of Ceilândia, DF, Brazil. Ceilândia contains the neighborhoods Ceilândia Centro, Ceilândia Sul, Ceilândia Norte, P Sul, P Norte, Setor O, Expansão do Setor O, QNQ, QNR, Pôr do Sol and Sol Nascente, plus an industrial zone and a construction materials zone and part of an INCRA (National Institute for Colonization and Agrarian Reform) land reform area. The sample size was estimated on the basis of the size of the population of Ceilândia reported by the 2013 District Survey of Households by Sample [10] (449,592 inhabitants).

The sample size estimated was 400 people, calculated to provide a 95% confidence interval based on statistical parameters. Residents from the industrial zone, the construction materials zone and the INCRA area were excluded from the sample, because they are designated as rural areas, as were residents of Pôr do Sol and Sol Nascente, because these neighborhoods are not yet officially recognized.

Sampling was conducted probabilistically, in multiple stages, as recommended by the authors of studies in which the probabilistic theory of the quantitative approach to research is employed. The sampling process comprised three stages. The sampling units in the first stage were the following 8 neighborhoods: Ceilândia Sul, Ceilândia Norte, P Sul, P Norte, Setor O, Expansão do Setor O, QNQ and QNR. In the second stage, 32 census sectors were chosen by lots, four from each of the neighborhoods selected in the first stage. In the third stage, households were selected in census sectors chosen in the previous stage. The addresses were selected from the National Register of Addresses for Statistical Purposes, maintained by the Brazilian Institute for Geography and Statistics (CNEFE-IBGE) [11].

Data were collected by survey during home visits from May to July of 2014, by administration of an instrument such as that described in the World Health Organization's "Household Survey to Measure Access and Use of Medicine: Guidelines and Questionnaire" [12], with certain modifications.

The instrument was designed to trace the profile of the hypertensive population in terms of sex, age, weight, height, age at which SAH was diagnosed, socioeconomic status and behavioral habits relating to smoking, diet and physical activity. With relation to these behavioral items, respondents were asked whether they smoked or had previously smoked regularly, whether they avoided eating salt and whether they engaged in sports, physical exercise or recreational activities such as walking, running, aerobics, football, cycling, basketball, volleyball, weight training, yoga, Pilates or martial arts for at least 10 consecutive minutes.

Access to medications for treatment of SAH was investigated in terms of specifications and quantities of products needed; difficulties with acquiring and methods of payment for medications needed by the user; geographic access to pharmacies that stock antihypertensive medications; and acceptability and user satisfaction with relation to the medications used to treat SAH.

The data collected during the home visits were stored in electronic files using EPI DATA version 3.1 and double checked against the originals to test for possible input errors. In order to guarantee interviewee confidentiality, all data were anonymized prior to analysis. Quality control was conducted with a sample of 10% of the people studied.

For statistical analyses, descriptive data were expressed as means, standard deviations and frequencies. The Chi-square test was used for inferential and qualitative data. The Monte Carlo method was employed for qualitative variables that did not have a minimum of 5% of the sample in each cell. The t test for independent samples was used for parametric data and when distributions were not normal the Mann-Whitney test was used, when a difference of 0.001 was detected.

The study was approved by the Research Ethics Committee at the University of Brasília's Faculty of Health under protocol number 29298814.0.0000.0030. Before interviews all participants signed free and informed consent forms which explained the guarantees of anonymity, confidentiality of information and their rights to non-participation and to withdrawal from the study at any time.

3. Results

Figure 1 illustrates the sample distribution and the profile of patients with hypertension in terms of their indications for antihypertensive drugs and the medications they take.

Table 1 lists the variables that comprise the epidemiological profile, socioeconomic status and behavioral of habits of the people with hypertension investigated in Ceilândia.

The weight variable revealed that 75% (n = 24) of the men and 58.3% (n = 63) of the women were over their ideal weight. The active smokers in the sample of people with hypertension had started smoking at around 18.3 years of age, 93.7% (n = 15) smoked every day and they smoked a mean of 15.2 cigarettes per day. The ex-smoker shad started smoking at a mean age of 18.4 and had quit at 38.6 years of age, which equates to an average of 22.2 years smoking. Reduced salt intake was reported by 90.7% of the sample of people with hypertension, 68.5% of whom had adopted this behavior in response to medical advice and 27.5% of whom had done so on their own initiative. Finally, 21.4% of the sample stated they engaged in physical activity and they exercised an average of 3 days per week, 60 minutes per day.

The questionnaire also contained items related to the SAH patients' access to antihypertensive medications. The responses to these questions were converted into indicators, which are shown in **Table 2**.

4. Discussion

Many studies dealing with access to medications focus on the physical availability of products and barriers that make it difficult for users to adhere to drug treatments [15]-[17]. However, there is research showing the importance of expanding this perspective of the dimensions of access to healthcare, including pharmacotherapy, particularly in low-income countries [18]. These dimensions were investigated in the present study, resulting in indicators that enabled identification of the barriers that make it difficult for users to access medications to treat SAH.

Indicators related to the physical accessibility of antihypertensive medications show that these users found it difficult to acquire their drugs on almost one third of occasions and in some cases were unable to access any of these products. It should be pointed out that the greatest difficulty was reported with relation to accessing Brazilian National Health Service (SUS) pharmacies, followed by access to drugs via the "People's Pharmacy" network.

There is evidence in the literature that the availability of antihypertensive medications in Brazilin creased after implementation of the "Health Has no Price" program [19] [20], but also shows that there has been a steady reduction in the availability of these products through pharmacies belonging to the SUS [21]-[23]. This finding may be in part due to problems related to management and application of financial resources in these pharmacies [24]. Issues with availability of medications are not restricted to antihypertensive drugs since studies conducted in Brazil have shown that, on average, 40% of medications prescribed to treat chronic disease within the public

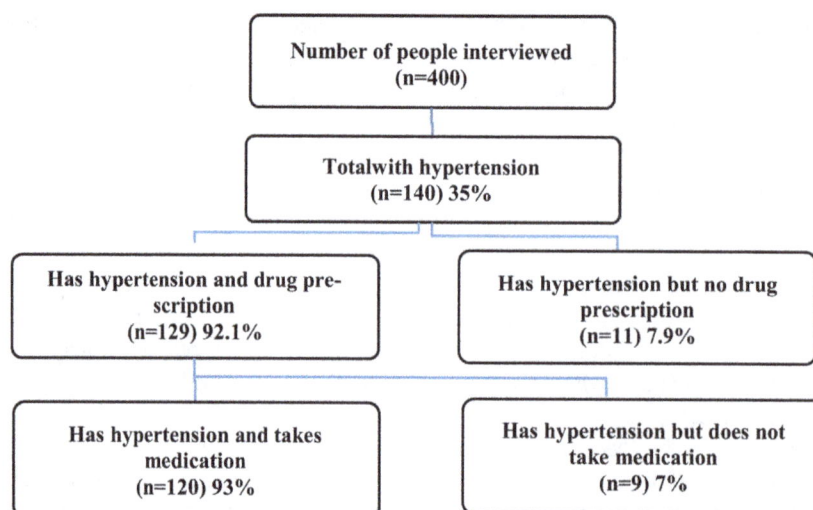

Figure 1. Sample distribution in terms of indications for and use of antihypertensive medication.

Table 1. Social, economic and behavioral profile of people with Systemic Arterial Hypertension in the city of Ceilândia, DF, Brazil.

	Men 22.9% (n = 32)		Women 77.1% (n = 108)		Total (n = 140)		P
Mean age ± SD (years)	56.21 ± 14		57.82 ± 13.6		57.45 ± 13.7		0.56
Age at SAH onset	46.03 ± 13.9		42.17 ± 11.7		43.08 ± 12.3		0.14
BMI [13]	%	n	%	n	%	n	
Underweight	3.1	1	1.9	2	2	3	
Normal weight	21.9	7	24.1	26	24	33	
Overweight	43.8	14	32.4	35	35	49	0.30
Obesity class I	21.8	7	16.7	18	18	25	
Obesity class II	9.4	3	7.4	8	8	11	
Obesity class III	0	0	1.9	2	1	2	
Did not answer	0	0	15.7	17	12	17	
Habits	%	n	%	n	%	n	
Smokers	6.2	2	12.9	14	11.4	16	0.30
Ex-smokers	40.6	13	25.9	28	29.2	41	0.23
Engages in physical activity	15.6	5	23.1	25	21.4	30	0.36
Reduces salt intake	78.1	25	94.4	102	90.7	127	0.005
Skin color/race	%	n	%	n	%	n	
Brown	34.4	11	56.5	61	51.4	72	
White	37.5	12	21.3	23	25	35	0.15
Black	15.6	5	16.7	18	16.4	23	
Asian	9.4	3	4.6	5	5.7	8	
Indigenous	3.1	1	0.9	1	1.4	2	
Educational level	%	n	%	n	%	n	
Never studied	9.4	3	6.5	7	7.1	10	
Up to 5 years in education	6.3	2	28.7	31	23.6	33	0.008
Up to 8 years in education	21.9	7	25	27	24.3	34	
Up to 11 years in education	37.5	12	33.3	36	34.3	48	
More than 11 years	25	8	6.5	7	10.7	15	
Per capita income (Mean)	R$1.535.68		R$662.55		R$862.12		0.001
Economic class [14]	%	n	%	n	%	n	
A	6.3	2	0.9	1	2.1	3	
B	68.8	22	36.1	39	43.6	61	0.001
C	18.8	6	49.1	53	42.1	59	
D	6.3	2	13.9	15	12	17	
Has health insurance	56.2	18	37.9	41	42.1	59	0.06

BMI: Body Mass Index.

health care system were not available when needed [25] [26].

This scenario is a challenge, since the majority of the Brazilian population has low incomes and is dependent on the public healthcare system for treatment and to dispense medications [27]. In common with the national situation, 88.8% of the population of Ceilândia use public health services and 98.6% seek care at healthcare centers in their own areas [10].

Table 2. Indicators of physical, financial and geographic access and acceptability of antihypertensive medications according to hypertensive residents of Ceilândia.

Indicators of physical accessibility of antihypertensive medications			
% of users with antihypertensive prescriptions who did not have access to their medication within the previous 30 days (n = 120)		14.1	(n = 17)
% of prescriptions for antihypertensive medications for which the recipient encountered some degree of difficulty in acquiring their medication (n = 198)		27.7	(n = 55)
% of the recipients who sought antihypertensive medication sat a pharmacy and could NOT obtain all the drugs they needed	SUS pharmacy (n = 68)	32.3	(n = 22)
	Private pharmacy (n = 95)	7.4	(n = 7)
	"People's Pharmacy" (n = 62)	17.7	(n = 11)
% of prescriptions for antihypertensive medications for which the recipient did not find the drug at the pharmacy (n = 163)	SUS pharmacy	12.8	(n = 21)
	Private pharmacy	2.4	(n = 4)
	"People's Pharmacy"	4.9	(n = 8)
% of responses that antihypertensive medications were not available at the pharmacy, including the responses "sometimes missing", "almost always missing" and "always missing"	SUS pharmacy (n = 67)	83.6	(n = 56)
	Private pharmacy (n = 94)	14.9	(n = 14)
	"People's Pharmacy" (n = 60)	33.3	(n = 20)
Indicators of financial accessibility of antihypertensive medications			
% of drugs for which recipient had to pay (n = 215)		35.3	(n = 76)
% of users who considered the price of medications "expensive" or "very expensive" (n = 120)		53.3	(n = 64)
% of users who did not take their medications because they were unable to pay for them (n = 120)		19.1	(n = 23)
% of users who stated that during the previous year they had been unable to buy a daily necessity, had to take out a loan or had to sell something to pay for costs incurred because of a health problem (n = 120)		12.5	(n = 15)
Indicators of geographical accessibility of antihypertensive medications			
% of users who did NOT consider it "difficult" to get to the pharmacy	SUS pharmacy (n = 68)	64.7	(n = 44)
	Private pharmacy (n = 93)	81.7	(n = 76)
	"People's Pharmacy" (n = 59)	81.4	(n = 48)
% of users who did not go to collect drugs because of difficulty of getting to pharmacy	SUS pharmacy (n = 68)	4.4	(n = 3)
	Private pharmacy (n = 94)	4.2	(n = 4)
	"People's Pharmacy" (n = 61)	3.3	(n = 2)
% of users who walk to pharmacy	SUS pharmacy (n = 68)	64.7	(n = 44)
	Private pharmacy (n = 94)	75.6	(n = 71)
	"People's Pharmacy" (n = 61)	70.5	(n = 43)
% of users who considered the pharmacy a long distance away	SUS pharmacy (n = 68)	14.7	(n = 10)
	Private pharmacy (n = 94)	3.2	(n = 3)
	"People's Pharmacy" (n = 61)	1.6	(n = 1)
Indicators of acceptability of and satisfaction with antihypertensive medications			
% of antihypertensive medications administered with which recipients stated they were satisfied (n = 203)		93.1	(n = 189)
% of antihypertensive medications administered with which recipients reported some type of discomfort or health problem related to taking the medication (n = 215)		4.7	(n = 10)

SUS = the Brazilian National Health Service (Sistema Único de Saúde).

Indicators related to financial accessibility of antihypertensive medications show that more than one third of this population pays for drugs with their own money. More than 50% of users stated that drug prices were "expensive" or "very expensive" with relation to their ability to pay, particularly for a population with an average per capita income that is close to the minimum wage. The finding that users are paying for drugs with their own money illustrates the lack of availability of these products in pharmacies belonging to the SUS and those on the "People's Pharmacy" network, which should be assured by the state since this is a right that is covered by applicable legislation and financed by the country's high rate of taxation.

As a result, almost 20% of the users failed to take the medications prescribed to treat SAH because they were unable to afford them. Access to medications can impose high costs on patients, to an extent that compromises basic requirements, if these medications cannot be acquired free of charge from the public health service [27]. Therefore, these findings are even more significant when the cost of drugs plays a decisive role on people's financial viability, whether subsidized by governments or healthcare systems, paid for by the end-user or distributed free of charge [28].

Another relevant fact is that 25% of all families in Brazil pay for private health insurance and the majority of the Brazilian population is dependent on health care provided by the Brazilian National Health Service [29]. Data from the 2008 to 2009 Family Budgets Survey (Pesquisa de Orçamentos Familiares) show that the poorest families in Brazil spend 12% of their monthly per capita income on medications, whereas the richest families spend 1.7% [30]. It was also observed that some of the residents of Ceilândia were compromising part of their family incomes to pay for private healthcare or to service loans taken out in order to recover their health, including to pay for drugs.

Data from the WHO global health report reveal that the Brazilian government's annual spending per citizen is less than the global average and that more than half of Brazilian health care spending is paid for directly from the pockets of the users [31]. On average, public spending in rich countries is more than five times what the Brazilian State spends [32]. Another finding in the WHO report is that in Brazil it is still the users who pay for health care, in the form of health insurance or private spending [31].

Inaccessibility of medications is also related to geographic barriers which are revealed by indicators of several obstacles to reaching the places where products are dispensed. Although in general the displacements required to reach pharmacies were not considered difficult by the majority of interviewees, it was among users of the pharmacies belonging to the SUS that the greatest dissatisfaction with traveling difficulties was observed, with the finding that 35% of these users are unable to get to the pharmacies on foot, which implies that they may must employ some form of transport, involving cost.

Recent studies that have investigated why people stop taking medication to treat chronic diseases found that the cost of transport and displacement is greater than the prices charged for the medications themselves and also revealed that if services and products are not available within an acceptable proximity, people decide not to use them, even if they are free [33]. Notwithstanding, it should be highlighted that the majority of the residents of Ceilândia with hypertension did not allow geographic barriers to prevent them accessing medications.

With regards to the indicators of acceptability of the antihypertensive medication and users' satisfaction with them, the great majority stated that they were satisfied with their drugs and little discomfort and few health problems related to their use were reported.

The barriers preventing access to antihypertensive medications identified in this study converge on the difficulty that the Brazilian government faces to maintain free distribution of these essential medications, in line with the goals that it has established. These factors provoked sporadic interruption or even abandonment of drug treatments. With regard specifically to antihypertensive treatments, the possibility of severe systemic repercussions are well known, such as, for example, increased risk of strokes, acute myocardial infarction and impairment of renal function leading to kidney failure, among others [34]-[36].

When correctly employed, antihypertensive medication is associated with avoidance of a large number of all causes of deaths and hospitalizations due to cardiovascular diseases [35] [36]. However, since the etiopathogenesis of hypertension is multi factorial, management of this disease is not restricted to drug treatment alone. In view of this, the epidemiological profile of residents of the city of Ceilândia who have hypertension indicates a need for additional interventions, since the majority are overweight or obese, a minority of them engage in physical activity and 40% are smokers or ex-smokers.

With regard to other variables investigated, the large imbalance in sex distribution was of note, with many more females, which may be because more women were at home and able to take part in the survey and also because they are more inclined to cooperate with research. We also found evidence that attempts to reduce dietary salt intake were more prevalent among women, while the men had higher incomes, had spent longer in education and had higher socioeconomic status. Notwithstanding, this significant difference in social and economic class was not enough to contribute to delaying onset of SAH among the men, when compared with the women, since both sexes were diagnosed with SAH in their fifth decades of life.

Several different studies have found a proportional relationship between obesity and SAH and according to the Ministry of Health, a reduction of 5% to 10% of body weight is enough to reduce blood pressure [37] [38]. Inactivity is another factor that contributes to elevated blood pressure and the correlation between inactivity, hypertension and cardiovascular mortality is well-established, which is why all guidelines on arterial hypertension recommend regular physical activity [39]. Many clinical trials have shown that reductions in blood pressure can be achieved with aerobic exercises and they are recommended for both prevention and treatment of SAH [38]. Smokers with hypertension are also more likely to develop severe forms of hypertension and they have twice the mortality of non-smokers [40].

The World Health Organization states that measures such as reducing salt intake, eating a balanced diet, practicing physical activities regularly and avoiding tobacco and harmful alcohol intake, can reduce the risk of hypertension [33]. Adopting healthy lifestyle habits contributes to prevention and treatment of chronic diseases and so the population should be encouraged to do so, in conjunction with ensuring continuous adherence to drug treatment.

Finally, there are limitations inherent to research employing population-based surveys. These are results based on self-reported measures and inaccuracies are possible. However, such surveys are an important mechanism for assessing the performance of health care systems, in dimensions such as access, utilization and degree of user satisfaction with health services.

The results reported here are an indication of the importance of investigating users' access to medications in a wider-reaching manner, considering additional dimensions that have an impact on the continuity of drug treatment. In view of the importance of the subject and of the need to improve understanding and the dimension of these issues, further similar studies should be conducted in order to support better targeting of activities in this area, expanding and improving access to medications, in order to contribute to improving the health conditions and the quality of life of the population that uses medications in this country.

5. Conclusions

Analysis of indicators of several different dimensions of access to antihypertensive medications, combined with epidemiological and behavioral data on people with SAH who are resident in Ceilândia revealed significant obstacles to the success of public health programs involving treatment of this morbidity.

Failure to keep the public health care system adequately supplied has had a negative impact on access to medications that are essential to treatment of hypertension and placed the costs on the users. Lack of access to medication results in discontinuation of treatment for hypertension, which can lead to the compensation of the disease and the serious consequences that this can have. This is a population that utilizes and is dependent on the Brazilian National Health Service for its healthcare and one which also has lifestyle habits considered to confer risk of exacerbation of the disease.

This scenario reveals a serious disconnect between pharmaceutical-based care and the social determinants of health and reveals a need for implementation of wider-ranging and more effective public policies that can ensure access to antihypertensive medications and will involve the participation of the users of the health care system in changing their habits and behaviors in order to achieve adequate and lasting control of systemic arterial hypertension.

References

[1]	Williams, B. (2009) The Year in Hypertension. *Journal of the American College of Cardiology*, **55**, 65-73. http://dx.doi.org/10.1016/j.jacc.2009.08.037

[2]	Cesarino C.B., Cipullo J.P., Martin J.F.V., *et al.* (2008) Prevalence and Sociodemographic Factors in a Hypertensive Population in São José do Rio Preto, São Paulo, Brazil. *Arquivos Brasileiros de Cardiologia*, **91**, 31-35.

[3]	Rosário T.M., Scala L.C.N.S., França G.V.A., Pereira M.R.G. and Jardim P.C.B.V. (2009) Prevalência, controle e tratamento da hipertensão arterial sistêmica em Nobres. *Arquivos Brasileiros de Cardiologia*, **93**, 672-678.

[4]   Andrade, J.P. and Nobre, F. (2010) VI Diretrizes Brasileiras de Hipertensão. *Arquivos Brasileiros de Cardiologia*, **95**, 1-51.

[5]   National Institute of Health (2012) 2012 NHLBI Morbidity and Mortality Chart Book. http://www.nhlbi.nih.gov/resources/docs/cht-book.htm

[6]   Leonel, R.B. (2010) Subsídios para a compreensão do acesso a medicamentos no Brasil. Monograph, Centro Universitário de Brasília, Brasília.

[7]   Leyva-Flores, R., Erviti-Erice, J., Kageyama-Escobar, M.L. and Arredondo, A. (1998) Prescripcion, acceso y gasto en medicamentos entre usuarios de servicios de salud en México. *Salud Publica de Mexico*, **40**, 24-31.

[8]   Lora A.P. (2004) Acessibilidade aos serviços de saúde: Estudo sobre o tema no enfoque da saúde da família no Município de Pedreira, São Paulo. Dissertation, Monograph, Universidade Estadual de Campinas, Faculdade de Ciencias Medicas, Campinas.

[9]   Penchansky, R. and Thomas, J.W. (1981) The Concept of Access: Definition and Relationship to Consumer Satisfaction. *Medical Care*, **19**, 127-140.

[10] Companhia de Planejamento do Distrito Federal (CODEPLAN) (2014) Pesquisa Distrital por Amostra de Domicílios— Distrito Federal—PDAD/DF 2013. http://www.codeplan.df.gov.br/images/CODEPLAN/PDF/pesquisa_socioeconomica/pdad/2013/Pesquisa%20PDAD-DF%202013.pdf

[11] Brasil. Censo 2010 (2010) Cadastro Nacional de endereços para fins estatísticos. http://www.censo2010.ibge.gov.br/cnefe/

[12] World Health Organization (WHO); HU(Harvard University—WHO Collaborating Center on Pharmaceutical Policies) (2007) Manual for the Household Survey to Measure Access and Use of Medicines. WHO, Geneva.

[13] World Health Organization (1998) Obesity—Presenting and Managing the Global Epidemic. Report of a WHO Consultation on Obesity, WHO, Geneve.

[14] Associação Brasileira de Empresas de Pesquisa (2002) Critério de classificação econômica do Brasil. Associação Brasileira de Empresas de Pesquisa, São Paulo.

[15] Bertoldi, A.D. (2006) Epidemiologia do acesso aos medicamentos e sua utilização em uma população assistida pelo Programa Saúde da Família. Universidade Federal de Pelotas, Pelotas.

[16] Miranda, E.S., Pinto Cdu, B., dos Reis, A.L., *et al.* (2009) Availability of Generic Drugs in the Public Sector and Prices in the Private Sector in Different Regions of Brazil. *Cadernos de Saúde Pública*, **25**, 2147-2158. http://dx.doi.org/10.1590/S0102-311X2009001000006

[17] Cameron, A., Ewen, M., Ross-Degnan, D., Ball, D. and Laing, R. (2009) Medicine Prices, Availability, and Affordability in 36 Developing and Middle-Income Countries: A Secondary Analysis. *The Lancet*, **373**, 240-249. http://dx.doi.org/10.1016/S0140-6736(08)61762-6

[18] Jacobs, B., Ir, P., Bigdeli, M., Annear, P.L. and Van Damme, W. (2012) Addressing Access Barriers to Health Services: An Analytical Framework for Selecting Appropriate Interventions in Low-Income Asian Countries. *Health Policy Plan*, **27**, 288-300. http://dx.doi.org/10.1093/heapol/czr038

[19] Helfer, A.P., Camargo, A.L., Tavares, N.U., Kanavos, P. and Bertoldi, A.D. (2012) Affordability and Availability of Drugs for Treatment of Chronic Diseases in the Public Health Care System. *Revista Panamericana de Salud Pública*, **31**, 225-232. http://dx.doi.org/10.1590/S1020-49892012000300007

[20] Araujo, J.L., Pereira, M.D., de Sa Del Fiol, F. and Barberato-Filho, S. (2014) Access to Antihypertensive Agents in Brazil: Evaluation of the "Health Has No Price" Program. *Clinical Therapeutics*, **36**, 1191-1195. http://dx.doi.org/10.1016/j.clinthera.2014.06.003

[21] Brasil. Ministério da Saúde (2014) National List of Essential Medicines: Rename. http://portalsaude.saude.gov.br/images/pdf/2015/julho/30/Rename-2014-v2.pdf

[22] Macedo, E.I., Lopes, L.C. and Barberato-Filho, S. (2011) A Technical Analysis of Medicines Request-Related Decision Making in Brazilian Courts. *Revista de Saúde Pública*, **45**, 706-713. http://dx.doi.org/10.1590/S0034-89102011005000044

[23] Santos-Pinto, C.D.B., Costa, N.R. and Osorio-de-Castro, C.G.S. (2011) Quem acessa o Programa Farmácia Popular do Brasil? Aspectos do fornecimento público de medicamentos. *Ciência & Saúde Coletiva*, **16**, 2963-2973. http://dx.doi.org/10.1590/S1413-81232011000600034

[24] Vieira, F.S. (2010) Pharmaceutical Assistance in the Brazilian Public Health Care System. *Revista Panamericana de Salud Pública*, **27**, 149-156. http://dx.doi.org/10.1590/S1020-49892010000200010

[25] Naves Jde, O. and Silver, L.D. (2005) Evaluation of Pharmaceutical Assistance in Public Primary Care in Brasilia, Brazil. *Revista de Saúde Pública*, **39**, 223-230. http://dx.doi.org/10.1590/S0034-89102005000200013

[26] Santos, V. and Nitrini, S.M. (2004) Prescription and Patient-Care Indicators in Healthcare Services. *Revista de Saúde Pública*, **38**, 819-826.

[27] Paniz, V.M.V., Fassa, A.G., Facchini, L.A., *et al.* (2008) Access to Continuous-Use Medication among Adults and the Elderly in South and Northeast Brazil. *Cadernos de Saúde Pública*, **24**, 267-280. http://dx.doi.org/10.1590/S0102-311X2008000200005

[28] Pan American Health Organization (PAHO) (2010) Access to High-Cost Medicines in the Americas: Situation, Challenges and Perspectives. http://apps.who.int/medicinedocs/documents/s19112en/s19112en.pdf

[29] Viacava, F., Souza-Junior, P.R. and Szwarcwald, C.L. (2005) Coverage of the Brazilian Population 18 Years and Older by Private Health Plans: An Analysis of Data from the World Health Survey. *Cadernos de Saúde Pública*, **21**, 119-128. http://dx.doi.org/10.1590/S0102-311X2005000700013

[30] Aurea, A.P., de Magalhães, L.C.G., Garcia, L.P., dos Santos, C.F. and de Almeida, R.F. (2011) Programas de Assistência Farmacêutica do Governo Federal: Evolução recente das compras diretas de medicamentos e primeiras evidências de sua eficiência, 2005-2008. http://repositorio.ipea.gov.br/bitstream/11058/1201/1/td_1658.pdf

[31] World Health Organization (WHO). Health Expenditure Ratios, All Countries, Selected Years Estimates by Country. http://apps.who.int/gho/data/view.main.HEALTHEXPRATIOLATESTv

[32] World Health Organization (WHO). Health Expenditure per Capita, All Countries, Selected Years Estimates by Country.

[33] Relatório Mundial de Saúde. Financiamento dos Sistemas de Saúde—O caminho para a cobertura universal. http://www.who.int/eportuguese/publications/WHR2010.pdf?ua=1

[34] Herttua, K., Tabak, A.G., Martikainen, P., Vahtera, J. and Kivimaki, M. (2013) Adherence to Antihypertensive Therapy Prior to the First Presentation of Stroke in Hypertensive Adults: Population-Based Study. *European Heart Journal*, **34**, 2933-2939. http://dx.doi.org/10.1093/eurheartj/eht219

[35] Degli Esposti, L., Saragoni, S., Benemei, S., *et al.* (2011) Adherence to Antihypertensive Medications and Health Outcomes among Newly Treated Hypertensive Patients. *ClinicoEconomics & Outcomes Research*, **3**, 47-54. http://dx.doi.org/10.2147/CEOR.S15619

[36] Sokol, M.C., McGuigan, K.A., Verbrugge, R.R. and Epstein, R.S. (2005) Impact of Medication Adherence on Hospitalization Risk and Healthcare Cost. *Medical Care*, **43**, 521-530. http://dx.doi.org/10.1097/01.mlr.0000163641.86870.af

[37] Reisin, E., Graves, J.W., Yamal, J., *et al.* (2014) Controle da pressão arterial e desfechos cardiovasculares em hipertensos com peso normal, sobrepeso e obesos tratados com três anti-hipertensivos diferentes no Estudo ALLHAT. *Revista Brasileira de Hipertensão*, **21**, 169-170.

[38] Weber, D., de Oliveira, K.R. and Colet, C.F. (2014) Adesão ao tratamento medicamentoso e não medicamentoso de hipertensos em Unidade Básica de Saúde. *Revista Brasileira de Hipertensão*, **21**, 114-121.

[39] Aziz, J.L. (2014) Sedentarismo e hipertensão arterial. *Revista Brasileira de Hipertensão*, **21**, 75-82.

[40] Virdis, A., Giannarelli, C., Neves, M.F., Taddei, S. and Ghiadoni, L. (2010) Cigarette Smoking and Hypertension. *Current Pharmaceutical Design*, **16**, 2518-2525. http://dx.doi.org/10.2174/138161210792062920

19

Prevalence of Frailty Syndrome in the Elderly and Associated Factors in Brazil

Anna Ferla Monteiro Silva Passos[1], Iris do Céu Clara Costa[2], Fábia Barbosa de Andrade[3], Maria do Carmo Eulálio[4], Anita Liberalesso Neri[5], Rômulo Lustosa Pimenteira de Melo[4], Adrianna Ribeiro Lacerda[1]

[1]Postgraduation Program in Health Sciences, Federal University of Rio Grande do Norte, Natal, Brazil
[2]Department of Dentistry, Federal University of Rio Grande do Norte, Natal, Brazil
[3]Nursing, Faculty of Health Sciencies of Trairi/Federal University of Rio Grande do Norte, Santa Cruz, Brazil
[4]Department of Psychology, State University of Paraíba, Campina Grande, Brazil
[5]Department of Educational Psychology, State University of Campinas, Campinas, Brazil
Email: annaferla@ig.com.br, iris_odontoufrn@yahoo.com.br, fabiabarbosabr@yahoo.com.br, carmitaeulalio@terra.com.br, anitalbn@uol.com.br, romulo.psiq@gmail.com, adriribeiro.cg@bol.com.br

Abstract

This paper aims to identify the prevalence of frailty syndrome and its association with demographic, economic, health, psychological and functional variables in Brazilian population. The study was cross-sectional and composed of 385 elderly aged from 65 years, an average age of 73.92 years. A multivariate Poisson regression was used to check for conditions associated with frailty and to determine the prevalence (α = 0.05). The prevalence of frailty was 8.7% and pre-frailty of 50.4%. The frail and pre-frail older adults showed larger and increasing prevalence ratios for marital status, difficulty performing instrumental activities of daily living, old age, involuntary loss of feces, depression and negative affections. These results can guide the establishment of preventive measures and the development of intervention strategies aimed at minimizing the adverse effects of frailty in elderly people.

Keywords

Aging, Frail Elderly, Frailty, Frailty Syndrome

1. Introduction

Numerous demographic and epidemiological studies have demonstrated the increasing elderly population worldwide, putting government and society on its own medical and socioeconomic challenges of population aging [1]. According to the World Health Organization (WHO) in 2025, Brazil will be the sixth country in number of elderly in the world, reaching about 32 million seniors. As a consequence, this will increase the impact on the social and economic sphere of the country, which promotes the interest of the scientific community, especially for those considered more fragile and vulnerable [2].

According to the national literature, the prevalence of frailty varies from 5% to 58%, and this increases proportionally with age [3]. Accordingly, a substantial portion of the elderly population is a carrier of health conditions that make them vulnerable to a large number of adverse events. These individuals are about to pass the barrier of cognitive and functional preservation, developing various frameworks of dependence, being classified as carriers of frailty syndrome—clinical syndrome identified by unintentional weight loss, decreased level of physical activity, reduced palm grip strength, sensation of fatigue and reduced gait velocity. Those characterized as fragile, suffering from three of these symptoms such as pre-frail of one or two non-frail those without symptoms [4].

Although there is no consensus on the definition of frailty in the elderly, there are common markers that indicate that this concept is broad and dynamic. It is characterized by both biomedical and psychosocial factors and is associated with age, decreased lean body mass, muscle strength and endurance, flexibility, balance, coordination, mobility, level of physical activity and cognitive function, increasing the risk for falls, functional decline, worsening of chronic and acute illness, hospitalization, absent or slow recovery from a clinical stage and death [3]-[6].

With the increasing elderly population, studies in health intensified, in particular those related to frailty, so that the identification of the instruments used to characterize the fragile state and enable the indication of relevant clinical markers [6] [7]. The prevalence of the elderly population's frailty has been stated in some studies through a descriptive analysis. In this study the multivariate analysis model was highlighted, in addition to increasing the association of frailty with psychological variables (negatives affections) and health variables (fecal incontinence). The early identification of characteristics associated with frailty syndrome can trigger measures to improve the quality of life of older people and prevent adverse events. Thus, the aim of this study was to identify the prevalence of Frailty Syndrome and its association with demographic, economic, health, psychological and functional variables in Brazilian population.

2. Methods

A cross-sectional study in 2009, conducted by Network FIBRA, acronym for "Frailty in Elderly Brazilians". The sample was randomly selected by cluster sampling, with the sampling unit of the urban census sectors a northeastern Brazilian city randomly selected. Subjects were recruited at their homes.

2.1. Sampling

We estimated the sample size needed to have a proportion of 50% of occurrence of a certain characteristic of the elderly population (value at which the sample size is the maximum possible for $p = 0.50$ and $q = 0.50$). The formula used was: $n = \left\{ z^2 \times \left[p \times q / (d)^2 \right] \right\}$ [8]. The calculation indicated a population of 385 elderly.

2.2. Data Collection Procedures

Data collection was performed at the agreed place during recruitment, lasting 40 - 80 minutes. Later, they were asked to sign a Statement of Form Informed Consent (SFIC). The project was approved by the Ethics Committee of the College of Medical Sciences, State University of Campinas No. 208/2007.

Through a structured questionnaire, demographics, self-reported health problems, variables functionality and psychological distress were collected. The Mini Mental State Examination (MMSE) [9], in order to identify seniors who presented cognitive deficits, which could adversely affect the reliability of answers - to the psychological measures of the cognitive screening test was used.

The criteria for inclusion and exclusion were the same used in the Cardiovascular Health Study and Women's Health and Aging Study [10] and based on studies by Fried *et al.* [11].

2.3. Techniques and Tools to Measure the Variables

To associate with the frailty phenotype four groups of variables were considered. The first demographic characteristics, with the following variables: sex, age, literacy, currently works. The second was composed of self-reported health problems, and asked if they have had a medical condition diagnosed as having hypertension and/or diabetes mellitus or if it happens to have involuntary loss of urine or feces frequently.

The third group of variables worked with tools from the Basic Activities of Daily Living (BADL) [12], Instrumental Activities of Daily Living (IADL) [13] and Advanced Activities of Daily Living (AADL) [14]. Finally, a last group of variables of psychological malaise composed by the Geriatric [15] Depression Scale and a measure of affections [16]. These instruments are described below.

The performance was evaluated using the BADL to the Independence in Activities of Daily Living developed by Sidney Katz [12], which consists of a list of six items organized hierarchically, which asked the seniors if they were totally independent, if they needed help or if they needed help to complete activities related to survival. For IADL, Instrumental Activities of Daily Living created by Lawton and Brody was used to scale on the maintenance of independent living in the household and neighborhood contexts, containing seven activities where the elderly were evaluated according to their performance and/or participation [13]. Already in assessing AADL, an inventory made based on the literature on Advanced Activities of Daily Living, which contained 12 self-report questions on the participation of older people in social roles and social life was more widely used [14].

The Geriatric Depression Scale (GDS) is recommended by the World Health Organization instrument that makes a survey of depressive disorder. His reduced form [15] consists of 15 items that verified the mood and the feeling of the subject in the last two weeks. Scores above 5 points suggests likely depression [16].

The scale of positive and negative affects consists of 14 adjectives, with response options ranging from 1 (nothing) to 5 (extremely). Six of the adjectives related to positive affects (eg. Happy, satisfied, fun, optimistic) and eight related to negative affective states (eg. Depressed, frustrated, angry). Thus, for example, the more the elderly person has experienced the negative affections in recent weeks, the higher their score. The sum of scores in positive affect could range between 5 and 30 and the sum of negative scores could range between 5 and 40 [17].

2.4. Techniques to Measure the Phenotype of Frailty

According to the Cardiovascular Health Study and the Women's Health and Aging Study [10], there are five elements of the operational or phenotype definition of frailty syndrome: 1) unintentional weight loss self-report: ≥ 4.5 kg or 5% of the body weight in the previous year; 2) assessed by self-report the fatigue evoked by two questions of a scale for depression screening, being considered the manifestation of fatigue assertion that in three or more days of the week, the elder felt it needed to make a lot of effort to account for the tasks; 3) low grip strength measured with a portable hydraulic dynamometer in the dominant hand, adjusted for sex and Body Mass Index (BMI); 4) low energy expenditure measured in metabolic equivalent (MET) and adjusted for gender, assessed from self-report physical exercise and housework performed in the last seven days, based on items from the Minnesota Leisure Time Activity Questionnaire validated for Brazil by Lustosa and adapted for this study; 5) Low gait speed indicated by the average time spent to complete three times the distance of 4.6 m, with adjustments for sex and height. For the last three criteria, frailty score for individuals that got results located between 20% of the sample [11] [18]-[22]. All self-reported measures were considered reliable, since the MMSE was used.

2.5. Data Analysis

The data were tabulated in Microsoft Excel software, being exported to the R language, version 2.15.1 and R Commander package, epicalc, lmtest and Sandwich. Initially, we tested the factor structure of the Geriatric Depression measures and Affections, with the use of measures adjustment (χ^2/gl; GFI; AGFI; CFI, RMSEA) and the internal consistency of the factors, verified by Cronbach's Alpha (α).

Subsequently, a bi-variant chi-square test (χ^2) was performed and a one way ANOVA with post hoc Tukey's test. The tests showed that less than or equal to 5% probability ($p \leq 0.05$) not to exclude the null hypothesis, were taken into account in a multivariate model, which was developed by two Poisson regressions, one where the dependent variable was not frail/pre-frail and another non frail/frail. For keeping variables in the multivariate model, we adopted the stepwise method. A robust estimator was used in the covariance matrix for more robust standards errors. The magnitude of the effects of the regressions was interpreted as a Prevalence Ratio (PR) with confidence intervals of 95%. Those who remained were in the multivariate model variables with less than or equal to 0.05 (α = 0.05) significance.

3. Results

Most of the sample is composed of females (70.12%) with an average age of 73.92 years. Regarding marital status, 46.58% of them were married and 38.23% widowed. In addition, 61.77% are literate and most (85.32%) reported they were employed.

3.1. Adjustment Measures of Affections and Geriatric Depression

Table 1 shows that the scale of affections exposes plausible fit (χ^2/gl = 2.00, GFI = 0.92, AGFI = 0.89, CFI = 0.94 and RMSEA = 0.064), corroborating the two-dimensional structure. The two factors (Positive and Negative Affections) had both alphas of α = 0.85. Similarly, the depression scale showed acceptable fit, even with the CFI Below that recommended by literature. The other parameters were within the recommended (χ^2/gl = 1.49, GFI = 0.93, AGFI = 0.91, CFI = 0.81 and RMSEA = 0.046). The alpha of the scale was of α = 0.68.

3.2. Description and Prevalence Ratios of the Frailty Phenotype

The sample exposed prevalence of pre-frail elderly of 50.4% [95% CI (45.63 - 55.36)] and the frail elderly of 8.7% [95% CI (6.33 - 11.87)]. **Table 2** presents the association between frailty profiles (non frail, pre-frail and frail) with the demographic profile. Of the five variables, only gender showed no significant association (p > 0.05) with the pre-frailty and frailty, even with women representing 71.4% of frail people. It adds to the pre-frail elderly, with significant gender being 0.07, approaching that which is accepted in this work and the majority of the literature in this area, still a consensus does not exist, it was decided by not including it in the multivariate models. The other variables, with the exception of marital status that provided no significance for the group of the pre-frail, showed significance for both groups of frailty (**Table 2**).

Table 1. Parameters of adjustment of the measurement of the affection and geriatric depression scales.

	Model	χ^2 (gl)	GFI	AGFI	CFI	RMSEA (IC 90%)
Scale of Affections	Bifactorial	150.68 (75)	0.92	0.89	0.94	0.064 (0.049 - 0.078)
Geriatric Depression Scale	Unifactorial	131.21 (88)	0.93	0.91	0.81	0.046 (0.028 - 0.062)

Notes: N = 785. χ^2 = chi-square, gl = degrees of liberty, GFI = Goodness-of-Fit Index, AGFI = Adjusted Goodness-of-Fit Index, CFI = Comparative Fit Index, RMSEA = Root-Mean-Square Error of Approximation, IC90% = Interal of Trust 90%.

Table 2. Association of the phenotype of frailty with demographic variables.

VARIABLES		NON FRAIL		PRE-FRAIL			FRAIL		
		F	%	F	%	p	F	%	p
Demographics and economics									
Sex	Male	55	35.0	53	26.1	0.07	10	28.6	0.46
	Female	102	65.0	150	73.9		25	71.4	
Age groups	65 - 69	63	40.1	48	23.6	<0.001	9	25.7	0.03
	70 - 74	50	31.8	64	31.5		8	22.9	
	75 - 79	24	15.3	40	19.7		7	20.0	
	≥80	20	12.7	51	25.1		11	31.4	
Marital Status	Maried of lives with companion	85	54.1	87	42.9	0.15	12	34.3	0.03
	Single	10	6.4	19	9.4		3	8.6	
	Divorced, separated	12	7.6	14	6.9		2	5.7	
	Widow	50	31.8	83	40.9		18	51.4	
Literate	Yes	111	70.7	118	58.1	0.01	15	42.9	0.002
	No	46	29.4	85	41.9		20	57.1	
Currently Working	Yes	31	19.7	25	12.3	0.05	2	5.7	0.05
	No	126	80.3	178	87.7		33	94.3	

Table 3 shows the association between the variables of health, functionality and psychological malaise. Those that were statistically significant were the involuntary loss of urine, involuntary loss of stool (specifically for the pre-frail phenotype), difficulties in IADL, depression, and positive and negative affections.

The variables that showed significance in the bi-variant tests were considered for the multivariate model. For the model with the outcome of non frail/pre-frail, with three variables remained significant (**Table 4**). The age

Table 3. Association of the phenotype of frailty with health, functional and psychological variables.

VARIABLES		NON FRAIL		PRE-FRAIL			FRAIL		
		F	%	F	%	p	F	%	p
Health Issues									
Hipertension	Yes	96	61.1	134	66.0	0.11	20	57.1	0.76
	No	60	38.2	65	32.0		15	42.9	
Diabetes Mellitus	Yes	17	10.8	22	10.8	0.60	7	20.0	0.098
	No	91	58.0	98	48.3		16	45.7	
Urinary Incontinence	Yes	18	11.5	41	20.2	0.002	9	25.7	0.015
	No	91	58.0	79	38.9		14	40.0	
Fecal Incontinence	Yes	3	1.9	18	8.9	0.001	3	8.6	0.065
	No	106	67.5	102	50.2		20	57.1	
Functional Capacity									
Dificulties in BADL	Little	97	61.8	101	49.8	0.18	19	54.3	0.48
	Much	12	7.6	21	10.3		4	11.4	
Dificulties in IADL	Little	104	66.2	107	52.7	0.038	13	37.1	<0.01
	Much	5	3.2	15	7.4		10	28.6	
AADL	0.00	17	10.8	20	9.9		3	8.6	
	1.00	25	15.9	24	11.8		4	11.4	
	2.00	22	14.0	27	13.3	0.49	6	17.1	0.36
	3.00	15	9.6	23	11.3		1	2.9	
	4.00	17	10.8	10	4.9		4	11.4	
	>5	13	8.3	18	8.9		5	14.3	
Psychological Variables									
Depression	m (dp)	2.72 (2.02)[a]		4.28 (2.55)[b]			5.39 (2.80)[b]		<0.001
Positive Affections	m (dp)	22.27 (3.63)[a]		21.16 (4.02)[a]			20.04 (3.22)[b]		0.013
Negative Affections	m (dp)	15.15 (5.11)[a]		17.74 (5.50)[b]			20 (5.13)[b]		<0.001

BADL: Basic Activities of Daily Living; IADL: Instrumental Activities of Daily Living; AADL: Advanced Activities of Daily Living; a, b, c: different letters, represent significant differences, verified by the post hoc Turkey test (p < 0.05).

Table 4. Multivariate model for the non frail/pre-frail outcomes.

Pre frAIl		B	Std. Error	Sig.	RP	95% IC	
						Lower	Upper
Age Group	Between 65 - 69 years	0[a]	.	.		.	.
	Between 70 - 74 years	0.10	0.05	0.05	1.10	1.00	1.21
	Between 75 - 79 years	0.15	0.05	0.01	1.16	1.037	1.30
	Less than 80 years	0.15	0.06	0.02	1.16	1.029	1.31
Literate	Yes	0[a]	.	.		.	.
	No	0.07	0.04	0.09	1.07	0.98	1.16
Fecal incontinence	No	0[a]	.	.		.	.
	Yes	0.13	0.05	0.01	1.14	1.029	1.26
Depression		0.03	0.01	0.01	1.03	1.017	1.05

0[a]: Parameter of Reference.

groups of older exposed higher prevalence of pre-frail group of the elderly between 65 and 69 years. The elderly who reported involuntary loss of feces also were significantly more prevalent, and finally, the data shows that the higher the scores on depression, the more frequent are the pre-frail.

The data relating to the multivariate model for non frail/frail outcome are shown in **Table 5**. In it, four variables remained statistically significant. The single, married and widowed had a higher prevalence of frailty compared to separate elderly. In addition, older people have more difficulty in IADL and showed a higher prevalence in frailty, as well as higher scores of depression and negative affections.

4. Discussion

Frailty Syndrome was found in 59.1% of the elderly studied. A systematic review [6] observed in the analysis of 18 studies, a wide variation in prevalence of frailty in general from 6.9% to 21% for the frail state and 33% to 55% for pre-frail state. The prevalence of frailty (8.7%) and pre-frailty (50.4%) values were slightly above those observed in a survey of elderly North Americans: pre-frail (7%) and frail (47%) [10]. An investigation on 993 Spanish elderly over 70 years showed much higher results for the weakness (16.9%) [23]. Similar numbers were found in a study involving 601 community-dwelling elderly in the Brazilian city of Belo Horizonte (8.7%) [24]. This wide variation may be attributed to the use of different models and methodology for identifying weak phenotypes, in addition to existing social and economic realities in different samples.

Among the demographic variables, a higher prevalence of pre-frailty in elderly people with older ages was identified. These data corroborate the national level [24] investigations and international [11] [23]-[25] linking the fragility of old age. Its association with advancing age has no explanation for the characteristic of the aging process, in which physiological changes in neuro-muscular-skeletal function and all body systems suffer losses and occur both in the structural and functional aspects [25]. It was also observed that poor socioeconomic and educational conditions, little formal education and low income characteristics are present in most debilitated people [26].

Association between frailty and marital status was found, since, single, widowed and married elderly had a higher prevalence to be a frail elderly when compared to separate ones. In the scientific literature, studies to a discussion of the relationship between these variables were not found.

The relationship between frailty and comorbidities can be determined by immunological dysfunction, neuro-endocrine deregulation and chronic inflammatory processes, as well as organic structural changes predisposing individuals to diseases such as hypertension, diabetes mellitus, cerebral vascular accident, renal failure, osteoarthritis and depression [4] [11].

Among the conditions associated with a significantly higher prevalence of frailty and pre-frailty have fecal incontinence and depression. Unpublished data found in this study was the association between frailty and involuntary loss of stool in the elderly indicating a significance not reported in the literature on the topic: high prevalence of pre-frailty (1.14 times) among the elderly who have fecal incontinence compared to elderly people who have the same condition. Among morbidities investigated in a cross-sectional descriptive Brazilian survey

Table 5. Multivariate model for the non frail/frail outcomes.

FRAILTY		B	Std. Error	Sig	RP	IC 95%	
						Lower	Upper
Marital Status	Separated	0[a]	.	.		.	.
	Single	0.50	0.18	0.01	1.64	1.16	2.32
	Married	0.34	0.11	0.01	1.41	1.13	1.75
	Widow	0.43	0.13	0.01	1.54	1.20	1.97
Fecal incontinence	No	0[a]	.	.		.	.
	Yes	0.27	0.18	0.10	1.31	0.93	1.84
Difficulty in IADL	Little	0[a]	.	.		.	.
	A lot	0.45	0.13	0.01	1.57	1.22	2.03
Depression		0.05	0.02	0.01	1.06	1.01	1.10
Negative Affections		0.02	0.01	0.04	1.02	1.00	1.03

0[a]: Parameter of Reference; IADL: Instrumental Activities of Daily Living.

[27] the following prevalence were found: 13.4% for depression and 5.6% for fecal incontinence.

The true incidence of this disorder channel is not accurate, however, it is estimated that may affect up to 5% of the general population, with higher prevalence in the elderly and women [28]. Chronic morbidities, particularly those associated with pain and/or loss of function, often added in the elderly and are most commonly involved with the occurrence of frailty [29].

More research is needed to examine the prevalence of fecal incontinence with frailty, since few studies have been found in the scientific literature and the pathogenesis of this condition may be present in old age or diseases associated with belonging to the clinical and surgical areas.

Depressive symptoms were strongly associated with frailty syndrome. Elderly people with depression had higher prevalence for frailty and pre-frailty compared with those who did not have depression. The growing trend of depression and weakness is reinforced by several studies [24] [30].

Depression is considered as one of the most frequent agents of emotional distress and significant decrease in the quality of life in old age. The occurrence of psychiatric symptoms increases with age and both levels of satisfaction with the levels of positive and negative emotions are influenced by biological, social and intra-psychic vulnerability inherent in the elderly [26].

In this sense, considering a possible psychosocial or psychological component as a predisposing factor of fragility, there seems to be a relationship between negative affections and the prevalence of the same. This study reveals an innovative way that elderly people that have a higher score in negative affections are more prevalent to be a frail elderly. Although negative affect components and frailty in the elderly has not been disclosed previously, it is remarkable that their respective theoretical concepts are different but interrelated.

The findings of this study corroborate international studies [5] [11] and national [24] the extent that they also found a significant association between difficulty in performing IADL with frailty. In a study in the United States, the results suggested that, the beginning of the frailty syndrome, it affects the more complex routine activities and less so the simplest routine activities [11]. In it the authors found 59.7% of frail elderly with difficulty to perform IADL.

In the current research, those with difficulty performing IADL showed a higher prevalence of frailty. The relationship between disability and frailty is evident primarily in IADL and a loss in these contributes to the reduction of advanced activities of daily living related to the social environment, cultural, religious, political and labor with tendency to isolation, corroborating research conducted in different populations [5] [24].

In the studied population, the prevalence of frailty in numbers is similar to other studies found. Among elderly surveyed, we identified factors associated with frailty syndrome, as that in the presence of it have higher chances for adverse health conditions.

5. Conclusions

Understanding relationships with certain variables that showed significance was limited. In this sense, it is suggested to conduct further research to allow other interpretations. Importantly, the investigation will continue, this is the first study of a longitudinal research on indicators of frailty. The multivariate model used shows that it is necessary to consider not only biological, but also psychological factors for understanding Frailty Syndrome.

The results show that the apprehension of signs and symptoms that are predictors of frailty in elderly aids in the development of strategies and interventions aimed at minimizing the adverse effects to the health of the elderly, which represents an essential step in the quest for improved quality of life.

Acknowledgements

The manuscript received financial support from the National Research Council—CNPq, the Coordination Development of Higher Education Personnel—CDHEP, the Foundation for Research Support of the State of São Paulo—FRSSSP and the Foundation for Research Support of the State of Rio Grande do Sul—FRSSRGS. All authors contributed to the completion of the study and participated in the analysis, interpretation of data, drafting and critical revision and agreed on the final version.

Disclosure

I declare that neither I nor the other authors or any first degree relative, possess financial and personal interests in the subject matter discussed in the manuscript. No potential conflicts of interest were disclosed.

References

[1] Veras, R. (2009) Envelhecimento populacional contemporâneo: Demandas, desafios e inovações. *Revista de Saúde Pública*, **43**, 548-554. http://dx.doi.org/10.1590/S0034-89102009000300020

[2] Ota, A., Yasuda, N., Horikawa, S., Fujimura, T. and Ohara, H. (2007) Differential Effects of Power Rehabilitation on Physical Performance and Higher-Level Functional Capacity among Community-Dwelling Older Adults with a Slight Degree of Frailty. *Journal of Epidemiology*, **17**, 61-67. http://dx.doi.org/10.2188/jea.17.61

[3] Sternberg, S.A., Wershof, S.A., Karunananthan, S., Bergman, H. and Mark, C.A. (2011) The Identification of Frailty: A Systematic Literature Review. *Journal of the American Geriatrics Society*, **59**, 2129-2138. http://dx.doi.org/10.1111/j.1532-5415.2011.03597.x

[4] Oliveira, D.R., Bettinelli, L.A., Pasqualotti, A., Corso, D., Brock, F. and Erdmann, A.L. (2013) Prevalence of Frailty Syndrome in Old People in a Hospital Institution. *Revista Latino Americana de Enfermagem*, **21**, 891-898. http://dx.doi.org/10.1590/S0104-11692013000400009

[5] Fried, P.L., Ferrucci, L., Darer, J., Williamson, J.D. and Anderson, G. (2004) Untangling the Concepts of Disability, Frailty, and Comorbidity: Implications for Improved Targeting and Care. *Journal of Gerontology: Medical Sciences*, **59**, 255-263. http://dx.doi.org/10.1093/gerona/59.3.m255

[6] Tribess, S. and Oliveira, R.J. (2011) Biological Fragility Syndrome in the Elderly: Systematic Review. *Revista de Salud Pública*, **13**, 853-864. http://dx.doi.org/10.1590/S0124-00642011000500014

[7] Remor, C.B., Bós, A.J.G. and Werlang, M.C. (2011) Características relacionadas ao perfil de fragilidade no idoso. *Scientia Medica*, **21**, 107-112.

[8] Silva, N.N. (2001) Amostragem probabilística: Um curso introdutório. 2nd Edition, EdUSP, São Paulo.

[9] Brucki, S.M.D., Nitrini, R., Caramelli, P., Bertolucci, P.H.F. and Okamoto, I.H. (2003) Sugestões para o uso do mini-exame do estado mental no Brasil. *Arquivos de Neuropsiquiatria*, **61**, 777-778. http://dx.doi.org/10.1590/S0004-282X2003000500014

[10] Ferrucci, L., Guralnik, J.M., Studenski, S., Fried, L.P., Cutler Jr., G.B. and Walston, J.D. (2004) Designing Randomized, Controlled Trials Aimed at Preventing or Delaying Functional Decline and Disability in Frail, Older Persons: A Consensus Report. *Journal of the American Geriatrics Society*, **52**, 625-634. http://dx.doi.org/10.1111/j.1532-5415.2004.52174.x

[11] Fried, L.P., Tangen, C.M., Walston, J., Newman, A.B., Hirsch, C., Gottdiener, J., *et al.* (2001) Frailty in Older Adults: Evidence for a Phenotype. *Journal of Gerontology: Medical Sciences*, **56**, 146-157. http://dx.doi.org/10.1093/gerona/56.3.m146

[12] Katz, S., Ford, A.B., Moskowitz, R.W., Jackson, B.A. and Jaffe, M.W. (1963) Studies of Illness in the Aged. The Index of ADL: A Standardized Measure of Biological and Psychosocial Function. *The Journal of the American Medical Association*, **185**, 914-919. http://dx.doi.org/10.1001/jama.1963.03060120024016

[13] Lawton, M.P. and Brody, E.M. (1969) Assessment of Older People: Self-Maintaining and Instrumental Activities of Daily Living. *Gerontologist*, **9**, 179-186. http://dx.doi.org/10.1093/geront/9.3_Part_1.179

[14] Reuben, D.B., Laliberte, L., Hiris, J. and Mor, V. (1990) A Hierarquical Exercise Scale to Measure Function at the Advanced Activities of Daily Living (AADL) Level. *Journal of the American Geriatrics Society*, **38**, 855-861. http://dx.doi.org/10.1111/j.1532-5415.1990.tb05699.x

[15] Yesavage, J.A., Brink, T.L., Rose, T.L., Lum, O., Huang, V., Adey, M. and Leirer, V.O. (1983) Development and Validation of a Geriatric Depression Screening Scale: A Preliminary Report. *Journal of Psychiatric Research*, **17**, 37-49. http://dx.doi.org/10.1016/0022-3956(82)90033-4

[16] Almeida, O.P. and Almeida, S.A. (1999) Confiabilidade da versão brasileira da Escala de Depressão em Geriatria (GDS) versão reduzida. *Arquivos de Neuropsiquiatria*, **57**, 421-426. http://dx.doi.org/10.1590/S0004-282X1999000300013

[17] Siqueira, M.M.M., Martins, M.C.F. and Moura, O.I. (1999) Construção e validação fatorial da EAPN: Escala de Ânimo Positivo e Negativo. *Revista da Sociedade de Psicologia do Triângulo Mineiro*, **2**, 34-40.

[18] Fried, L.P. and Walston, J.M. (2003) Frailty and Failure to Thrive. In: Hazzard, W.R., Blass, J.P., Ettinger Jr., W.H., Halter, J.B. and Ouslander, J., Eds., *Principles of Geriatric Medicine and Gerontology*, 5th Edition, MacGraw-Hill, New York, 1487-1502.

[19] Batistoni, S.S.T., Neri, A.L. and Cupertino, A.P.F.B. (2010) Validade e confiabilidade da versão Brasileira da Center for Epidemiological Scale-Depression (CES-D) em idosos Brasileiros. *Psico-USF*, **15**, 13-22. http://dx.doi.org/10.1590/S1413-82712010000100003

[20] Rauen, M.S., Moreira, E.A.M., Calvo, M.C.M. and Lobo, A.S. (2008) Avaliação do estado nutricional de idosos institucionalizados. *Revista de Nutrição*, **21**, 303-310. http://dx.doi.org/10.1590/S1415-52732008000300005

[21] Ainsworth, B.E., Haskell, W.L., Whitt, M.C., Irwin, M.L., Swartz, A.M., Strath, S.J., *et al.* (2000) Compendium of Physical Activities: An Update of Activity Codes and MET Intensities. *Medicine and Sciences in Sports and Exercise*, **32**, S498-S516. http://dx.doi.org/10.1097/00005768-200009001-00009

[22] Guralnik, J.M., Simonsick, E.M., Ferrucci, L., Glynn, R.J., Berkman, L.F. and Blazer, D.G. (1994) A Short Physical Performance Battery Assessing Lower Extremity Function: Association with Self-Reported Disability and Prediction of Mortality and Nursing Home Admission. *Journal of Gerontology: Medical Sciences*, **49**, 85-94. http://dx.doi.org/10.1093/geronj/49.2.M85

[23] Abizanda, P., Romero, L., Sánchez-Jurado, P.M., Martínez-Reig, M., Gómez-Arnedo, L. and Alfonso, S.A. (2013) Frailty and Mortality, Disability and Mobility Loss in a Spanish Cohort of Older Adults: The FRADEA Study. *Maturitas*, **74**, 54-60. http://dx.doi.org/10.1016/j.maturitas.2012.09.018

[24] Vieira, R.A., Guerra, R.O., Giacomin, K.C., de Souza Vasconcelos, K.S., de Souza Andrade, A.C., Pereira, L.S.M., *et al.* (2013) Prevalência de fragilidade e fatores associados em idosos comunitários de Belo Horizonte, Minas Gerais, Brasil: dados do estudo FIBRA. *Cadernos de Saúde Pública*, **29**, 1631-1643. http://dx.doi.org/10.1590/S0102-311X2013001200015

[25] Lenardt, M.H., Carneiro, N.H.K., Betiolli, S.E., de Melo Neu Ribeiro, D.K. and Wachholz, P.A. (2013) Prevalence of Pre-Frailty for the Component of Gait Speed in Older Adults. *Revista Latino Americana de Enfermagem*, **21**, 734-741. http://dx.doi.org/10.1590/S0104-11692013000300012

[26] Neri, A.L. (Orgs.) (2013) Fragilidade e Qualidade de Vida na Velhice. Editora Alínea, Campinas.

[27] Faria, C.A., Lourenço, R.A., Ribeiro, P.C.C. and Lopes, C.S. (2013) Desempenho cognitivo e fragilidade em idosos clientes de operadora de saúde. *Revista de Saúde Pública*, **47**, 923-930. http://dx.doi.org/10.1590/S0034-8910.2013047004451

[28] Fruehauf, H. and Fox, M.R. (2012) Anal Manometry in the Investigation of Fecal Incontinence: Totum pro parte, not pars pro toto. *Digestion*, **86**, 75-77. http://dx.doi.org/10.1159/000339633

[29] Lang, P.O., Michel, J.P. and Zekry, D. (2009) Frailty Syndrome: A Transitional State in a Dynamic Process. *Gerontology*, **55**, 539-549. http://dx.doi.org/10.1159/000211949

[30] Guerrero-Escobedo, P., Tamez-Rivera, O., Amieva, H. and Avila-Funes, J.A. (2014) Frailty Is Associated with Low Self-Esteem in Elderly Adults. *Journal of the American Geriatrics Society*, **62**, 396-398. http://dx.doi.org/10.1111/jgs.12679

20

Determinants of Treatment Delays among Pulmonary Tuberculosis Patients in Enugu Metropolis, South-East, Nigeria

Omotowo Ishola Babatunde[1*], Eke Christopher Bismark[2], Nwobi Emmanuel Amaechi[1], Eyisi Ifeanyi Gabriel[1], Agwu-Umahi Rebecca Olanike[1]

[1]Department of Community Medicine, College of Medicine, University of Nigeria, Enugu, Nigeria
[2]Department of Paediatrics, College of Medicine, University of Nigeria, Enugu, Nigeria
Email: *babatundeomotowo@yahoo.com

Abstract

Introduction: Globally, the burden of Tuberculosis is escalating. Early diagnosis and prompt initiation of treatment are essential to achieve an effective tuberculosis control programme. Objective: To investigate the duration of delay for treatment and assess the determinants of treatment delays among pulmonary tuberculosis patients in Enugu metropolis, South-East, Nigeria. Methods: This cross sectional study was conducted among 219 pulmonary tuberculosis patients in six randomly selected DOTS centres in the three LGAs in Enugu metropolis. Data were analysed using SPSS version 17, and statistical significance of association between variables was assessed using Chi-square test at p < 0.05. STATA version 13.1 was used to calculate the positive predictors of TB treatment delays using logistic regression. Ethical clearance was obtained from the Health Research Ethics Committee of UNTH and verbal informed consent was obtained from the participants. Results: Overall, 291 respondents took part in the study, 55.7% were males, 84.4% were aged between 16 to 60 years, while their mean age was 35.4 ± 12.6 years. Most of the participants 32.9%, 26.9%, 15.5% were traders, civil servants, and students respectively. Among the respondents, 3.6% knew that Mycobacterium tuberculosis is the cause of tuberculosis. Among the participants, only 23.3% presented for first appropriate treatment consultation within 1 - 30 days of onset of symptoms. The reasons given by the respondents for the delay are: ignorance of necessity treatment (36.1%), Lack of money (24.2%), no health facility close to the house (13.2%), and other reasons 26.5%. Delay in treatment was found to be significantly associated with HIV status (X^2 = 23.412, df = 8, p = 0.003), knowledge of the cause of TB (X^2 = 42.322, df = 28, p = 0.040), TB symptoms experienced (X^2 = 46.857, df = 20, p = 0.001), occupation (X^2 = 34.217, df = 20, p = 0.025), and distance of the health facility from the respondents' residence (X^2 = 34.908, df = 8, p = 0.000). The positive predictors of delayed treatment, using logistic regression, were first presentation at: patent medicine

---

*Corresponding author.

dealer (OR 12.3 CI: 3.22 - 36.23), private hospital (OR 10.6 CI: 5.73 - 17.94), prayer house (OR 7.2 CI: 2.75 - 23.64), and traditional healer (OR 11.9 CI: 6.87 - 32.85). Conclusion: Majority of TB patients in this study did not present early to health facilities. The positive predictors of delayed presentation for appropriate PTB treatment were first presentations at inappropriate treatment centres. There is need to intensify public health awareness among potential TB patients on the associated risks of treatment delay to prevent transmission. Unskilled health care providers should refer suspected PTB patients promptly to facilitate their treatment.

Keywords

Determinants, Delay, Tuberculosis

1. Introduction

Approximately one third of the world's population are infected with tuberculosis bacilli and at risk of developing active tuberculosis (TB) [1]. In 2012, there were an estimated 13 million TB cases, including 8.6 million incident cases and 1.3 million died from the disease [1]. Smear-positive pulmonary TB, the most likely source of TB transmission in the community constitutes 35% of new TB cases.

Most tuberculosis patients were not visiting health facility but transmit disease to healthy individuals in the community for longer time in Nigeria [2] [3]. Nigeria is ranked 13th among the 22 high burden countries for TB in the world and 3rd in Africa [1] [2]. The 2012 national TB prevalence survey in Nigeria revealed that 75% of the previously undetected cases had sputum smear positive [1] [2].

Early diagnosis of the disease and prompt initiation of treatment are essential for an effective tuberculosis control programme. Delay in the diagnosis may worsen the disease, increase the risk of death and enhance tuberculosis transmission in the community [4]. Also, it is estimated that an untreated smear-positive patient can infect between ten and fifteen contacts annually, and over 20 during the natural history of the disease until death [2] [5]-[7]. The importance of having effective methods of early detection and prompt treatment of the cases in the communities cannot be ignored [7].

Studies conducted in several countries have shown that patient and health care delay are major problems in the control of tuberculosis. The study conducted at the North Middlesex University, London, UK reported median patient related delay between 34.5 and 54 days, median health related delay was 29.5 days [8]. Considerable delays were observed in the studies done in Japan [9] [10]. Median patient delay of 60 days was documented in a study conducted in Tanzania [11].

Studies conducted in Ibadan and Lagos in South-West, Nigeria revealed high prevalence of treatment delay among pulmonary TB patients [3] [12]. These delays are attributable to patients and doctors. Another study from Nigeria showed that the mean patient delay was 13.2 ± 7.4 weeks [13]. Causes of these delays should be investigated to be able to control TB effectively. Our study was aimed at estimating duration of delay for treatment by pulmonary TB patients in Enugu metropolis and assessing the determinants of patient related factors associated with the treatment delays.

2. Methods

2.1. Background

The study was conducted among pulmonary tuberculosis patients in Enugu metropolis. Enugu is the capital of old Eastern region, and current Enugu state in south-east, Nigeria, with estimated population of 722,664 people. The metropolis has three Local Government Areas which are Enugu east, Enugu south and Enugu north. There are sixteen DOTS centres in Enugu metropolis. In Enugu state, tuberculosis is treated free. Diagnosis and treatment of TB patients are according to the National Tuberculosis Control Programme guidelines. All the DOTS centres treat both sputum smear positive and sputum smear negative pulmonary TB cases. All presumptive TB cases (TB suspects) submit two sputum samples by using spot-early morning approach for sputum smear microscopy, and also do HIV counselling. A sputum smear positive TB case is when one or two samples are positive [2]. The laboratory diagnosis of TB rests mainly on the identification of the tubercle bacilli in a clinical specimen by using any of the following laboratory methods available; microscopy, culture or new molecular tests e.g. Gene Xpert MTB/RIF and line probe assays [2]. Smear negative cases are diagnosed on clinical findings, and chest x ray. All new pulmonary TB patients who were diagnosed were recruited into our study.

2.2. Study Design

A cross sectional study was conducted among all new pulmonary tuberculosis patients who were diagnosed and commenced treatment during February 1 to October 30, 2014 in six randomly selected among the sixteen DOTS centres in the three local government areas in Enugu metropolis. All patients that participated in the study are new as part of the inclusion criteria, while all extra-pulmonary tuberculosis patients were excluded. All the subjects were interviewed using structured questionnaire. The questions were pretested and the interviewers were supervised regularly throughout the duration of the study. All the questions were closed and included socio-demographic characteristics, knowledge of pulmonary tuberculosis which includes tuberculosis symptoms, transmission and treatment. Also, they were asked duration of symptoms before first visit to the health facility, places they sought for treatment before first visit to the health facility, reasons for delay before visit to the health facility and distance from their residence to the health facility.

2.3. Definitions of Different Types of Delays

Patient delay is when the time interval from the appearance of the major pulmonary TB symptoms until the first visit to a medical facility exceeds 30 days. Health facility referral delay is when the time interval between the first visit to a health facility and the time the patient is seen at any health facility with DOTS services exceed two days. Diagnosis delay is when the time between first consultation at a health facility with DOTS services and a time when a definitive diagnosis of tuberculosis is made exceeded three days. Treatment delay is when interval between the time of diagnosis and treatment initiation exceeded one day. Health facility delay is when the time interval from when the patients were first seen at health facility with DOTS and treatment initiation exceeded five days. Total delay is the sum of patient delay and health service delay [11] [14].

2.4. Ethical Approval

Ethical approval was obtained from Health Research Ethics Committee of University of Nigeria Teaching Hospital (UNTH), Enugu. Permission was obtained from National TB Control Programme, Enugu State, Heads of all the health centres, and DOTS providers in the facilities used for the study.

Verbal informed consent was obtained from all study participants after explaining benefits of the study and assurance of confidentiality.

2.5. Data Analysis

Data collected from 219 pulmonary TB patients was analysed using SPSS version17 and statistical significance of association between variables was assessed using Chi-square test at $p < 0.05$. The positive predictors of delayed treatment were calculated by STATA version 13.1. Also, the Odds Ratio and Confidence Interval were calculated to identify the factors associated with the delay in seeking treatment using bivariate and multivariate logistic regression analysis. Variables that were significant at a level of up 10% on bivariate analysis were included in multivariate logistic regression.

3. Results

3.1. Socio-Demographic Characteristics of the Study Participants

A total of 219 newly diagnosed pulmonary tuberculosis patients (PTB) were enrolled in the 10 months study period, of which 122 (55.7%) were males and 97 (44.3%) were females. The mean age was 35.4 ± 12.6 years. Among the study participants, One hundred and fifty nine (72.6%) had sputum smear positive, while 60 (27.3%) were HIV positive. Most of the participants: 72 (32.9%), 59 (26.9%), 34 (15.5%) were traders, civil servants, and students respectively, while 15 (6.8%) were unemployed. With regards to education 15 (6.8%) had no formal education, 33 (15.1%) completed primary education, while 83 (37.9%) and 88 (40.2%) had secondary and tertiary education respectively. Majority of the participants 177 (80.8%) are Igbos, while Yorubas and Hausas were 19 (8.7%) and 11 (5%) respectively. Also, majority of the participants 94 (42.9%) had income of less than

N40,000 ($200) per annum, while only 3 (1.4%) had income >1,000,000 naira (>$5000) per annum. The most prominent religion among the participants is Christianity 183 (83.6%), while 20 (9.1%) and 15 (6.8%) were Muslims and African traditional worshipers respectively. One hundred and three participants (47%) had more than 5 individuals per household, while 30 (13.7%) and 86 (39.3%) had between 1 - 2 and 3 - 5 individuals per household (**Table 1**).

Table 1. Socio-demographic characteristics of the participants and duration of delay.

VARIBLES	CATEGORY	DELAYED DURATION (>30 Days)		DURATION (≤30 Days)		TOTAL	
		N	%	N	%	N	%
Sex	Male	92	75.4	30	24.6	122	55.7
	Female	61	62.9	36	37.1	97	44.3
Age grp (Years)	0 - 15	5	71.5	2	28.5	7	3.2
	>15 - 30	46	68.6	21	31.4	67	30.6
	>30 - 45	76	92.7	6	7.3	82	37.4
	>45 - 60	24	66.7	12	33.3	36	16.4
	>60	20	74.1	7	25.9	27	12.3
Marital Status	Single	65	90.3	7	9.7	72	32.9
	Married	98	77.8	28	22.2	126	57.5
	Divorced	3	60.0	2	40.0	5	2.3
	Widowed	11	73.3	4	26.7	15	6.8
	Not Documented	1	100	0	0	1	0.5
Occupation	Student	21	61.8	13	38.2	34	15.5
	Civil Servant	31	52.6	28	47.3	59	26.9
	Trader	57	79.2	15	20.8	72	32.9
	House wife	3	42.8	4	57.2	7	3.2
	Unemployed	9	60.0	6	40.0	15	6.8
	Others	21	65.6	11	34.4	32	14.7
Education Level	No formal education	13	86.7	2	13.3	15	6.8
	Primary	28	84.8	5	15.2	33	15.1
	Secondary	59	71.1	24	28.9	83	37.9
	Tertiary	68	77.3	20	22.7	88	40.2
Tribe	Igbo	143	80.8	34	19.2	177	80.8
	Yoruba	8	42.1	11	57.9	19	8.7
	Hausa	8	72.7	3	27.3	11	5.0
	Others	7	58.3	5	41.7	12	5.4
Religion	Christianity	98	53.6	85	46.4	183	83.6
	Islam	12	60.0	8	40.0	20	9.1
	African traditional religion	7	46.7	8	53.3	15	6.8
	Others	1	100	0	0	1	0.5
Annual income	<N40,000	46	48.9	48	51.1	94	42.9
	>N40,000 - 80,000	28	62.2	17	37.8	45	20.5
	>N80,000 - 1000,000	39	50.6	38	49.4	77	35.2
	>N1000,000	2	66.7	1	33.3	3	1.4
No of individual per household	1 - 2	17	56.7	13	43.3	30	13.7
	3 - 5	37	43.0	49	57.0	86	39.3
	>5	74	71.8	29	28.2	103	47.0

3.2. Knowledge and Symptoms Experienced by the Study Participants.

Table 2 shows that majority of the participants 30.6%, 21.9% and 21.9% believed that alcohol, smoking and dust are the causes of TB respectively, while only 0.9% knew that mycobacterium tuberculosis is the cause. Also, most of the participants (93.1%) knew that cough is a symptom. Among the participants, 83.1%, 11.8% and 0.9% knew that TB can be transmitted through cough, sneezing and talking respectively, while 4.2% believed sharing of spoons or cups could transmit it. Majority of the participants (94.9%) experienced cough, but 0.9%, 0.55 and 1.9% experienced haemoptysis, weight loss and night fever respectively.

3.3. Facilities First Attended and Delay by TB Patients

The facilities patients first visited included patent medicine dealer: 75 (34.2%), hospital: 83 (37.9%), prayer house: 14 (6.4%), traditional healers: 19 (8.7%), while those that visited other places were 28 (12.8%) (**Table 3**).
Among the study participants, 168 (76.7%) delayed presentation to the DOTS facilities. The study also

Table 2. Knowledge and symptoms experienced by the study participants.

VARIBLES	CATEGORY	DELAYED DURATION (>30 Days)		DURATION (≤30 Days)		TOTAL	
		N	%	N	%	N	%
Causes of TB	Alcohol	40	59.7	27	40.3	67	30.6
	Smoking	29	60.4	19	39.6	48	21.9
	Mycobacterium TB	0	0	2	100	2	0.9
	Dust	18	37.5	30	62.5	48	21.9
	Witchcraft	5	33.3	10	66.7	15	6.9
	Others	24	61.5	15	38.5	39	17.8
Symptoms of TB	Cough	106	51.9	98	48.1	204	93.1
	Cough up of blood	4	66.7	2	33.3	6	2.8
	Weight loss	1	33.3	2	66.7	3	1.4
	Fever at night	1	25.0	3	75.0	4	1.8
	Difficulty in breathing	1	50.0	1	50.0	2	0.9
Spread of Tb	Coughing	72	45.1	110	54.9	182	83.1
	Sneezing	12	46.2	14	53.8	26	11.8
	Speaking	0	0	2	100	2	0.9
	Sharing spoons or cups	6	66.7	3	33.3	9	4.2
TB is always associated with HIV	No	50	65.8	26	34.2	76	34.7
	Yes	29	30.5	66	69.5	95	43.4
	Don't Know	26	54.2	22	45.8	48	21.9
Symptoms experienced	Cough	76	36.5	132	63.5	208	94.9
	Coughing up blood	1	50.0	1	50.0	2	0.9
	Weight loss	1	100	0	0	1	0.5
	Fever at night	1	25	3	75	4	1.9
	Fatigue	1	50	1	50	2	0.9
	Chest pain	0	0	2	100	2	0.9

Table 3. Facilities TB patients go first.

VARIBLES	CATEGORY	DELAYED DURATION (>30 Days)		DURATION (≤30 Days)		TOTAL	
		N	%	N	%	N	%
Facilities they go first	Patent medicine dealer	52	69.3	23	30.7	75	34.2
	Hospital	49	59.0	34	41	83	37.9
	Prayer house	6	42.9	8	57.1	14	6.4
	Traditional healers	10	52.6	9	47.4	19	8.7
	Others	15	53.6	13	46.4	28	12.8

revealed that 75 (34.3%), 32 (14.6%), and 24 (10.9%) delayed treatment for 6 weeks, 8 weeks, and 12 weeks respectively; while 37 (16.9%) delayed for more than 16 weeks.

Reasons given by the respondents for delay included lack of money 53 (24.2%), long distance of health facility from residence 79 (36.1%), Thirty eight (17.3%) felt it was not necessary to seek treatment. Lack of awareness of DOTS 24 (10.9%), while those that gave other reasons were 25 (11.5%) (**Table 4**).

Patient's delay was found to be significantly associated with HIV status (X^2 = 23.412, P = 0.003), distance of DOTS facility from the patient's residence (X^2 = 34.908, P = 0.000), symptoms experienced by TB patients (X^2 = 46.857, P = 0.001), knowledge about the causes of TB (X^2 = 42.322, P = 0.040) and occupation of the participants (X^2 = 34.217, P = 0.025). However, the study revealed that patients' delays were not significantly associated with age (X^2 = 24.057, P = 0.088), level of educational (X^2 = 20.194, P = 0.064) and sex of the patients (X^2 = 1.310, P = 0.861) (**Table 5**).

3.4. Predictors of TB Treatment Delay

The positive predictors of delayed treatment, using logistic regression, were first presentation at: patent medicine dealer (OR 12.3 CI: 3.22 - 36.23), private hospital (OR 10.6 CI: 5.73 - 17.94), prayer house (OR 7.2 CI: 2.75 - 23.64), and traditional healer (OR 11.9 CI: 6.87 - 32.85), distance of DOTS facility from the residence (OR 3.6, CI: 1.41 - 16.35), HIV (OR 2.4 CI: 1.0 - 15.5), Occupation (OR 5.3 CI: 1.1 - 14.3) and symptoms experienced (OR 7.6 CI: 2.9 - 20.8) (**Table 6**).

3.5. Delay of Seeking Treatment by TB Patients

Among the study participants, 168 (76.7%) of patients delayed seeking treatment at the DOTS facility. The mean delay from onset of symptoms to first visit to the DOTS facility was 10.2 ± 7.3 weeks. The maximum patient delays was found in 37 (16.9%) patients who first presented at DOTS facility after 12 weeks, while 131 (59.8%) presented between 4 - 12 weeks after the onset of symptoms (**Table 7**).

4. Discussion

Understanding the factors associated with patient delays is vital for the achievement of the Global Plan to Stop TB, which aims to halve the prevalence and deaths from TB by 2015 [15]. It is also known that early detection and treatment of TB patients are one of the strategies of WHO to reduce the diseases morbidity and mortality throughout the world. Our study estimated the duration of delay in seeking treatment at DOTS facilities, and factors associated with the delay. The overall median delay among TB patients in our study was 10 weeks. The median delay in this study is longer than in the studies conducted by Fatiregun and Ejeckam in Nigeria, Odusanya and Babafemi in Nigeria, Endalew et al. in Ethiopia, Tegegn et al. in Ethiopia, and Alexis et al. in Cameroon where 60 days, 60 days, 30 days, 63 days, and 30 days were found respectively [3] [11] [16]-[18]. However, the delay is shorter than in the study done in Tanzania [19] where 120 days was found, but similar to a study done in Ethiopia [11] where duration of 78 days was reported. The long delay might be due to the fact that the symptoms mostly experienced by TB patients are thought to be mild that could be treated by traditional healers and other non medical facilities. Some symptoms experienced may be taken for mild chest infections which they just take self medication or visit patent medicine dealers. More than 60% of the patients first went to patent medicine dealers, prayer houses, and traditional healers for treatment after the onset of the symptoms. Most of the patients (69.3%) that went for treatment at patent medicine dealers delayed seeking treatment at DOTS facility. This could be as a result of poor collaboration between the National TB control programme and patent medicine dealers in the study area. There is need to improve public private partnership with National TB control programme so that TB suspects will be referred early to DOTS facilities for sputum smear microscopy and other investigations necessary for confirmation of tuberculosis. However, the proportion of patients (76.7%) who delayed presentation at the DOTS facility in this study are similar to studies conducted in Tanzania, and Ethiopia [11] [19], but slightly less than 83%, and 81% found in the studies done in Lagos, Nigeria [12] [20].

In our study, the major reasons for delay are far distance of the DOTS facility (36.1%) and poor socio-economic conditions (24.2%). Other reasons that contributed to the delay include lack of awareness of DOTS, and some felt it was not necessary. These reasons were similar to those reported in the study in Syrian Arab Republic conducted among 800 new smear positive pulmonary TB patients, and in Zambia where lack of

Table 4. Reasons for delay for more than 30 days before presentation at DOTS facility.

Reasons:	N	%
Poor socio-economic condition	53	24.2
Distance of health facility far	79	36.1
Felt not necessary	38	17.3
Lack of awareness of DOTS	24	10.9
Others	25	11.5

Table 5. Relationship of different variables with treatment delay.

VARIBLES	CATEGORY	DELAYED DURATION (>30 Days)		DURATION (≤30 Days)		TOTAL		Chi-square	P-Value
		N	%	N	%	N	%	X^2	P
HIV status	Positive	65	76.5	20	23.5	85	38.8		
	Negative	68	73.1	25	26.9	93	42.5	23.412	0.003
	Unknown	35	85.4	6	14.6	41	18.7		
Level of Education	No formal education	13	86.7	2	13.3	15	6.8		
	Primary	28	84.8	5	15.2	33	15.1		
	Secondary	59	71.1	24	28.9	83	37.9	20.194	0.064
	Tertiary	68	77.3	20	22.7	88	40.2		
Distance of DOTS Center	<5 km	51	61.4	32	38.6	83	37.9		
	5 - 10 km	83	83.8	16	16.2	99	45.2	34.908	0.000
	>10 km	34	91.9	3	8.1	37	16.9		
Symtoms experienced	Cough	106	51.9	98	48.1	204	93.1		
	Haemoptysis	4	66.7	2	33.3	6	2.8		
	Weight loss	1	33.3	2	66.7	3	1.4	46.857	0.001
	Night fever	1	25.0	3	75.0	4	1.8		
	Breathing difficulty	1	50.0	1	50.0	2	0.9		
Knowledge about causes of TB	Alcohol	40	59.7	27	40.3	67	30.6		
	Mycobacterium Tuberculosis	0	0	2	100	2	0.9		
	Smoking	29	60.4	19	39.6	48	21.9	42.322	0.040
	Witch craft	5	33.3	10	66.7	15	6.9		
	Dust	1	50.0	1	50.0	48	21.9		
	Others	24	61.5	15	38.5	39	17.8		
Occupation	Student	22	64.7	12	35.3	34	15.5		
	Civil servant	48	81.4	11	18.6	59	26.9		
	Trader	50	69.4	20	30.6	72	32.9	34.217	0.025
	House wife	7	100	0	0	7	3.2		
	Unemployed	13	86.7	2	13.3	15	6.8		
	Others	26	81.3	6	18.7	32	14.7		
Sex	Male	92	75.4	30	24.6	122	55.7	1.310	0.861
	Female	76	78.4	21	21.6	97	44.3		
Age (Years)	0 - 15	4	57.1	3	42.9	7	3.2		
	>15 - 30	40	59.7	20	40.3	67	30.6		
	>30 - 45	65	79.3	17	20.7	82	37.4	24.057	0.088
	>45 - 60	28	77.7	8	22.3	36	16.4		
	>60	24	88.9	3	11.1	27	12.3		

Table 6. Binary logistic regression analysis for positive predictors of TB treatment delay.

Variables	Odds Ratio	95% Confidence Interval	
Patent medicine dealer	12.3	3.22	36.23
Private hospital	10.3	5.73	17.94
Prayer house	7.2	2.75	23.64
Traditional healer	11.9	6.87	32.85
Distance of DOTS facility	3.6	1.41	16.35
HIV status	2.4	1.0	15.0
Occupation	5.3	1.1	14.3
Symptoms experienced	7.6	2.9	20.8

Table 7. Period of TB patients presentation at the DOTS facility after onset of symptoms.

Period (Weeks)	Frequency	Percent
1 - 4	51	23.3
>4 - 6	75	34.3
>6 - 8	32	14.6
>8 - 12	24	10.9
>12 weeks	37	16.9

money was a major contributing factor to the patient delay [21] [22]. Factors that are significant predictors of patient delay in our study are HIV status, distance of DOTS facility, symptoms experienced, knowledge of the patients, and occupation of patients. All these factors are reported in the studies done in Ghana, Tanzania, and Gambia [4] [19] [23], while other factors reported to be significant in the studies such as educational level, sex, and age could not be found in our study. This could be due to the fact that our study was conducted in the state capital, and majority of the study participants are students (15.5%), and civil servants (26.9%).

Our findings in this study showed that there was relationship between patient's delay in seeking treatment and their knowledge of causes, transmission, and symptoms of TB experienced. This is similar to findings in the study done among rural Vietnamese adults, while the study done in Ibadan, Nigeria found no relationship [3] [24]. The low knowledge in our study might be due to low health education on TB through radio and television to the public by the National TB control programme.

The association of patient's delay with sex in the studies done in Ibadan, Nepal, and Bangladesh [3] [25] [26] were different from our findings in this study where there was no association, but the results were similar to studies done in Lagos, Ethiopia and India [12] [21] [27]. The proportion of females that delayed treatment were more than males in this study, which is comparable to the results reported in studies in Ghana, Nigeria, South Africa, and Tanzania [4] [28]-[30]. This difference could be attributed to socio-economic inequality between males and females in our study area. These findings indicate the need to increase tuberculosis awareness among females attending health facilities for other reasons such as ante-natal clinics, maternal and child health clinics for immunization and other services. The result in our study is different from what was observed in a study done in Southern India that employed men face difficulties to get a leave of absence from work to visit health services [31]. This delay was attributed to male behaviour which is socialization and care process that is detached from male practice [32]. All these reasons might be why more males delayed seeking treatment compared to females. However, more males (55.7%) compare to females (44.3%) were TB patients in our study. This is similar to reported cases in the studies conducted in Ibadan, Nigeria [3] [28].

In this study, patients with no formal and primary education delayed presentation at DOTS facilities compare to those who had secondary and tertiary education. This result is similar to findings reported in other studies conducted in Ethiopia and China where illiterate patients are 3.73 times more likely delay when compared with patients who had college and above education level [16] [33]-[35]. Also in Yemen, illiterate patients experienced much longer delay than literate patients. This could be due to the fact that those with secondary and tertiary education might have better information about TB, and may likely seek care early.

The limitations of this study include recall bias, and perception of disease by the patients. However, only newly registered TB cases were included in our study, and the questionnaire were pretested.

5. Conclusion

Majority of TB patients in this study did not present early to health facilities. The positive predictors of delayed presentation for appropriate PTB treatment were first presentations at inappropriate treatment centers. There is need to intensify public health awareness among potential TB patients on the associated risks of treatment delay to prevent transmission. Collaboration between NTBLCP and unskilled health care providers should be intensified so that they could refer suspected PTB patients promptly to facilitate their treatment.

Acknowledgements

The authors would like to show appreciation to DOTS providers who participated in this study. We thank Oyiga Arinze, Thompson Nosgie, Ozogbo Stanley and Uche Chukwuemeka that collected the data for their commitment, and also study participants for their willingness to participate in the study.

Conflict of Interests

The authors declare that there is no conflict of interests regarding the publication of this paper.

References

[1] WHO (2013) Global Tuberculosis Control Report. WHO/HTM/TB/2013.16, Geneva. http://www.who.int/tb/publications/global_report/en

[2] Federal Ministry of Health, Nigeria (2015) National Tuberculosis and Leprosy Control Programme Workers Manual Revised 6th Edition, 1-5.

[3] Fatiregun, A.A. and Ejeckam, C.C. (2010) Determinants of Patient Delay in Seeking Treatment among Pulmonary Tuberculosis Cases in a Government Specialist Hospital in Ibadan, Nigeria. *Tanzania Journal of Health Research*, **12**, 1-9. http://dx.doi.org/10.4314/thrb.v12i2.56398

[4] Lawn, S.D., Afful, B. and Acheampong, J.W. (1999) Pulmonary Tuberculosis in Adults: Factors Associated with Mortality at a Ghanaian Teaching Hospital. *West African Journal of Medicine*, **18**, 270-274.

[5] World Health Organization (2006) The Stop TB Strategy, Building on and Enhancing DOTS to Meet the TB-related Millennium Development Goals. WHO, Geneva.

[6] Storla, D.G., Yimer, S. and Bjune, G.A. (2008) A Systematic Review of Delay in the Diagnosis and Treatment of Tuberculosis. *BMC Public Health*, **8**, 15. http://dx.doi.org/10.1186/1471-2458-8-15

[7] World Health Organization (2006) Diagnostic and Treatment Delay in Tuberculosis an In-Depth Analysis of the Health-Seeking Behaviour of Patients and Health System Response in Seven Countries of the Eastern Mediterranean Region. WHO, Geneva.

[8] Paynter, S., Hayward, A., Wilkinson, P., Lozewicz, S. and Coker, R. (2004) Patient and Health Service Delays in Initiating Treatment for Patients with Pulmonary Tuberculosis: Retrospective Study. *International Journal of Tuberculosis and Lung Disease*, **8**, 180-185.

[9] Aoki, M., Mori, T. and Shimao, T. (1985) Studies on Factors Influencing Patient's, Doctor's and Total Delay of Tuberculosis Case-Detection in Japan. *Bulletin of the International Union against Tuberculosis*, **60**, 128-132.

[10] Ohmori, M., Ozasa, K., Mori, T., *et al.* (2005) Trends of Delays in Tuberculosis Case Finding in Japan and Associated Factors. *International Journal of Tuberculosis and Lung Disease*, **9**, 999-1005.

[11] Demissie, M., Lindtjorn, B. and Berhance, Y. (2002) Patient and Health Service Delay in the Diagnosis of Pulmonary Tuberculosis in Ethiopia. *BMC Public Health*, **2**, 23-31. http://dx.doi.org/10.1186/1471-2458-2-23

[12] Odusanya, O.O. and Babafemi, J.O. (2004) Patterns of Delays amongst Pulmonary Tuberculosis Patients in Lagos, Nigeria. *BMC Public Health*, **4**, 46-51.

[13] Falodun, O.I., Cadmus, E.O., Alabi, P., *et al.* (2014) Delayed Treatment Seeking Behaviours and Associated Factors among Tuberculosis Patients in Ibadan, Nigeria. *African Journal of Epidemiology*, **2**, 27-33.

[14] Mfinanga, S.G., Mutayoba, B.K., Kahwa, A., *et al.* (2008) The Magnitude and Factors Associated with Delays in Management of Smear Positive Tuberculosis in Dar es Salam, Tanzania. *BMC Public Health*, **8**, 158.

[15] Raviglione, M. and Uplekar, M. (2006) WHO's New Stop TB Strategy. *The Lancet*, **367**, 952-955.

http://dx.doi.org/10.1016/S0140-6736(06)68392-X

[16] Endalew, G., Muluken, A. and Gedefaw, A. (2014) Factors Associated with Patient's Delay in Tuberculosis Treatment in Bahir City Administration, Northwest Ethiopia. *BioMed Research International*, **2014**, Article ID: 701429.

[17] Alexis, C., Andy, R., Mohammed, A.Y. and Luis, E.C. (2007) Duration and Associated Factors of Patient Delay during Tuberculosis Screening in Rural Cameroon. *Tropical Medicine and International Health*, **12**, 1309-1314. http://dx.doi.org/10.1111/j.1365-3156.2007.01925.x

[18] Tegegn, A. and Yazachew, M. (2009) Delays in Tuberculosis Treatment and Associated Factors in Jimma Zone, Southwest Ethiopia. *Ethiopian Health Science Journal*, **19**, 29-37.

[19] Wandwalo, E.R. and Morkve, O. (1998) Delay in Tuberculosis Case Finding and Treatment in Mwanza, Tanzania. *International Journal of Tuberculosis and Lung Disease*, **2**, 635-640.

[20] Enwuru, C.A., Idigbe, E.O., Ezeobi, N.V. and Otegbeye, A.F. (2002) Care-Seeking Behavioural Patterns, Awareness and Diagnostic Processes in Patients with Smear and Culture-Positive Pulmonary Tuberculosis in Lagos, Nigeria. *Transactions of the Royal Society of Tropical Medicine and Hygiene*, **96**, 614-616. http://dx.doi.org/10.1016/S0035-9203(02)90328-7

[21] Mesfin, M.M., Newell, J.N., Walley, J.D., Gessessew, A. and Madeley, R.J. (2009) Delayed Consultation among Pulmonary Tuberculosis Patients: A Cross Sectional Study of 10 DOTS Districts of Ethiopia. *BMC Public Health*, **9**, 53. http://dx.doi.org/10.1186/1471-2458-9-53

[22] Needham, D.M., Godfrey, F.P. and Foster, S.D. (1998) Barriers to Tuberculosis Control in Urban Zambia: Economic Impact and Burden on Patients Prior to Diagnosis. *International Journal of Tuberculosis and Lung Disease*, **2**, 811-817.

[23] Lienhardt, C., Rowley, J., Manneh, K., *et al.* (2001) Factors Affecting Time Delay to Treatment in a Tuberculosis Control Programme in a Sub-Saharan African Country: The Experience of the Gambia. *International Journal of Tuberculosis and Lung Disease*, **5**, 233-239.

[24] Hoa, N.P., Thorson, A.E.K., Long, N.H. and Diwan, V.K. (2003) Knowledge of Tuberculosis Associated Health-Seeking Behaviour among Rural Vietnamese Adults with a Cough for at Least Three Weeks. *Scandinavian Journal of Public Health*, **31**, 59-65. http://dx.doi.org/10.1080/14034950310015121

[25] Yamasaki, N.M., Ozasa, K., Yamada, N., *et al.* (2001) Gender Difference in Delays to Diagnosis and Health Care Seeking Behaviour in a Rural Area of Nepal. *International Journal of Tuberculosis and Lung Disease*, **5**, 24-31.

[26] Giasuddin, A. and Jalaluddin, A. (2004) Gender Difference in Treatment Seeking Behaviours of Tuberculosis Cases in Rural Communities of Bangladesh. National TB Control Programme, Ministry of Health and FW, Dhaka.

[27] Rajeswari, R., Chandrasekaran, V., Suhadev, M., *et al.* (2002) Factors Associated with Patient and Health System Delays in the Diagnosis of Tuberculosis in South India. *International Journal of Tuberculosis and Lung Disease*, **6**, 789-795.

[28] Falodun, O.I., Cadmus, E.O., Alabi, P., *et al.* (2014) Delayed Treatment Seeking Behaviours and Associated Factors among Tuberculosis Patients in Ibadan, Nigeria. *African Journal of Epidemiology*, **2**, 27-33.

[29] Pronyk, R.M., Makhubele, M.B., Hargreaves, J.R., Tollman, S.M. and Hausler, H.P. (2001) Assessing Health Seeking Behaviour among Tuberculosis Patients in Rural South Africa. *International Journal of Tuberculosis and Lung Disease*, **5**, 619-627.

[30] Sayoki, G.M., Beatrice, K.M., Amos, K., *et al.* (2008) The Magnitude and Factors Associated with Delays in Management of Smear Positive Tuberculosis in Dar es Salam, Tanzania. *BMC Health Services Research*, **8**, 8-15.

[31] Balasubramanian, R., Garg, R., Santha, T., *et al.* (2004) Gender Disparities in Tuberculosis: Report from a Rural DOTS Programme in South India. *International Journal of Tuberculosis and Lung Disease*, **8**, 323-332.

[32] Courtenay, W.H. (2000) Constructions of Masculinity and Their Influence on Men's Well-Being: A Theory of Gender and Health. *Social Science & Medicine*, **50**, 1385-1401. http://dx.doi.org/10.1016/S0277-9536(99)00390-1

[33] Zhou, C., Tobe, R.G., Chu, J., *et al.* (2012) Detection Delay of Pulmonary Tuberculosis Patients among Migrants in China: A Cross-Sectional Study. *International Journal of Tuberculosis and Lung Disease*, **16**, 1630-1636. http://dx.doi.org/10.5588/ijtld.12.0227

[34] Hussen, A., Biadgilign, S., Tessema, F., *et al.* (2012) Treatment Delay among Pulmonary Tuberculosis Patients in Pastoralist Communities in Bale Zone, South-East Ethiopia. *BMC research Notes*, **5**, 7-11.

[35] Date, J. and Okita, K. (2005) Gender and Literacy: Factors Related to Diagnostic Delay and Unsuccessful Treatment of Tuberculosis in the Mountainous Area of Yemen. *International Journal of Tuberculosis and Lung Diseases*, **9**, 680-685.

Abbreviations

UNTH: University of Nigeria Teaching Hospital
DOTS: Direct Observe Treatment Short Course
OR: Odds Ratio
CI: Confidence Interval
SPSS: Statistical Packages for Social Science
TB: Tuberculosis
MTB/RIF: Mycobacterium Tuberculosis/Rifampicin Resistant
HIV: Human Immunodeficiency Virus
NTBLCP: National Tuberculosis and Leprosy Control Programme

21

Development of the Diabetes Oral Health Assessment Tool © for Nurses

Yumi Kuwamura[1], Masuko Sumikawa[2], Tetsuya Tanioka[1], Toshihiko Nagata[3],
Eijiro Sakamoto[3], Hiromi Murata[4], Munehide Matsuhisa[5], Ken-ichi Aihara[6],
Daisuke Hinode[7], Hirokazu Uemura[8], Hirokazu Ito[1], Yuko Yasuhara[1], Rozzano Locsin[1]

[1]Department of Nursing, Institute of Biomedical Sciences, Tokushima University Graduate School, Tokushima, Japan
[2]Sapporo Medical University School of Health Sciences, Hokkaido, Japan
[3]Department of Periodontology and Endodontology, Institute of Biomedical Sciences, Tokushima University Graduate School, Tokushima, Japan
[4]Former Tokushima University Hospital, Tokushima, Japan
[5]Diabetes Therapeutics and Research Center, Tokushima University, Tokushima, Japan
[6]Department of Community Medicine for Diabetes and Metabolic Disorders, Institute of Biomedical Sciences, Tokushima University Graduate School, Tokushima, Japan
[7]Department of Hygiene and Oral Health Science, Institute of Biomedical Sciences, Tokushima University Graduate School, Tokushima, Japan
[8]Department of Preventive Medicine, Institute of Biomedical Sciences, Tokushima University Graduate School, Tokushima, Japan
Email: kuwamura.yumi@tokushima-u.ac.jp

Abstract

Although some studies have suggested a bidirectional relationship between diabetes and periodontal disease, there were no appropriate tools for nurses to evaluate oral status and oral health behaviors in patients with diabetes. Therefore, the Diabetes Oral Health Assessment Tool (DiOHAT©) was developed with items contributed by health care professionals (diabetologists, periodontal specialists, a preventive dentist, a Certified Nurse in Diabetes Nursing, a national registered dietitian, registered nurses, a dental hygienist, and nursing researchers) who were involved in the medical care of patients with diabetes. Subsequently, a survey of 700 Diabetes Nurse Specialists (DNS) was conducted to determine their score of recognition and implementation of the DiOHAT©, however, 304 participants (43.4%) responded. Constructive concept validation and the Cronbach's alpha coefficient for all assessment items was 0.932, indicating high reliability: Factor 1, Patient's oral health status ($\alpha = 0.874$); Factor 2, Implementation of oral health behaviors ($\alpha = 0.890$); Factor 3, Information transmission regarding dental visits ($\alpha = 0.862$); and Factor 4, Perceptions and knowledge of oral health behaviors ($\alpha = 0.793$). Although the mean score of recognition of DiOHAT© was 3.5 ± 0.4 points, the mean value of the implementation score was 1.5 ± 0.5

points (obtained using a 4-grade scale). The implementation scores were significantly lower than the recognition scores for all items ($p < 0.001$). The findings suggested that the DNS were not inclined to implement all items of DiOHAT©, despite recognizing their importance.

Keywords

Diabetes, Oral Health Behavior, Oral Status, Nursing Assessment, Diabetes Nurse Specialist

---

1. Introduction

It is becoming increasingly important worldwide to take critical measures to manage diabetes. In Japan, there are no signs of a decreasing prevalence of diabetes [1]. The continuing goal of treatment is to prevent or delay complications [2], which can be achieved via patients with diabetes (hereafter referred to as patients) self-care interventions. Patients need not only amend their diet, exercise, and medication but also consider how they can maintain their overall health. Diet therapy is a requirement for all patients. There have been many studies about the relationship between postprandial blood glucose levels and mastication [3]-[5]; eating vegetables before carbohydrate [6]; and higher masticatory performance and slow eating [7]. To implement these behavioral activities, patients need good oral health. The 2011 Survey of Dental Diseases [8] conducted in Japan showed that the percentages of those with the highest community periodontal index codes in permanent teeth were 74.2% (in total) and 86.7% (within the age group of 45 - 49 years old). In particular, patients are often susceptible to periodontal disease [9], which can be easily exacerbated [10] by oral health disease conditions. Periodontal disease is referred to as the sixth complication of diabetes [11] and its exacerbation has a negative influence on diabetes [12] [13]. It is therefore important that patients maintain good oral health behaviors to prevent periodontal disease from developing or if existing, from worsening.

In Japan, some attempts have been made to share patient information among medical staffs (e.g., internists, ophthalmologists, and dentists), who treat patients with diabetes by utilizing a diabetes information sharing notebook [14] [15]. Patients bring these notebooks to the medical staffs to report their physical conditions (e.g., hemoglobin A1c levels, retinopathy stage, periodontal disease stage). These surveys by a cooperative medical and dental team also clarified the association between periodontal disease and glycemic control [16].

In a study by nurses aimed to determine support of patients with difficulty maintaining good oral health, in addition to identifying the oral health behaviors and associated factors of the patients [17], the result indicated that it was important for nurses to understand both the perceptions [18] [19] and behaviors of their patients. To prevent severe diabetic complications, such as ischemic heart disease, the goal of oral health behaviors is to prevent the onset and/or worsening of oral diseases, including periodontal disease and dental caries, and their associated diseases [20]. It is also effective to ensure that patients receive appropriate dental care considering their current diabetic therapies.

Clarification of nurses' assessments of patient oral health behaviors will facilitate the provision of support to patients to conduct appropriate oral health behavioral assessments. Current oral health care assessments by Eilers' Oral Assessment Guide [21] and its revised versions [22]-[24] are often used as references. These are assessment methods for the oral cavity, especially for detecting mucositis in patients undergoing chemotherapy [25]-[27] or radiotherapy [28]. However, for nurses' use, there are no existing guidelines for assessing oral status and oral health behaviors of patients that consider diabetes treatment goals and current oral physical status.

The aims of this study were to develop the Diabetes Oral Health Assessment Tool (DiOHAT©) which enabled nurses to evaluate patients' oral status and oral health behaviors easily and simply, and to clarify how diabetes nurse specialists recognize the contents of DiOHAT© and the frequency of its use in the real world.

2. Methods

2.1. The Process to Develop the Diabetes Oral Health Assessment Tool (DiOHAT©) for Nurses

2.1.1. Identification of Items to Develop the DiOHAT©

From the literature reviews and preliminary survey interviews conducted, sources of items describing the oral health status and oral health behaviors were identified to initiate the development of the DiOHAT©. Information derived from interviews with internists, dentists, and nurses who were working in medical or dental departments regarding patients' oral health status and oral health behaviors, were analyzed. From these sources, the draft DiOHAT© was developed.

2.1.2. Discussions among Interdisciplinary Team of Professionals

Discussions among members of the interdisciplinary team of professionals focused on determining the validity of the assessment items of the DiOHAT©. In a meeting conducted by health care professionals (including diabetologists, periodontal specialists, a preventive dentist, a Certified Nurse in Diabetes Nursing, a national registered dietitian, registered nurses, a dental hygienist, and nursing researchers), interdisciplinary approaches to support oral health behaviors for patients, and recognition of effective assessment ways were discussed. From this meeting, the assessment items were identified including terms depicting situations that predict periodontal disease and characteristics of diabetes treatments. Consequently, the draft of the assessment items was modified such that it would be possible for any nurses to easily conduct an efficient bedside assessment. There were more than 50 items in the initial assessment tool. However, after careful discussion and focused consideration, the final assessment items of the DiOHAT© were reduced to 21, comprising four assessment areas of concern, namely, "Patient's oral health status", "Patient's implementation of oral health behaviors", "Patient's visit to dental clinic", and "Patient's perceptions and knowledge of oral health behaviors".

2.1.3 Detailed Description of the Assessment Items

The items included in the area of "Patient's oral health status" are related to the main functions of the teeth and the oral cavity. These are basic items intended to assess mastication and swallowing, vocalization and pronunciation, facial appearance, and saliva secretion.

The items pertaining to "Patient's implementation of oral health behaviors" focused on whether patients are able to perform two critical actions for oral health by themselves: cleaning dental plaque (biofilms) from the surface of teeth (oral self-care), undergoing regular dental examinations and cleanings performed by dentists or dental hygienists (professional oral health care) for the prevention of cavities and periodontal disease.

The items pertaining to "Patient's visit to dental clinic" assessed whether or not patients are able to visit dentists and offer information regarding their therapies from the internists to dentists, and to relay that information to their medical staffs. The common complications of diabetes are incomplete healing of wounds [29] due to hyperglycemia associated with the onset and exacerbation of infectious disease and hypoglycemia caused by delayed or missed meals after the dental therapy, for example during interventions involving the use of anesthesia. In addition, when patients are given an anti-platelet agent, it is often difficult for bleeding to stop. It is also crucial that patients inform their dentists before therapy if they have any diabetes-related complications, such as hypertension and heart disease.

The items pertaining to "Patient's perceptions and knowledge of oral health behaviors" assessed how well the patients understand the close link between periodontal disease and diabetes, and the importance of oral health behaviors.

2.2. Diabetes Nurse Specialists' Recognition and Implementation of the Diabetes Oral Health Assessment Tool (DiOHAT©)

2.2.1. Participants of the Study

Three hundred four Certified Nurses in Diabetes Nursing and Certified Nurse Specialists in Chronic Care Nursing were recognized as Diabetes Nurse Specialists (DNS) in Japan. Seven-hundred self-administered questionnaires by anonymous form were mailed to the DNS. They agreed to participate in the survey and returned the questionnaires containing the demographic data sheet and the DiOHAT©. The data were collected from December 2014 to January 2015.

2.2.2. Instruments

In the questionnaire participants were asked to include their personal data such as age, gender, years of experience as a nurse, certifications as DNS, years passed since the acquisition of certifications, and presence or absence of a specialty outpatient department for diabetes in the clinics where they work.

A five-point Likert scale questionnaire was used with responses for each of the items of the DiOHAT©.

These items were focused on the necessity of patients' oral health behaviors. Recognition scores were set as follows: "not necessary at all, one point", "not very necessary, two points", "cannot determine, three points", "a little necessary, four points", and "very necessary, five points". Participants were asked to answer the frequency of implementation of the assessment within the last two weeks, by choosing one of four alternatives. Implementation scores were set as follows: "never, one point", "sometimes, two points", "often, three points", and "always, four points". It was found that the higher the score, the more the participants implemented and recognized the necessity of the assessment.

2.2.3. Methods of Analysis

The Kaiser-Meyer-Olkin (KMO) measures of sampling adequacy for the factor analysis of the 21 items were calculated, and confirmed an appropriate value of 0.923. In addition, Bartlett's test of sphericity was used to confirm the validation of the factor analysis (chi-squared test value of 3702.6, $p < 0.001$). The factor analysis was conducted by adopting the principal factor analysis. Regarding the rotation method, the varimax rotation method supplemented with Kaiser Normalization test was used. The analysis was conducted by setting the four factors with the corresponding factor loadings of greater than 0.30 being adopted.

To compare the scores obtained for the recognition of the necessity of each assessment item (five-point scale) and those for implementation of the item (four-point scale), the modified scores for the recognition of necessity were obtained by multiplying these scores by 0.8. These scores were divided by the number of factors to obtain an average score, which was taken as the score for each factor. In order to compare the recognition and implementation of each assessment item, these were compared using paired t-test. The significance level was set at 5%. The IBM SPSS Statistics 19.0, 23.0 were used for the statistical analyses.

2.3. Ethical Considerations

This research was conducted with the approval of the clinical research ethics review board at Tokushima University Hospital Clinical Trial Center for Developmental Therapeutics (reference number 2042). The approval document states that cooperation with this research is on a voluntary basis, where completing the questionnaire is considered as approval, and cancellation of a response is not permitted because all responses are anonymous. Information for distribution of the questionnaires was obtained from the website of the Japan Nursing Association.

3. Results

3.1. Demographic Data (Table 1)

Out of the 700 questionnaire copies distributed to prospective participants, only 304 were returned and received. The return rate was 43.4%. The mean age of the participants was 41.7 ± 6.6 years. Most of them (74.7%) worked at the clinic/hospital with a specialty outpatient clinic for patients with diabetes. Although there were 277 Certified Nurses in Diabetes Nursing (CNDN), only 262 responded about the years of work after acquiring their certification. There were 29 Certified Nurse Specialists in Chronic Care Nursing (CNSCCN), but only 24 provided information about years or practice after acquisition of certification.

3.2. Factor Analysis of the ©Diabetes Oral Health Assessment Tool (Table 2)

Cronbach's alpha coefficient was 0.932, showing a high degree of reliability. As a result of the factor analysis, the following classifications were confirmed for the assessment items: Factor 1, Patient's oral health status ($\alpha = 0.874$), seven items; Factor 2, Patient's implementation of oral health behaviors ($\alpha = 0.890$), six items; Factor 3, Patient's information transmission regarding dental visits ($\alpha = 0.862$), five items; and Factor 4, Patient's perceptions and knowledge of oral health behaviors ($\alpha = 0.793$), three items. Additionally, the researchers further considered the following points: whether the assessment items were easy to use and whether the content regarding professional oral health care was adequate.

3.3. Differences between Diabetes Nurse Specialists' Recognition and Implementation to Assess Patients' Oral Health Status and Behaviors (Table 3)

The average score for all items pertaining to recognition was 3.5 ± 0.4 points out of a possible 4. In particular,

Table 1. Characteristics of participants.

		n	(%)	
Gender	Male/Female	13 / 290	4.3 / 95.4	
	No description	1	0.3	
Department (can be plural)	Ward	127	41.8	
	Outpatient	132	43.4	
	Diabetes nursing outpatient	68	22.4	
	Others	39	12.8	
Number of beds in the facility	1 - 19 beds	6	2.0	
	20 - 199 beds	41	13.5	
	200 - 499 beds	127	41.8	
	More than 500 beds	123	40.5	
	No description	7	2.3	
Clinics opened in the hospital	Specialty outpatient clinic for diabetes	227	74.7	
		n	M	SD
Age (years old)		295	41.7	6.6
Experience as a nurse (years)		301	18.6	6.5
Experience working as a nurse for diabetes patients (years)		295	11.6	4.6
After the acquisition (years) (can be plural)	Certified Nurses in Diabetes Nursing (N=277)	262	3.3	2.9
	Certified Nurse Specialists in Chronic Care Nursing (N=29)	24	3.5	2.4

N = 304, M: Mean, SD: Standard Deviation.

the items regarding "knowledge of a relationship between periodontal disease and systemic disease including diabetes (3.8 ± 0.4)" and "dental visiting more than once a year (3.7 ± 0.5)" scored very highly. In contrast, "counting the patient's total number of teeth (3.0 ± 0.8)", "checking the one's inside of mouth with a mirror by oneself (3.3 ± 0.6)", "biting firmly on molar or dentures (3.3 ± 0.6)", and "toothbrushing one by one very carefully (3.3 ± 0.6)", showed lower scores compared with the others.

The average total implementation score was 1.5 ± 0.5 points out of a possible 4. Those items with very low scores were as follows: "counting the patient's total number of teeth (1.2 ± 0.5)", "biting firmly on molar or dentures (1.3 ± 0.6)", "toothbrushing around the border between the teeth and marginal gingiva (1.3 ± 0.6)", "checking the one's inside of mouth with a mirror by oneself (1.3 ± 0.6)", and "toothbrushing one by one very carefully (1.3 ± 0.7)". In contrast, those items showing higher scores were as follows: "dentures (2.3 ± 1.1)", "knowledge of a relationship between periodontal disease and systemic disease including diabetes (2.0 ± 1.0)"; "dental visiting more than once a year (1.9 ± 1.0)"; and "showing diabetes information-sharing notebook to the dentist (1.7 ± 1.0)".

In the comparison between recognition scores and implementation scores, the latter were significantly lower for all factors ($p < 0.001$). Furthermore, for all items of the implementation scores were very low ($p < 0.001$).

4. Discussion

For all assessment items, Cronbach's alpha coefficient of reliability was 0.932, with the α coefficients of the four factors ranked below ranging from 0.793 to 0.890, suggesting a rather high level of reliability of the items. The assessment items were confirmed to be reliable from a statistical point of view. In addition, it was considered clinical validity of the DiOHAT© is likely to be sufficient, because its items were developed based on agree-

Table 2. Result of factor analysis for assessment items for nurses (Row of factors after rotation).

Assessment Items	Factor 1	Factor 2	Factor 3	Factor 4
Factor 1: Patient's oral health status ($\alpha = 0.874$)				
Bleeding during toothbrushing	0.706	0.309	0.183	0.184
Abscess on gingiva	0.697	0.315	0.238	0.175
Awareness of halitosis	0.670	0.351	0.183	0.128
Dentures (partial or full)	0.633	0.134	0.081	0.283
Biting firmly on molar or dentures	0.603	0.237	0.239	0.188
Checking the patient's inside of mouth	0.555	0.263	0.073	0.255
Counting the patient's total number of teeth (dentures, bridges and implants are excluded)	0.446	0.136	0.104	0.135
Factor 2: Patient's implementation of oral health behaviors ($\alpha = 0.890$)				
Toothbrushing around the border between the teeth and marginal gingiva	0.302	0.853	0.160	0.230
Toothbrushing one by one very carefully	0.284	0.815	0.173	0.224
Supplementary tools (e.g., interdental brush, dental floss.)	0.346	0.762	0.152	0.095
Checking the one's inside of mouth (teeth, gums, buccal mucosa, and tongues) with a mirror by oneself	0.385	0.583	0.221	0.178
Experience being given dentists' instructions for brushing	0.366	0.400	0.368	0.143
Dental visiting more than once a year	0.169	0.333	0.270	0.243
Factor 3: Patient's information transmission regarding dental visits ($\alpha = 0.862$)				
Showing medicine information-sharing notebook to the dentist	0.090	0.100	0.761	0.089
Showing diabetes information-sharing notebook to the dentist	0.110	0.107	0.745	0.069
Showing self-monitoring blood glucose notebook to the dentist	0.079	0.186	0.728	0.124
Telling dental treatment to the diabetes doctor	0.241	0.154	0.685	0.190
Telling dental treatment to the diabetes nurse	0.354	0.142	0.595	0.240
Factor 4: Patient's perceptions and knowledge of oral health behaviors ($\alpha = 0.793$)				
Perceptions of one's oral health status	0.362	0.245	0.212	0.717
Perceptions of oral care efficacy regardless of timing of care initiation	0.300	0.271	0.239	0.578
Knowledge of a relationship between periodontal disease and systemic disease including diabetes	0.334	0.158	0.195	0.545
Square sum of loading after rotation — Fixed value	3.847	3.321	3.168	1.769
Cumulative rate (%)	18.321	34.133	49.217	57.640
Correlation factor between contents: significance probability (one sided test) Spearman — Factor 1	1.000			
Factor 2	0.692	1.000		
Factor 3	0.468	0.541	1.000	
Factor 4	0.626	0.589	0.488	1.000

Method to select factors: Primary factor method. Barimax rotation method supplemented by a normalization of Kaiser rotation method. Cronbach's alpha coefficient (α) 0.932 for all assessment items.

Table 3. Comparison between recognitions and implementation of nursing specialists.

Assessment Items	Recognition		Implementation		t value[1]	p value[2]
	Mean	SD	Mean	SD		
Total score	3.5	0.4	1.5	0.5	54.4	**
Factor 1: Patient's oral health status	3.4	0.5	1.5	0.5	51.4	**
Bleeding during toothbrushing	3.5	0.6	1.5	0.7	42.8	**
Abscess on gingiva	3.4	0.6	1.4	0.7	42.6	**
Awareness of halitosis	3.3	0.7	1.4	0.7	40.8	**
Dentures (partial or full)	3.6	0.5	2.3	1.1	20.6	**
Biting firmly on molar or dentures	3.3	0.6	1.3	0.6	44.8	**
Checking the patient's inside of mouth	3.6	0.6	1.6	0.8	41.1	**
Counting the patient's total number of teeth (dentures, bridges and implants are excluded)	3.0	0.8	1.2	0.5	40.4	**
Factor 2: Patient's implementation of oral health behaviors	3.4	0.5	1.5	0.6	48.0	**
Toothbrushing around the border between the teeth and marginal gingiva	3.4	0.6	1.3	0.6	44.2	**
Toothbrushing one by one very carefully	3.3	0.6	1.3	0.7	43.0	**
Supplementary tools (e.g., interdental brush, dental floss)	3.3	0.7	1.4	0.7	39.0	**
Checking the one's inside of mouth (teeth, gums, buccal mucosa, and tongues) with a mirror by oneself	3.3	0.6	1.3	0.6	45.0	**
Experience being given dentists' instructions for brushing	3.4	0.6	1.5	0.8	37.4	**
Dental visiting more than once a year	3.7	0.5	1.9	1.0	31.1	**
Factor 3: Patient's information transmission regarding dental visits	3.5	0.5	1.6	0.7	42.5	**
Showing medicine information-sharing notebook to the dentist	3.5	0.6	1.6	0.9	36.0	**
Showing diabetes information-sharing notebook to the dentist	3.6	0.6	1.7	1.0	34.9	**
Showing self-monitoring blood glucose notebook to the dentist	3.3	0.7	1.5	0.8	35.8	**
Telling dental treatment to the diabetes doctor	3.6	0.6	1.7	0.9	34.1	**
Telling dental treatment to the diabetes nurse	3.4	0.6	1.4	0.8	38.8	**
Factor 4: Patient's perceptions and knowledge of oral health behaviors	3.7	0.4	1.7	0.7	44.2	**
Perceptions of one's oral health status	3.6	0.5	1.6	0.7	43.5	**
Perceptions of oral care efficacy regardless of timing of care initiation	3.5	0.6	1.5	0.7	42.3	**
Knowledge of a relationship between periodontal disease and systemic disease including diabetes	3.8	0.4	2.0	1.0	32.1	**

[1]Paired t-test. [2]**: $p < 0.001$.

ments among the diabetes health care professionals.

The DNS recognized most of the items to be "necessary". In particular, the following items were also found to be necessary: "knowledge of a relationship between periodontal disease and systemic diseases including diabetes", "dental visiting more than once a year", "perception of one's oral health status", "showing diabetes information-sharing notebook to the dentist", and "telling dental treatment to the diabetes doctor".

It was considered by DNS that communication with dentists is an important, and recognizing the importance of periodontal disease. In addition, for items such as "dentures (full/partial)", "knowledge of a relationship between periodontal disease and systemic disease including diabetes", and "dental visiting more than once a year", almost half of the DNS answered "yes". However, most of DNS didn't assess about patient's dental status and functions, such as "counting the patient's total number of teeth", "checking the one's inside of mouth with a mirror by oneself", and "biting firmly on molar or dentures". Similarly, the items assessing the actual status of the implementation of oral health behaviors, such as "toothbrushing around the border between the teeth and marginal gingiva" and "toothbrushing one by one very carefully", showed lower scores. This showed that although they understood the basic concept of oral health behaviors, they have not yet confirmed what to do to avoid aggravation of dental status. Therefore oral education for nurses is important and oral assessment items are needed.

Regarding patients' feet, nurses often watch, care, and educate [30] patients to prevent foot ulcers. Similar to the case of foot care, it is easy to obtain information about the oral cavity by direct visual observation with penlight. Nurses' counting the number of teeth [31] is a useful method to assess the health of the oral cavity without any expertise required. It is possible to determine the trajectory of oral illness by the loss of teeth, due to periodontal disease or dental caries, which enables us to acquire important information to evaluate oral functions such as mastication. The loss of teeth reduces mastication ability, alters the senses in the oral cavity, and affects physical appearance. By counting the patients' total number of teeth, nurses can watch the position of the teeth and they can get the data of cleanliness of the oral cavity, too. Then it is possible to estimate the mastication function and implementation of oral health behavior. In addition, it is also reported that "total number of teeth" is linked to dementia [32], mortality [33], and quality of life [34].

Nurses are positively involved in solving problems associated with the oral cavity, as caused by systemic diseases. For example, when patients' suffering from chemotherapy induced oral mucositis [25]-[27], stroke care settings [35], in these patients situation, nurses have to provide oral care for such patients. In the textbooks used in fundamental nursing courses, there are few descriptions on dental mastication, which is a basic oral function, but there are instructions for classic tooth brushing. It is obvious that there is a need to strengthen the basic information on oral health assessment [36], which included occlusion and mastication.

Further discussions from the viewpoint of nursing education are necessary. Nurses need to assess the oral cavity of patients. Self-monitoring [37], (e.g., blood glucose, body weight, diet) is important for the patients. A positive involvement in oral care by nurses might provide good effects through patients' self-care. In addition, oral care by nurses is not appreciated enough in the Japanese medical insurance system; and foot care is rewarded by medical service fees to nurses: this is not the case for oral care. As Costello et al. [38] pointed out, while nurses appreciate the need for oral care, in reality they lack knowledge and experience about this area of care.

In the consideration of the oral health behavior of patients, it is essential to evaluate the number of existing teeth. Based on the results obtained, loss of any teeth increased the importance of the remaining teeth. Nurses need to collect comprehensive data to provide patients with appropriate oral care using evidence-based assessment tools. In checking the patients' oral cavity, the nurses evaluate their oral functions.

The findings of the study further showed that although the DNS recognized the usefulness of the assessment items, they were not inclined to perform them. These warrant further investigation.

5. Limitations

In this research study the response rate for returning the questionnaire was 43.4%, this was not satisfactory. In the future, it is necessary to clarify the problems occurring on the clinical sites clearer by utilizing these assessment items of DiOHAT© as a trial for examining the patients' oral health status and behaviors.

6. Conclusion

The DiOHAT© was developed with the four factors: Patient's oral health status, Patient's implementation of oral health behaviors, Patient's information transmission regarding dental visits, and Patient's perceptions and knowledge of oral health behaviors. These four factors were determined reliable and valid by factor analysis, and Cronbach's alpha coefficient of reliability of 0.932. However, DNS did not assess all items of oral health behaviors in the DiOHAT© despite being aware of the importance of the assessment items.

Acknowledgements

This work was supported by Japan Society for the Promotion of Science (JSPS), JSPS KAKENHI Grant Number 26463305, and Grant-in-Aid for Scientific Research (C). We are grateful to the nurses who participated in this study and we appreciate clinicians: Dr. Hamada Y., MD, Ms. Ishida N., RN, Ms. Takikawa I., RN, Ms. Yamato H., RN, and Ms. Kikui S. helping this study.

Competing Interests

The authors declare that they have no competing interests for this article.

References

[1]   Ministry of Health, Labour and Welfare. Health Japan 21 (The Second Team): Analysis and Assessment project. Annual Changes in Current Data, Table 2 Targets of the Prevention of Onset and Progression of Life-Style Related Disease: Diabetes.
       http://www.mhlw.go.jp/seisakunitsuite/bunya/kenkou_iryou/kenkou/kenkounippon21/en/kenkounippon21/data02.html#c0

[2]   American Diabetes Association: Living with Diabetes. http://www.diabetes.org/living-with-diabetes/

[3]   Suzuki, H., Fukushima, M., Okamoto, S., Takahashi, O., Shimbo, T., Kurose, T., Yamada, Y., Inagaki, N., Seino, Y. and Fukui, T. (2005) Effect of Thorough Mastication on Postprandial Plasma Glucose Concentration in Nonobese Japanese Participants. *Metabolism Clinical and Experimental*, **54**, 1593-1599.
       http://dx.doi.org/10.1016/j.metabol.2005.06.006

[4]   Ranawana, V., Henry, C.J. and Pratt, M. (2010) Degree of Habitual Mastication Seems to Contribute to Interindividual Variations in the Glycemic Response to Rince But Not to Spaghetti. *Nutrition Research*, **30**, 382-391.
       http://dx.doi.org/10.1016/j.nutres.2010.06.002

[5]   Sonoki, K., Iwase, M., Takata, Y., Nakamoto, T., Masaki, C., Hosokawa, R., Murakami, S., Chiwata, K. and Inoue, H. (2013) Effects of Thirty-Times Chewing per Bite on Secretion of Glucagon-Like Peptide-1 in Healthy Volunteers and Type 2 Diabetic Patients. *Endocrine Journal*, **60**, 311-319. http://dx.doi.org/10.1507/endocrj.EJ12-0310

[6]   Imai, S., Matsuda, M., Hasegawa, G., Fukui, M., Obayashi, H., Ozasa, N. and Kajiyama S. (2011) A Simple Meal Plan of "Eating Vegetables before Carbohydrate" Was More Effective for Achieving Glycemic Control than an Exchange-Based Meal Plan in Japanese Patients with Type 2 Diabetes. *Asia Pacific Journal of Clinical Nutrition*, **20**, 161-168.
       http://apjcn.nhri.org.tw/server/APJCN/20/2/161.pdf

[7]   Yamazaki, T., Yamori, M., Asai, K., Nakano-Araki, I., Yamaguchi, A., Takahashi, K., Sekine, A., Matsuda, F., Kosugi, S., Nakayama, T., Inagaki, N. and Bessho, K., Nagahama Study Collaboration Group (2013) Mastication and Risk for Diabetes in Japanese Population: A Cross-Sectional Study. *PLoS ONE*, **8**, e64113.
       http://dx.doi.org/10.1371/journal.pone.0064113

[8]   Ministry of Health, Labour and Welfare: Statisticaltables of the Survey of Dental Diseases. (In Japanese with English)
       http://www.mhlw.go.jp/toukei/list/62-17c.html

[9]   Nelson, R.G., Shlossman, M., Budding, L.M., Pettitt, D.J., Saad, M.F., Genco, R.J. And Knowler, W.C. (1990) Periodontal Disease and NIDDM in Pima Indians. *Diabetes Care*, **13**, 836-840. http://dx.doi.org/10.2337/diacare.13.8.836

[10]   Seppälä, B., Seppälä, M. and Ainamo, J. (1993) A Longitudinal Study on Insulin-Dependent Diabetes Mellitus and Periodontal Disease. *Journal of Clinical Periodontology*, **20**, 161-165.
       http://dx.doi.org/10.1111/j.1600-051X.1993.tb00338.x

[11]   Löe, H. (1993) Periodontal Disease: The Sixth Complication of Diabetes Mellitus. *Diabetes Care*, **16**, 329-334.
       http://dx.doi.org/10.2337/diacare.16.1.329

[12]   Collin, H.L., Uusitupa, M., Niskanen, L., Kontturi-Närhi, V., Markkanen, H., Koivisto, A.M. and Meurman, J.H. (1998) Periodontal Findings in Elderly Patients with Non-Insulin Dependent Diabetes Mellitus. *Journal of Periodontology*, **69**, 962-966. http://dx.doi.org/10.1902/jop.1998.69.9.962

[13]   Choi, Y.H., McKeown, R.E., Mayer-Davis, E.J., Liese, A.D., Song, K.B. and Merchant, A.T. (2011) Association between Periodontitis and Impaired Fasting Glucose and Diabetes. *Diabetes Care*, **34**, 381-386.
       http://dx.doi.org/10.2337/dc10-1354

[14]   Japan Association for Diabetes Education and Care. (In Japanese)
       http://www.nittokyo.or.jp/patient/goods/handbook.html

[15]   Kishimoto, I., Ashida, Y., Omori, Y., Nishi, H., Hagiwara, Y., Fujimoto, T., Makino, H., Ohata, Y., Iwane, M., Iinuma, K., Maeda, K. and Sato, S. (2013) Surveillance and Evaluation of Diabetes Management in the Toyono Medical District. *Journal of the Japan Diabetes Society*, **56**, 543-550. (In Japanese, abstract in English)
       http://doi.org/10.11213/tonyobyo.56.543

[16]   Strauss, S.M., Rosedale, M.T., Pesce, M.A., Rindskopf, D.M., Kaur, N., Juterbock, C.M., Wolff, M.S., Malaspina, D.

and Danoff, A. (2015) The Potential for Glycemic Control Monitoring and Screening for Diabetes at Dental Visits Using Oral Blood. *The American Journal of Public Health*, **105**, 796-801. http://dx.doi.org/10.2105/AJPH.2014.302357

[17] Kuwamura, Y. and Matsuda, N. (2013) Oral Health Behaviors and Assosiated Factoers in Patients with Diabetes. *Bulletin of Health Sciences in Kobe*, **29**, 1-16. http://www.lib.kobe-u.ac.jp/handle_kernel/81005509

[18] Broadbent, E., Donkin, L. and Stroh, J.C. (2011) Illness and Treatment Perceptions Are Associated with Adherence to Medications, Diet, and Exercise in Diabetic Patients. *Diabetes Care*, **34**, 338-340. http://dx.doi.org/10.2337/dc10-1779

[19] Redman, B.K. (2004) Chapter 2: Advances in Learning Theory for Patient Education. Springer Publishing Company, New York, 17-37.

[20] Saremi, A., Nelson, R.G., Tulloch-Reid, M., Hanson, R.L., Sievers, M.L., Taylor, G.W., Shlossman, M., Bennett, P.H., Genco, R. and Knowler, W.C. (2005) Periodontal Disease and Mortality in Type 2 Diabetes. *Diabetes Care*, **28**, 27-32. http://dx.doi.org/10.2337/diacare.28.1.27

[21] Eilers, J., Berger, A.M. and Petersen, M.C. (1988) Development, Testing, and Application of the Oral Assessment Guide. *Oncology Nursing Forum*, **15**, 325-330.

[22] Andersson, P., Hallberg, I.R. and Renvert, S. (2002) Inter-Rater Reliability of an Oral Assessment Guide for Elderly Patients Residing in a Rehabilitation Ward. *Special Care in Dentistry*, **22**, 181-186. http://dx.doi.org/10.1111/j.1754-4505.2002.tb00268.x

[23] Ribeiro, M.T., Ferreira, R.C., Vargas, A.M. and e Ferreira, E.F. (2014) Validity and Reproducibility of the Revised Oral Assessment Guide Applied by Community Health Workers. *Gerodontology*, **31**, 101-110. http://dx.doi.org/10.1111/ger.12014

[24] Sjögren, R. and Nordström, G. (2000) Oral Health Status of Psychiatric Patients. *Journal of Clinical Nursing*, **9**, 632-638. http://dx.doi.org/10.1046/j.1365-2702.2000.00380.x

[25] Miller, M., Taylor, A., Kearney, N., Paterson, G., Wells, M., Roe, L., Hagen, S. and Maguire, R. (2007) Evaluation of the Feasibility and Acceptability of an Oral Care Diary by Patients during Chemotherapy. *International Journal of Nursing Studies*, **44**, 693-701. http://dx.doi.org/10.1016/j.ijnurstu.2006.01.009

[26] Berger, A.M. and Eilers, J. (1998) Factors Influencing Oral Cavity Status during High-Dose Antineoplastic Therapy: A Secondary Data Analysis. *Oncology Nursing Forum*, **25**, 1623-1629.

[27] Chen, C.F., Wang, R.H., Cheng, S.N. and Chang, Y.C. (2004) Assessment of Chemotherapy—Induced Oral Complications in Children with Cancer. *Journal of Pediatric oncology Nursing*, **21**, 33-39. http://dx.doi.org/10.1177/1043454203259947

[28] Knöös, M. and Ostman, M. (2010) Oral Assessment Guide—Test of Reliability and Validity for Patients Receiving Radiotherapy to the Head and Neck Region. *European Journal of Cancer Care*, **19**, 53-60. http://dx.doi.org/10.1111/j.1365-2354.2008.00958.x

[29] Markuson, M., Hanson, D., Anderson, J., Langemo, D., Hunter, S., Thompson, P., Paulson, R. and Rustvang, D. (2009) The Relationship between Hemoglobin A1c Values and Healing Time for Lower Extremity Ulcers in Individuals with Diabetes. *Advances in Skin & Wound Care*, **22**, 365-372. http://dx.doi.org/10.1097/01.ASW.0000358639.45784.cd

[30] Nemcová, J. and Hlinková, E. (2014) The Efficacy of Diabetic Foot Care Education. *Journal of Clinical Nursing*, **23**, 877-882. http://dx.doi.org/10.1111/jocn.12290

[31] Warren, J.J., Levy, S.M. and Hand, J.S. (1999) The Accuracy of Tooth Loss Data Collected by Nurses. *Special Care in Dentistry*, **19**, 75-78. http://dx.doi.org/10.1111/j.1754-4505.1999.tb01372.x

[32] Luo, J., Wu, B., Zhao, Q., Guo, Q., Meng, H., Yu, L., Zheng, L., Hong, Z. and Ding, D. (2015) Association between Tooth Loss and Cognitive Function among 3063 Chinese Older Adults: A Community-Based Study. *PLoS ONE*, **10**, e0120986. http://dx.doi.org/10.1371/journal.pone.0120986

[33] Liljestrand, J.M., Havulinna, A.S., Paju, S., Männistö, S., Salomaa, V. and Pussinen, P.J. (2015) Missing Teeth Predict Incident Cardiovascular Events, Diabetes, and Death. *Journal of Dental Research*, **94**, 1055-1062. http://dx.doi.org/10.1177/0022034515586352

[34] Huang, D.L., Chan, K.C. and Young, B.A. (2013) Poor Oral Health and Quality of Life in Older U.S. Adults with Diabetes Mellitus. *Journal of the American Geriatrics Society*, **61**, 1782-1788. http://dx.doi.org/10.1111/jgs.12452

[35] Brady, M.C., Stott, D., Weir, C.J., Chalmers, C., Sweeney, P., Donaldson, C., Barr, J., Barr, M., Pollock, A., McGowan, S., Bowers, N. and Langhorne, P. (2015) Clinical and Cost Effectiveness of Enhanced Oral Healthcare in Stroke Care Settings (SOCLE II): A Pilot, Stepped Wedge, Cluster Randomized, Controlled Trial Protocol. *International Journal of Stroke*, **10**, 979-984. http://dx.doi.org/10.1111/ijs.12530

[36] Munoz, N., Touger-Decker, R., Byham-Gray, L. and Maillet, J.O. (2009) Effect of an Oral Health Assessment Education Program on Nurses' Knowledge and Patient Care Practices in Skilled Nursing Facilities. *Special Care in Dentistry*,

29, 179-185. http://dx.doi.org/10.1111/j.1754-4505.2009.00084.x

[37] Wing, R.R., Hamman, R.F., Bray, G.A., Delahanty, L., Edelstein, S.L., Hill, J.O., Horton, E.S., Hoskin, M.A., Kriska, A., Lachin, J., Mayer-Davis, E.J., Pi-Sunyer, X., Regensteiner, J.G., Venditti, B. and Wylie-Rosett, J. (2004) Achieving Weight and Activity Goals among Diabetes Prevention Program Lifestyle Participants. *Obesity Research*, **12**, 1426-1434. http://dx.doi.org/10.1038/oby.2004.179

[38] Costello, T. and Coyne, I. (2008) Nurses' Knowledge of Mouth Care Practices. *British Journal of Nursing*, **17**, 264-268. http://dx.doi.org/10.12968/bjon.2008.17.4.28716

22

Fidelity of Intervention Implementation: A Review of Instruments

Sarah Ibrahim[1], Souraya Sidani[2]

[1]Arthur Labatt School of Nursing, University of Western Ontario, London, Canada
[2]Daphne Cockwell School of Nursing, Ryerson University, Toronto, Canada
Email: sibrah25@uwo.ca, ssidani@ryerson.ca

Abstract

Background: Interventions, whether simple or complex, are increasing in health care in response to the growing complexity and acuity of patient's conditions. Monitoring the fidelity of implementing interventions is challenging. A common method to assess and monitor fidelity of intervention implementation is through a structured, reliable and valid instrument. Purpose: The purpose of this paper is to examine existing instruments measuring fidelity of intervention implementation in order to determine aspects of fidelity that have been assessed and reported on the reliability and validity of these instruments. Design: A descriptive review was conducted. Studies were included if they described and reported on the fidelity of intervention implementation instruments, their psychometric properties were published between 1980 and 2015. Methods: Data were extracted on the study characteristics, levels and aspects of fidelity and the psychometric properties, specifically the reliability and validity of the fidelity of intervention implementation instruments. Results: In total, 21 studies were included in the review. Overall results showed that some aspects and levels of fidelity of intervention implementation are included in the instruments. At the theoretical level, fidelity of intervention implementation is not accounted for majority of the studies and few explicitly reports on the use of instruments to evaluate intervention differentiation. At the operational level, interventionists' adherence and competence are included in the instruments; however, participants' engagement, exposure and enactment are not. The instruments demonstrate acceptable level of validity and reliability. Conclusion: Sustained focus on developing psychometrically sound instruments that account for all levels (*i.e.* theoretical and operational) and aspects of fidelity of intervention implementation is imperative to strengthen the methodological literature for interventions research; and for researchers to correctly interpret research findings and to arrive at valid conclusions on the effectiveness of interventions, whether simple or complex.

Keywords

Interventions, Intervention Fidelity, Intervention Fidelity Instrument

1. Introduction

Historically, intervention fidelity received little attention in intervention research because of the assumption that interventions were delivered in a standardized and consistent manner by interventionists who strictly followed the treatment protocol and manual [1]. However, concerns over intervention fidelity arose in various fields of research, most notably in psychotherapy, as brought forth by Eysenck (1952) [2]. Eysenck critiqued the vague descriptions provided for psychotherapy treatments in the 1960s and the report on overall effectiveness, disregarding evidence on the contribution of different components and actual implementation of treatments [3]. In the 1970s, a shift in intervention research emerged with an emphasis on collecting data on the implementation of treatment. This was done as a means of ensuring the interventionists adhered to the treatment protocol and determining whether contamination took place, that is, the extent to which the experimental treatment was disseminated to the control arm of the study. This emphasis on examining the implementation of the experimental and comparison treatments occurred at a time when there was ambiguous information and descriptions of the nature and dose of treatments; this in turn, affected the ability to replicate interventions and to reach valid conclusions on their effects [4].

Over the past three decades, there has been growing recognition of the importance to monitor and assess fidelity of implementing health interventions [5]. Intervention fidelity, also referred to as implementation fidelity and treatment integrity in the literature, is the competent and reliable delivery of an intervention as intended in the original design [6]-[8]. This ensures the intervention is carried out in the selected dose and mode to initiate the mechanisms that are responsible for producing the desired changes in the outcomes [1].

Intervention fidelity is conceptualized at two levels: theoretical and operational. At the theoretical level, intervention fidelity is related to the process of developing and designing an intervention. It refers to the correspondence between the intervention's active ingredients and its components and activities. The active ingredients are identified in the intervention theory as the elements that characterize the intervention and are responsible for producing the changes in outcomes. The active ingredients are reflected in the components and activities comprising the intervention. At the operational level, intervention fidelity refers to the degree to which the intervention is delivered according to the original design and plan. The interventionists' performance in delivering the intervention and the client's exposure, engagement, and adherence to the intervention are necessary for ensuring successful implementation of its components and activities and in turn, effectiveness in instigating the desired changes [1].

Intervention fidelity affects the external and internal validity and statistical conclusions in intervention research [1] [9]. Specific to external validity, a clear and detailed description of the intervention's active ingredients, components, activities and mode and dose of delivery, and protocol for carrying out the intervention allow for reproducibility of the intervention [4]. Specific to internal validity, the lack of information on the fidelity of intervention implementation impedes the ability to know whether the effects are due to the intervention itself or to a Type III error, that is, failure to implement the intervention as planned [10]. Specific to statistical conclusions, variations in the delivery of an intervention result in differences in participants' exposure to the intervention components and dose, leading to variability in outcome achievement. Such variability inflates error variance in posttest outcomes and decreases the statistical power to detect significant effects, potentially leading to incorrect conclusions about the effectiveness of the intervention [1] [9] [11] [12]. In general, failure to monitor and assess fidelity of intervention implementation precludes researchers from concluding what was actually responsible for the significant or non-significant effects [6] [13].

A common strategy to monitor and assess for fidelity of intervention implementation is through a structured, valid and reliable instrument. The development and use of such instruments to assess the quality of the implementation of an intervention has been widely accepted in health intervention research. Although efforts have been made to develop instruments to assess fidelity of intervention implementation, limited research has been conducted on identifying the aspects of fidelity that are captured in these measures. In this descriptive review, we examined existing instruments measuring fidelity of intervention implementation to determine aspects of fidelity that they assess, and reported on the reliability and validity of these instruments.

2. Methods

2.1. Selection Criteria

Studies were included in the review if they met these criteria: original research study reporting on an instrument measuring fidelity of intervention implementation and its psychometric properties, published in the English language in peer-reviewed journals, dissertations or theses, between 1980 and 2015. The start date of 1980 provided a time period for publication of relevant papers, following the emphasis in the 1960s and 1970s on data collection, assessment, and reporting of intervention fidelity [4].

2.2. Search Strategies

The databases used to identify the literature were: Health and Psychological Instruments (HAPI), Cumulative Index to Nursing and Allied Health Literature (CINAHL), Medline, Educational Resources Information Center (ERIC), Web of Science, Proquest Dissertations and Theses, and Google Scholar. The following keywords and Boolean operators were used to combine and refine the searches: ("fidelity" OR "integrity" OR "adherence" OR "implementation fidelity" OR "fidelity to treatment" OR "intervention fidelity" OR "intervention integrity" OR "intervention adherence") AND (tool* OR instrument* OR questionnaire OR survey*) AND (valid* OR reliab*) AND (measure* OR evaluat* OR assess*). Also, reference lists of the selected articles were reviewed to identify additional publications.

2.3. Data Extraction

Data were extracted from full papers on study characteristics, aspects of fidelity assessed by the instruments and psychometric properties of the instruments. Information presented in relevant sections of the papers was summarized and coded by the authors. Any difference was resolved through consensus. High level of agreement (> 80%) was attained.

2.3.1. Study Characteristics
The following information specific to the study characteristics was extracted: (a) author's last name and year of publication; (b) discipline; (c) target population; (d) type of intervention under evaluation; and (e) number of components comprising the intervention.

2.3.2. Aspects of Fidelity Assessed
Information was gathered on elements of theoretical and operational fidelity assessed and on strategies or items used to conduct the assessment. The information was derived from relevant methodological literature [1] [6] [13].

Two strategies have been proposed to examine theoretical fidelity. The first is applied when designing the intervention and consists of generating a matrix to link the intervention's active ingredients with its components and activities; the matrix forms the basis for developing the items for measuring the implementation of the intervention's activities [1]. The second strategy refers to intervention differentiation [6]; it involves the use of the items to monitor the performance of the specified activities when implementing the intervention and the non-engagement in these activities in the control or comparison group.

Operational fidelity is assessed at two levels: interventionist and participant. For the interventionists, two elements of operational fidelity are examined: adherence and competence [4] [10] [14]. Adherence refers to the degree to which the interventionists carried out the intervention in a way that is consistent with the original design and plan as delineated in the treatment protocol and manual [1] [8] [14]. To assess interventionists' adherence, the instruments should contain a list of activities to be performed and allow documentation of the extent to which they are being followed during intervention implementation [15]. Competence refers to the extent to which the interventionists possess the skills and knowledge required to deliver the intervention [16].

For participants, the elements of operational fidelity are: exposure, engagement and enactment. Exposure refers to the extent to which the participant is in contact with the intervention's content. Exposure is often documented as the number of intervention sessions attended and duration of each session. Engagement is the extent to which the participants are involved in the intervention activities and captured through participants' self-report and or interventionists' observation of the activities completed during the intervention sessions (e.g. participation in group discussion). Adherence refers to the extent to which participants apply the activities or recommendations in the context of daily life such as exercising for 30 minutes five times per week [1] [6].

2.3.3. Psychometric Properties
The psychometric properties of instruments measuring fidelity of intervention implementation were evaluated

using the methodological framework of Streiner and Norman (2008) [17]. Reliability demonstrated the ability of an instrument to yield consistent and reproducible results [18] [19]. Three types of reliability were examined in this review: test-retest, inter-rater, and internal consistency. Validity refers to the extent to which an instrument measures what it is intended to measure [19] [20]. Two aspects of validity of the instruments were examined: construct and content.

2.4. Data Analysis

The data pertaining to the study characteristics, identification of the aspects of fidelity and the psychometric properties of the instruments were analyzed descriptively using the Statistical Package for the Social Sciences (SPSS) Version 22.

3. Results

3.1. Literature Search

The literature search yielded a total of 104,143 titles and abstracts (**Figure 1**). All abstracts were reviewed and 104, 117 were excluded because they did not meet the selection criteria; nine articles were duplicates. A total of 20 articles were selected for full review, and of these, 18 met all selection criteria. A hand search of the reference lists of the selected articles yielded three additional articles for full review. A total of 21 publications were reviewed.

3.2. Study Characteristics

The studies were published between 1996 and 2015. The reported disciplines included: nursing ($n = 4$, 19%), psychology ($n = 4$, 19%), psychiatry ($n = 3$, 14.2%), social work ($n = 1$, 4.8%), public health ($n = 1$, 4.8%), behavioral medicine ($n = 1$, 4.8%), rehabilitation science (specifically Occupational Therapy) ($n = 2$, 9.5%), education ($n = 3$, 14.3%), and health services ($n = 2$, 9.5%). The target population included: persons living with addictions ($n = 4$, 19%), pre-mature infants ($n = 1$, 4.8%), children ($n = 4$, 19%), older adults ($n = 1$, 4.8%), persons living with mental health challenges ($n = 5$, 24%), persons living with physical health challenges ($n = 2$, 10%), homeless persons ($n = 1$, 4.8%); couples ($n = 1$, 4.8%), parents of lower socioeconomic status ($n = 1$, 4.8%), and teachers providing social-emotional competence and behavioral support ($n = 1$, 4.8%). The type of interventions comprised of two or more components, such as educational (*i.e.* provision of information on addictions, mental health, and child safety) and behavioral (*i.e.* targeting behaviors related to addictions) and included: psychotherapy ($n = 3$, 14.3%); psycho-education ($n = 1$, 4.8%); cognitive behavioral therapy (CBT) ($n = 2$, 9.5%); emotion-focused therapy ($n = 1$, 4.8%); educational ($n = 1$, 4.8%) behavioral therapy ($n = 6$, 28.9%);

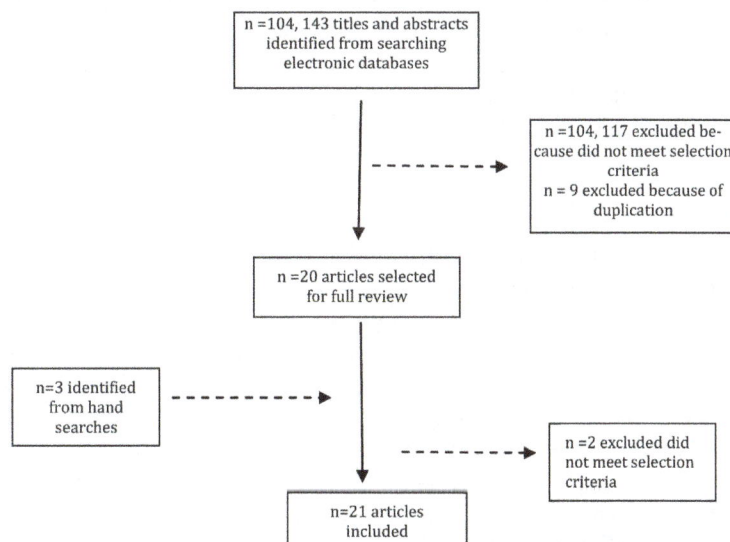

Figure 1. Flow diagram of literature selection.

prevention-related (*i.e.* hospital related functioning decline among older adults) (n = 4, 19%); and technology (n = 3, 14.3%).

3.3. Assessment of Intervention Fidelity

To examine theoretical fidelity, the authors of all studies (n = 21, 100%) generated a matrix to construct the items measuring fidelity. The active ingredients of the interventions were identified through various means, separately or in combination: experts, literature and review of the treatment protocol. In addition the content of the items was validated in majority of the studies (as reported in a later section). However, intervention differentiation was assessed in only three studies (14.3%).

Different elements of operational fidelity were represented in the instruments. Interventionists' competency and adherence in delivering the intervention were most commonly assessed (n = 12, 57%). Specifically, interventionists' adherence was measured by the respective instruments used in five studies (24%); interventionists' general behavior was assessed in one study (4.8%); and the remaining three studies (14.3%) did not clearly indicate whether or not interventionists' competency and adherence were measured. In the majority (n = 20, 95%) of the studies, participants' exposure, engagement and enactment of the intervention were not accounted for in the instruments measuring the fidelity of intervention implementation. One study assessed participant's engagement in the intervention through report by a third party and direct and indirect observations by the interventionist.

3.4. Psychometric Properties

3.4.1. Reliability

In the majority (n = 19, 91%) of the studies, the reliability of the intervention fidelity instruments was evaluated.

Internal consistency. Of the 19 studies, 13 (68.4%) reported on internal consistency of the intervention fidelity instruments using Cronbach's alpha (α), and the remaining four did not provide empirical evidence. The Cronbach's alpha ranged from 0.70 - 0.72 (acceptable) for nursing interventions; 0.70 - 0.99 (acceptable to excellent) for rehabilitation science interventions; 0.47 - 0.98 (unacceptable to excellent) for psychological interventions; 0.62 - 0.95 (acceptable to excellent) for psychiatry interventions; and 0.721 - 0.91 (good-excellent) for education interventions.

Inter-rater reliability. A total of 13 studies (68.4%) reported on inter-rater reliability using different coefficients. The Krippendorff's α coefficient was 0.70 and 0.81 (good to excellent) for social work interventions. The Intra-class Correlation Coefficient ranged from 0.35 - 0.79 (unacceptable to acceptable) for psychiatry interventions; 0.71 - 0.95 (acceptable to excellent) for psychological interventions; 0.60 - 0.74 (questionable to acceptable) for nursing interventions; and 0.99 (excellent) for rehabilitation science interventions. The value of the Cohen's Kappa coefficient was reported at 0.69 (good) for psychological interventions; 0.72 - 0.87 (good to very good) for behavioral interventions; and 0.66 - 0.96 (good to very good) for nursing interventions. The G coefficients ranged from 0.75 - 0.87 (acceptable) for rehabilitation science and education interventions. The percent of agreement ranged from 78.8% - 98% (acceptable) for nursing and education interventions.

Test re-test reliability. None of the 21 studies reported on test re-test reliability of the intervention fidelity instruments.

3.4.2. Validity

The majority (n = 18, 86%) of the studies reported on the validity of the intervention fidelity instruments.

Construct validity. About half of the studies (11 of 18, 61.1%) reported on construct validity of the instruments measuring fidelity of implementing psychology, psychiatry, health services, education, and rehabilitation interventions. However, not all provided empirical evidence to support the claim of construct validity. Of those that did, results demonstrated the instruments were able to discriminate between the different conditions (e.g. Cognitive Therapy and Supportive Expressive Dynamic Therapy; Twelve Step Facilitation, Clinical Management, and Cognitive Behavioral Therapy). Further, six studies (33.3%) reported on the relationships between the instruments' subscales which captured the different aspects of fidelity with other measures of interventionists' adherence to interventions such as Twelve Step Facilitation, Clinical Management scales; the association were relatively small in magnitude (Pearson's r = −0.29 to −0.10; 0.23 - 0.63; 0.18 - 0.36; Spearman's rho Correlation: r_s 0.14 and 0.33).

Content validity. Most studies (10 of 18, 56%) reported on content validity of the instruments. This was done through expert judgment of the content of the items ($n = 4$, 22.2%). Agreement among experts was quantified in terms of the Cohen's Kappa Coefficient (κ) in one study, and the Content Validity Index (CVI) in three studies. Overall, the CVIs were high (82.2% - 100%) implying the majority of the experts rated the items as relevant in capturing the key ingredients of the interventions.

4. Discussion

This study represents a first attempt to examine and identify the aspects of fidelity that are represented in existing instruments measuring fidelity of intervention implementation and to report on the validity and reliability of these measures.

Overall, the findings of this review showed that majority of the instruments were developed to measure the fidelity of implementing a specific intervention. Although advantageous in explicitly representing the active ingredients, components and activities that characterize a particular intervention, specific measures have limited applicability to similar or different interventions [21] [22]. This situation creates the need to develop multiple instruments; this precludes meaningful comparisons of fidelity with which the interventions were implemented. Therefore, it would be useful to develop generic instruments, as proposed by Breitenstein *et al.* (2010) [21] and Di Rezze *et al.* (2012) [22] to assess fidelity. Generic instruments assess the adherence to the protocol of interventions that have the same theoretical underpinning, consist of similar components (such as cognitive-behavioral therapy), and target a particular population (e.g. substance use) or practice (e.g. nursing) [21]. The advantage of these generic instruments is that they can be broadly applied to theoretically consistent interventions and or adapted to a specific target population [22]. For example, the main components of Cognitive Behavioral Therapy (CBT) can be implemented in a similar manner for persons with insomnia, depression, and anxiety. This in turn, standardizes the assessment of the fidelity with which these interventions are delivered [21] [22].

4.1. Assessment of Fidelity of Intervention Implementation

Although there has been a proliferation of instruments for measuring fidelity of intervention implementation, the findings of this review pointed to several gaps. Theoretical fidelity was addressed primarily when developing the instruments by following a systematic process, which strengthens the validity and utility of the instruments. The process involved the identification of the active ingredients, components and activities, as well as the generation of a matrix, which was used to operationalize the intervention and guide the statement of items. However, a few of the studies explicitly reported use of the instrument to evaluate intervention differentiation. This finding may not be surprising as theoretical fidelity is often perceived as important during the stage of intervention design more so than implementation and evaluation. Assessment of intervention differentiation should be done in future research in order to determine the extent of contamination or dissemination of the intervention under evaluation to the control or comparison group, which may account for non-significant effects.

The findings of this review indicated that not all aspects of operational fidelity were captured in the instruments. Most instruments contained items that assessed interventionists' competence or adherence, but not both. According to Hogue *et al.* (1996) [23], attainment of high levels of fidelity of intervention implementation requires assessment of adherence and competence. This is because adherence and competence are interrelated, that is, an interventionist cannot be competent in implementing an intervention without adhering to its protocol and adherence alone is not sufficient for the delivery of the intervention competently [23]-[26]. In contrast, the instruments did not capture aspects of operational fidelity pertaining to participants' exposure, engagement and enactment. The extent to which participants carry out the intervention activities and or recommendations is equally important for the success of an intervention in producing the desired outcomes [1] [27].

The overall findings of this review have demonstrated that although some aspects of fidelity (*i.e.* interventionists' adherence and competence) have been accounted for in instruments measuring fidelity of intervention implementation instruments, not all levels (*i.e.* theoretical) and aspects (*i.e.* participant engagement, exposure, and enactment) have been captured in the existing measures. Implementation of interventions, whether simple of complex, is one that requires the actions of both participants and interventionists in order to successfully attain the intervention goals and achieve the desired changes [1].

4.2. Psychometric Properties

The instruments measuring fidelity of intervention implementation have shown acceptable levels of reliability and validity. This finding is consistent with a narrative review of generic intervention fidelity instruments for paediatric rehabilitation [22]. Reliability testing yielded fair to excellent internal consistency and inter-rater reliability. Not all studies provided empirical evidence supporting construct validity; those that did reported significant association between theoretically related concepts, primarily the association between fidelity and outcomes. The majority of the instruments were subjected to content validity by experts in the field. However none of the instruments were examined for test re-test reliability. Test re-test reliability examines stability of instruments over time and is often conducted for measures of stable concepts [17]. The examination of test re-test reliability is not feasible or meaningful for intervention fidelity instruments because one cannot administer the same intervention to the same group of participants at two separate points in time (usually between two and 14 days).

5. Implications for Practice and Research and Conclusion

The results of this review highlight key implications for research and practice. First, the review can inform researchers and clinicians of the current reliable and valid intervention fidelity instruments to monitor and assess the implementation of theoretically similar interventions (*i.e.* CBT for persons with depression and anxiety). This will decrease the burden of developing new instruments [22] and build the science of interventions research [21]. Second, the review identifies gaps related to limited assessment of theoretical fidelity and non-inclusion of all aspects of operational fidelity in the instruments used to evaluate fidelity of implementing a range of health interventions. Though there are different terms used across disciplines (e.g. psychology and nursing) to refer to aspects of theoretical and operational fidelity, researchers and clinicians are recommended to account for interventionists' adherence and competence, participants' exposure, engagement and enactment and intervention differentiation for assessing and monitoring fidelity of intervention implementation. Frameworks describing types and aspects of intervention fidelity are available [6] [7] [13] [28] and have the potential to support the development of instruments to conduct comprehensive assessment of the fidelity with which interventions are implemented, as well the valid interpretation of findings.

There are several limitations that are noteworthy in this review. First, despite the extensive search strategy, only a limited number of papers that report on the development and use of instruments for measuring fidelity are found. Additional papers, published in languages other than English may have been missed. Second, there is variability in the reported reliability and validity of the instruments by researchers; some authors do not provide empirical evidence to support their claims, which limit information needed to inform researchers and clinicians intending to use the instrument of its psychometric prosperities.

There is a need for the development and use of objective, reliable and valid fidelity of intervention implementation instruments that capture all aspects of fidelity and enhance the validity of findings in interventions research [8]. This is because healthcare providers to implement appropriate, efficient, effective, and safe complex interventions in clinical practice, it is important for them to understand the goal, essential and non-essential elements, mode of delivery, and dose of the intervention. Such an understanding provides direction for the operationalization of the intervention, and the implementation of the intervention with fidelity to produce changes in outcomes and to improve patient health and care [29]. This review examines and identifies the aspects of fidelity that are included in fidelity of intervention implementation and are reported on the psychometric properties of the measures. Sustained focus on developing psychometrically sound instruments that account for all aspects of fidelity (*i.e.* theoretical and operational level) as a method to assess and monitor implementation of interventions is imperative to strengthen the methodological literature for interventions and health research and for researchers to correctly interpret research findings and arrive to valid conclusions on the interventions effectiveness.

References*

[1]   Sidani, S. and Braden, C.J. (2011) Design, Evaluation, and Translation of Nursing Interventions. Wiley-Blackwell, Ames.

[2]   Eysenck, H. (1952) The Effects of Psychotherapy, an Evaluation. *Journal of Consulting Psychology*, **16**, 319-324. http://dx.doi.org/10.1037/h0063633

[3]   VandenBos, G.R. (1980) Psychotherapy: Practice, Research, Policy. Sage, Beverly Hills.

*Full list of the references are available by the authors upon request.

[4] Moncher, F.J. and Prinz, R.J. (1991) Treatment Fidelity in Outcome Studies. *Clinical Psychology Review*, **11**, 247-266. http://dx.doi.org/10.1016/0272-7358(91)90103-2

[5] Gearing, R.E., El-Bassel, N., Ghesquiere, A., Baldwin, S., Gillies, J. and Ngeow, E. (2011) Major Ingredients of Fidelity: A Review and Scientific Guide to Improving Quality of Intervention Research Implementation. *Clinical Psychology Review*, **31**, 79-88. http://dx.doi.org/10.1016/j.cpr.2010.09.007

[6] Bellg, A.J., Borrelli, B., Resnick, B., Hecht, J., Minicucci, D.S., Ory, M., *et al.* (2004) Enhancing Treatment Fidelity in Health Behavior Change Studies: Best Practices and Recommendations from the NIH Behaviour Change Consortium. *Health Psychology*, **23**, 443-451. http://dx.doi.org/10.1037/0278-6133.23.5.443

[7] Carroll, C., Patterson, M., Wood, S., Booth, A., Rick, J. and Balain, S. (2007) A Conceptual Framework for Implementation Fidelity. *Implementation Science*, **2**, 40. http://dx.doi.org/10.1186/1748-5908-2-40

[8] Stein, K.F., Sargent, J.T. and Rafaels, N. (2007) Intervention Research: Establishing Fidelity of the Independent Variable in Nursing Clinical Trials. *Nursing Research*, **56**, 54-62. http://dx.doi.org/10.1097/00006199-200701000-00007

[9] Shadish, W.R., Cook, T.D. and Campbell, D.T. (2002) Experimental and Quasi-Experimental Designs for Generalized Causal Inference. Houghton Mifflin Company, Boston.

[10] Dusenbury, L., Brannigan, R., Falco, M. and Hansen, W.B. (2003) A Review of Research on Fidelity of Implementation: Implications for Drug Abuse Prevention in School Settings. *Health Education Research*, **18**, 237-256. http://dx.doi.org/10.1093/her/18.2.237

[11] Brandt, P.A., Kirsch, S.D., Lewis, F.M. and Casey, S.M. (2004) Assessing the Strength and Integrity of an Intervention. *Oncology Nursing Forum*, **31**, 833-837. http://dx.doi.org/10.1188/04.ONF.833-837

[12] Dumas, J.E., Lynch, A.M., Laughlin, J.E., Smith, P.E. and Prinze, R.J. (2001) Promoting Intervention Fidelity: Conceptual Issues, Methods, and Preliminary Results from the EARLY ALLIANCE Prevention Trial. *American Journal of Preventive Medicine*, **20**, 38-47. http://dx.doi.org/10.1016/S0749-3797(00)00272-5

[13] Borrelli, B., Sepinwall, D., Ernst, D., Bellg, A.J., Czajkowski, S., Breger, R., *et al.* (2005) A New Tool to Assess Treatment Fidelity and Evaluation of Treatment Fidelity across 10 Years of Health Behaviour Research. *Journal of Consulting and Clinical Psychology*, **73**, 852-860. http://dx.doi.org/10.1037/0022-006X.73.5.852

[14] Santacroce, S.J., Maccarelli, L.M. and Grey, M. (2004) Intervention Fidelity. *Nursing Research*, **53**, 63-66. http://dx.doi.org/10.1097/00006199-200401000-00010

[15] Mowbray, C.T., Holter, M.C., Teague, G.B. and Bybee, D. (2003) Fidelity Criteria: Development, Measurement, and Validation. *American Journal of Evaluation*, **24**, 315-340. http://dx.doi.org/10.1016/S1098-2140(03)00057-2

[16] Faiburn, C.G. and Cooper, Z. (2011) Therapist Competence, Therapy Quality and Therapist Training. *Behavioral Research and Therapy*, **49**, 373-378. http://dx.doi.org/10.1016/j.brat.2011.03.005

[17] Streiner, D.L. and Norman, G.R. (2008) Health Measurement Scales: A Practical Guide to Their Development and Use. 4th Edition, Oxford University Press Inc., New York. http://dx.doi.org/10.1093/acprof:oso/9780199231881.001.0001

[18] DeVon, H.A., Block, M.E., Moyle-Wright, P., Ernst, D.M., Hayden, S.J., Lazzara, D.J., *et al.* (2007) A Psychometric Toolbox for Testing Validity and Reliability. *Journal of Nursing Scholarship*, **39**, 155-164. http://dx.doi.org/10.1111/j.1547-5069.2007.00161.x

[19] Fayers, P.M. and Machin, D. (2007) Quality of Life. 2nd Edition, John Wiley & Sons Inc., Hoboken. http://dx.doi.org/10.1002/9780470024522

[20] Eigenmann, C.A., Colagiuri, T.C., Skinner, T.C. and Trevena, L. (2009) Are Current Psychometric Tools Suitable for Measuring Outcomes for Diabetes Education? *Diabetes Medicine*, **26**, 425-436. http://dx.doi.org/10.1111/j.1464-5491.2009.02697.x

[21] Breitenstein, S.M., Fogg, L., Garvey, C., Hill, C., Resnick, B. and Gross, D. (2010) Measuring Implementation Fidelity in a Community-Based Parenting Intervention. *Nursing Research*, **59**, 158-165. http://dx.doi.org/10.1097/NNR.0b013e3181dbb2e2

[22] Di Rezze, B., Law, M., Gorter, J.W., Eva, K. and Pollock, N. (2012) A Narrative Review of Generic Intervention Fidelity Measures. *Physical and Occupational Therapy in Pediatrics*, **32**, 430-446. http://dx.doi.org/10.3109/01942638.2012.713454

[23] Hogue, A., Liddle, H.A. and Rowe, C. (1996) Treatment Adherence Process Research in Family Therapy: A Rationale and Some Practical Guidelines. *Psychotherapy*, **33**, 332-345. http://dx.doi.org/10.1037/0033-3204.33.2.332

[24] Barber, J.P. and Crits-Christoph, P. (1996) Development of a Therapist Adherence/Competence Rating Scale for Supportive-Expressive Dynamic Psychotherapy: A Preliminary Report. *Psychotherapy Research*, **6**, 81-94. http://dx.doi.org/10.1080/10503309612331331608

[25] Perepletchikova, F., Treat, T.A. and Kazdin, A.E. (2007) Treatment Integrity in Psychotherapy Research: Analysis of the Studies and Examination of the Associated Factors. *Journal of Consulting and Clinical Psychology*, **75**, 829-841.

http://dx.doi.org/10.1037/0022-006X.75.6.829

[26] Waltz, J., Addis, M., Koerner, K. and Jacobson, N.S. (1993) Testing the Integrity of a Psychotherapy Protocol: Assessment of Adherence and Competence. *Journal of Consulting and Clinical Psychology*, **61**, 620-630. http://dx.doi.org/10.1037/0022-006X.61.4.620

[27] Leventhal, H. and Friedman, M.A. (2004) Does Establishing Fidelity of Treatment Help in Understanding Treatment Efficacy? Comment on Bellg *et al.* (2004). *Health Psychology*, **23**, 452-456. http://dx.doi.org/10.1037/0278-6133.23.5.452

[28] Lichstein, K.L., Riedel, B.W. and Grieve, R. (1994) Fair Tests of Clinical Trials: A Treatment Implementation Model. *Advances in Behaviour Research and Therapy*, **16**, 1-29. http://dx.doi.org/10.1016/0146-6402(94)90001-9

[29] Sidani, S. (2015) Health Intervention Research: Understanding Research Design and Methods. Sage, Thousand Oaks.

Permissions

List of Contributors

Athanassios Vozikis and Maria Siganou
Economics Department, University of Piraeus, Piraeus, Greece

Maria Hassandra
University of Jyväskylä, Jyväskylä, Finland

Marios Goudas and Yiannis Theodorakis
Department of Physical Education and Sport Science, University of Thessaly, Karyes, Greece

Melis Naçar, Fevziye Çetinkaya, Zeynep Baykan and Mehmet Sağiroğlu
Department of Medical Education, School of Medicine, Erciyes University, Kayseri, Turkey

Gökmen Zararsiz
Department of Biostatistics, School of Medicine, Erciyes University, Kayseri, Turkey

Gülay Yilmazel
Department of Nursery, School of Health, Hitit University, Çorum, Turkey

Samuel Ambapour and Hylod Armel Moussana
Institut National de la Statistique, Brazzaville, République du Congo

Jean Christophe Okandza
Faculté des Sciences Economiques, Université Marien Ngouabi, Brazzaville, République du Congo

María J. Miranda Velasco
Department of Educational Sciences, University of Extremadura, Coordinator of Research Group Education and Health Innovation, Cáceres, Spain

Maria Gloria Solís Galán
Department of Educational Sciences, University of Extremadura, Research Group Education and Health Innovation, Cáceres, Spain

Enma Domínguez Martín
Research Group Education and Health Innovation, Cáceres, Spain

Koji Harada
Graduate School of Health Sciences, Hiroshima University, Hiroshima, Japan

Michiko Moriyama, Mariko Uno and Toshio Kobayashi
Institute of Biomedical & Health Sciences, Hiroshima University, Hiroshima, Japan

Takefumi Yuzuriha
Hizen Psychiatric Center, Saga, Japan

Dilip C. Nath and Bhushita Patowari
Department of Statistics, Gauhati University, Guwahati, India

Athanassios Vozikis
Economics Department, University of Piraeus, Piraeus, Greece

Lina Stavropoulou and George P. Patrinos
Department of Pharmacy, School of Health Sciences, University of Patras, Patras, Greece

Víctor Patricio Díaz-Narváez
Facultad de Odontología, Universidad San Sebastián, Santiago, Chile
Universidad Autónoma de Chile, Santiago, Chile

Ana María Erazo Coronado
Universidad Metropolitana, Barranquilla, Colombia

Jorge Luis Bilbao
Facultad de Medicina, Universidad Libre Seccional Barranquilla y Fundación Universitaria San Martín Sede Puerto Colombia, Barranquilla, Colombia

Farith González
Facultad de Odontología, Universidad de Cartagena, Cartagena, Colombia

Mariela Padilla and Robert Utsman
Universidad Latinoamericana de Ciencia y Tecnología, San José, Costa Rica

Madeline Howard
Facultad de Odontología, Universidad de Costa Rica, San José, Costa Rica

Guadalupe Silva and Joel Arboleda
Universidad Central del Este, San Pedro de Macorís, República Dominicana

Mirian Bullen
Facultad de Odontología, Universidad de Panamá, Ciudad de Panamá, República de Panamá

Elizabeth Fajardo
Faculty of Health Sciences, Universidad del Tolima, Ibagué, Colombia

Luz Marina Alonso
División de Salud, Universidad del Norte, Barranquilla, Colombia

Marcos Cervantes
Facultad de Ciencias Sociales, Universidad del Norte, Barranquilla, Colombia

Mary Hassandra
Department of Sports, University of Jyväskylä, Jyväskylä, Finland

Athanasios Kolovelonis, Marios Goudas and Yiannis Theodorakis
Department of Physical Education & Sport Science, University of Thessaly, Trikala, Greece

Stiliani Ani Chroni
Department of Sports & Physical Education, Hedmark University College, Elverum, Norway

Alkistis Olympiou
School of Sport and Exercise Science, College of Social Science, University of Lincoln, Lincoln, UK

Víctor Patricio Díaz-Narváez
School of Dentistry, Universidad San Sebastián, Santiago, Chile
Associate Investigator, Universidad Autónoma de Chile, Santiago, Chile

Ana María Erazo Coronado
Universidad Metropolitana, Barranquilla, Colombia

Jorge Luis Bilbao
School of Medicine, Universidad Libre Seccional Barranquilla y Fundación Universitaria San Martín Sede Puerto Colombia, Barranquilla, Colombia

Farith González
School of Dentistry, Universidad de Cartagena, Campus de la Salud Barrio Zaragocilla, Cartagena, Colombia

Mariela Padilla
School of Health Sciences, Universidad Latinoamericana de Ciencia y Tecnología, San José, Costa Rica

Madeline Howard
School of Dentistry, Universidad de Costa Rica, San Pedro de Montes de Oca, San José, Costa Rica

María Guadalupe Silva
Institute for Scientific Research, Universidad Central del Este, San Pedro de Macorís, Dominican Republic

Mirian Bullen
School of Dentistry, Universidad de Panamá, Panama City, Panama

Fredy Gutierrez
Facultad de Estomatología Roberto Beltrán, Universidad Peruana Cayetano Heredia, Lima, Peru

Teresa Varela de Villalba
School of Medicine, Universidad Católica de Córdoba, Córdoba, Argentina

Mercedes Salcedo Rioja
Department of Pediatric Dentistry, School of Dentistry, Universidad Nacional Mayor de San Marcos, Lima, Peru

Joyce Huberman
School of Dentistry, Faculty of Clinical Medicine, Universidad del Desarrollo, Santiago, Chile

Doris Carrasco
School of Dentistry, Universidad de Concepción, Concepción, Chile

Robert Utsman
Investigation of the School of Health Sciences, Universidad Latinoamericana de Ciencia y Tecnología, San José, Costa Rica

Estela Maria Leite Meirelles Monteiro
Graduate Program in Nursing, Federal University of Pernambuco (UFPE), Recife, Brazil
Graduate Program in Child and Adolescent Health, Centre of Health Sciences, Federal University of Pernambuco, Recife, Brazil

Amanda Araújo das Mercês, Amanda Carla Borba de Souza Cavalcanti and Ana Catarina Torres de Lacerda
Nursing Department at the Federal University of Pernambuco, Recife, Brazil

Ana Márcia Tenório de Souza Cavalcanti and Andrea Rosane Sousa Silva
Graduate Program in Nursing, Federal University of Pernambuco (UFPE), Recife, Brazil

Rosália Daniela Medeiros da Silva and Waldemar Brandão Neto
Graduate Program in Child and Adolescent Health, Centre of Health Sciences, Federal University of Pernambuco, Recife, Brazil

Angelika Anita Schlarb, Merle Claßen and Frank Neuner
Faculty of Psychology and Sports, University of Bielefeld, Bielefeld, Germany

E.-S. Schuster and Martin Hautzinger
Faculty of Science, University of Tuebingen, Tuebingen, Germany

Hiroshi Fujioka
Department of Nursing, Faculty of Health Sciences, Tsukuba International University, Tsuchiura-Shi, Japan

Rie Wakimizu
Department of Child Health Care Nursing, Division of Health Innovation and Nursing, Faculty of Medicine, University of Tsukuba, Tsukuba-Shi, Japan

Ryuta Tanaka and Tatsuyuki Ohto
Department of Child Health, Graduate School of Comprehensive Human Sciences, University of Tsukuba, Tsukuba-Shi, Japan

Atsushi Ieshima
Aiseikai Kinen Ibaraki Welfare & Medical Center, Mito-Shi, Japan

Akira Yoneyama
National Rehabilitation Center for Children with Disabilities, Itabashi-Ku, Japan

Kiyoko Kamibeppu
Department of Family Nursing, School of Health Sciences and Nursing, Graduate School of Medicine, The University of Tokyo, Bunkyo-Ku, Japan

Hussein Salman Mohammed
Dermatology and Venereology, OIU, Khartoum, Sudan

Jahelrasoul Abdalla Edriss
Dermatology and Venereology, KTHDV, Khartoum, Sudan

P. Cougar Hall, Josh H. West, Benjamin T. Crookston and Yvonne Allsop
Department of Health Science, Brigham Young University, Provo, UT, USA

Rosa M. Limiñana-Gras
Research Group Personality and Health: A Intercultural and Gender Perspective, Murcia, Spain
Universidad de Murcia, Murcia, Spain

María del Pilar Sánchez-López
Universidad Complutense de Madrid, Madrid, Spain
Red Hygeia (Health & Gender International Alliance), Madrid, Spain

María Teresa Calvo-Llena and Francisco Javier Corbalán
Universidad de Murcia, Murcia, Spain

Fabiana Xavier Cartaxo Salgado, Dayani Galato, Aline Gomes de Oliveira, Letícia Farias Gerlack and Margô Gomes de Oliveira Karnikowski
Graduate Program in Health Sciences and Technology, Campus of Ceilândia, University of Brasília (FCE/UnB), Brasília, Brazil

Gislane Ferreira de Melo and Marileusa Dosolina Chiarello
Graduate Program in Gerontology, Catholic University of Brasília (UCB), Brasília, Brazil

Micheline Marie Milward de Azevedo Meiners
Graduate Program in Public Health, University of Brasília (UnB), Brasília, Brazil

Anna Ferla Monteiro Silva Passos and Adrianna Ribeiro Lacerda
Postgraduation Program in Health Sciences, Federal University of Rio Grande do Norte, Natal, Brazil

Iris do Céu Clara Costa
Department of Dentistry, Federal University of Rio Grande do Norte, Natal, Brazil

Fábia Barbosa de Andrade
Nursing, Faculty of Health Sciencies of Trairi/Federal University of Rio Grande do Norte, Santa Cruz, Brazil

Maria do Carmo Eulálio and Rômulo Lustosa Pimenteira de Melo
Department of Psychology, State University of Paraíba, Campina Grande, Brazil

Anita Liberalesso Neri
Department of Educational Psychology, State University of Campinas, Campinas, Brazil

Omotowo Ishola Babatunde, Nwobi Emmanuel Amaechi, Eyisi Ifeanyi Gabriel and Agwu-Umahi Rebecca Olanike
Department of Community Medicine, College of Medicine, University of Nigeria, Enugu, Nigeria

Eke Christopher Bismark
Department of Paediatrics, College of Medicine, University of Nigeria, Enugu, Nigeria

Yumi Kuwamura, Tetsuya Tanioka, Hirokazu Ito, Yuko Yasuhara and Rozzano Locsin
Department of Nursing, Institute of Biomedical Sciences, Tokushima University Graduate School, Tokushima, Japan

Masuko Sumikawa
Sapporo Medical University School of Health Sciences, Hokkaido, Japan

Toshihiko Nagata and Eijiro Sakamoto
Department of Periodontology and Endodontology, Institute of Biomedical Sciences, Tokushima University Graduate School, Tokushima, Japan

Hiromi Murata
Former Tokushima University Hospital, Tokushima, Japan

Munehide Matsuhisa
Diabetes Therapeutics and Research Center, Tokushima University, Tokushima, Japan

Ken-ichi Aihara
Department of Community Medicine for Diabetes and Metabolic Disorders, Institute of Biomedical Sciences, Tokushima University Graduate School, Tokushima, Japan

Daisuke Hinode
Department of Hygiene and Oral Health Science, Institute of Biomedical Sciences, Tokushima University Graduate School, Tokushima, Japan

Hirokazu Uemura
Department of Preventive Medicine, Institute of Biomedical Sciences, Tokushima University Graduate School, Tokushima, Japan

Sarah Ibrahim
Arthur Labatt School of Nursing, University of Western Ontario, London, Canada

Souraya Sidani
Daphne Cockwell School of Nursing, Ryerson University, Toronto, Canada